Cybersecurity and the Digital Health: An Investigation on the State of the Art and the Position of the Actors

Cybersecurity and the Digital Health: An Investigation on the State of the Art and the Position of the Actors

Editor

Daniele Giansanti

MDPI • Basel • Beijing • Wuhan • Barcelona • Belgrade • Manchester • Tokyo • Cluj • Tianjin

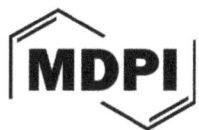

Editor
Daniele Giansanti
Centro TISP
Istituto Superiore di Sanità
Rome
Italy

Editorial Office
MDPI
St. Alban-Anlage 66
4052 Basel, Switzerland

This is a reprint of articles from the Special Issue published online in the open access journal *Healthcare* (ISSN 2227-9032) (available at: www.mdpi.com/journal/healthcare/special_issues/cybersecurity_digital_health).

For citation purposes, cite each article independently as indicated on the article page online and as indicated below:

LastName, A.A.; LastName, B.B.; LastName, C.C. Article Title. *Journal Name* **Year**, *Volume Number*, Page Range.

ISBN 978-3-0365-4388-8 (Hbk)
ISBN 978-3-0365-4387-1 (PDF)

© 2022 by the authors. Articles in this book are Open Access and distributed under the Creative Commons Attribution (CC BY) license, which allows users to download, copy and build upon published articles, as long as the author and publisher are properly credited, which ensures maximum dissemination and a wider impact of our publications.

The book as a whole is distributed by MDPI under the terms and conditions of the Creative Commons license CC BY-NC-ND.

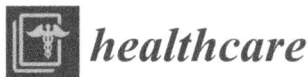

Editorial

Cybersecurity and the *Digital-Health*: The Challenge of This Millennium

Daniele Giansanti

Centre Tisp, Istituto Superiore di Sanità, Via Regina Elena 299, 00161 Roma, Italy; daniele.giansanti@iss.it; Tel.: +39-06-4990-2701

Citation: Giansanti, D. Cybersecurity and the *Digital-Health*: The Challenge of This Millennium. *Healthcare* **2021**, *9*, 62. https://doi.org/10.3390/healthcare9010062

Received: 25 December 2020
Accepted: 5 January 2021
Published: 11 January 2021

Publisher's Note: MDPI stays neutral with regard to jurisdictional claims in published maps and institutional affiliations.

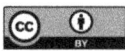

Copyright: © 2021 by the author. Licensee MDPI, Basel, Switzerland. This article is an open access article distributed under the terms and conditions of the Creative Commons Attribution (CC BY) license (https://creativecommons.org/licenses/by/4.0/).

1. Cybersecurity

The problem of computer security is as old as computers themselves and dates back decades. The transition from: (a) a single-user to multi-user assignment to the resource and (b) access to the computer resource of the standalone type to one of the types distributed through a network made it necessary to start talking about computer security. All network architectures, from *peer to peer* to *client-server* type, are subject to IT security problems.

The term *Cybersecurity* has recently been introduced to indicate the set of procedures and methodologies used to defend computers, servers, mobile devices, electronic systems, networks and data from malicious attacks. *Cybersecurity* [1–3] is therefore applied to various contexts, from the economic one to that relating to mobile technologies and includes various actions:

- *Network security*: the procedures for using the network safely;
- *Application Security*: the procedures and solutions for using applications safely;
- *Information security*: the management of information in a secure way and in a privacy-sensitive manner in accordance with pre-established regulations;
- *Operational security*: the security in IT operations, such as, for example, in bank-type transactions;
- *Disaster recovery and operational continuity*: the procedures for restarting after problems that have affected the regular/routine operation of a system and to ensure operational continuity. For example, using informatic solutions such as an efficient disk mirroring and/or backup policy;
- *End-user training*: specific training for the actors involved in the use of the systems, which where necessary, must also include the citizen.

2. Cybersecurity and Health Care

The recent decade has seen a growing interest in information security. *Cyber attacks* in the industry and consumer sectors have been widely echoed in the past and recent *cyber attacks* in the healthcare sector are of concern. Recently, for example, at the center of the debate were the attacks on health systems and the potential vulnerabilities that have come to light for some types of critical medical device (mostly active implantable) that can be connected to the network [1,2]. In several nations, there has generally been a delay in addressing *cybersecurity* issues compared to other nations, for example, the US. This is due to the fact that in the US, the world of health is undoubtedly an industry, not only in terms of perception, but in practice: the approach to the problem in the US has, in fact, been identical to that taken in general towards the world of industry and consumption. Only recently, however, has the problem begun to be given due attention. In the current healthcare sector, the criticality relating to the extraordinary diffusion of innovative technologies (e.g., artificial pancreas, pacemakers) connected to the network in the healthcare sector (over 300,000 classes of Medical Devices) are inevitably intertwined with the safety and efficacy characteristics of the services provided and the protection of the data processed, creating a context of high attention.

The *cybersecurity* in the healthcare:
- Includes all the general actions listed and described in the previous paragraph (Network Security, Application Security, Information Security, Operational Security, Disaster Recovery and Operational Continuity, End-User Training) tuned and specialized for the health-care sector;
- Faces *four main aspects* in the *cyber-system* that can either be a complex medical device (e.g., wearable pumps; wearable stimulators; pacemakers; artificial pancreas) and/or a complex interoperable and heterogeneous system (e.g., A Hospital Information System; a Radiology Information System; a dedicated medical network) comprehending several components of *elaboration systems, informatics, biomechatronics, bioengineering, electronics, networks, eHealth, mHealth* [1].

The data preservation

The procedures assuring the data for a prolonged period remains reachable and functioning. These procedures must respect adequate specifications and use informatic resources that are adequate for the purpose, such as adequate and stable filing systems.

The data access and modification

Refers to those typical functionalities such as storing and recovering data stored in databases or other archives. The implementation of these actions is obtained by means of specific designed procedures for the authentication and authorization of the regulated access.

The data exchange

Data exchange can be carried out either internally (for example, in the Hospital LAN) or externally (from the Hospital Lan to the external actors, such as, for example, the citizen and/or other practitioners, and/or other healthcare bodies). It is evident that the data exchange should take in a safe way place, in compliance with defined security specifics, with the application of suitable measures of data protection.

The interoperability and compliance

The *Interoperability* allows both a health-care worker and a citizen to exchange the data among several systems and devices in a shared manner. Two systems are considered interoperable when they are able to exchange data and later present that data so that they are comprehensible by all the involved actors. The *compliance refers* to the world of regulations. It deals, for example, both with the use of the same standards (e.g., Dicom in the radiology information systems) and with adherence to national and international regulations (e.g., the GPRS in Europe) concerning the usage of health information.

3. Specific Healthcare Sectors to Be Faced with Particular Attention in the Cybersecurity

3.1. Wearable Medical Device

The wearable medical devices [2–6], and, in particular, the implantable ones, are part of a heterogeneous system (e.g., pacemakers, artificial pancreas). In a heterogeneous system, the wireless connection allows the components to communicate with each other, and creates an environment potentially susceptible to *cyber attacks*. If the connection between the *wearable device* for continuous monitoring and the external elaborator is potentially unsafe, an attacker could send deliberately incorrect data to the control algorithm. For the *artificial pancreas*, for example, this could cause the release of a high amount of insulin, resulting in a situation of hypoglycemia in the patient; the body would respond to a hypoglycemic situation through the release of glucagon and epinephrine and continuing the situation would compromise the brain, motor and cognitive functions, even leading to death. For the *pacemaker*, this could cause the generation of an incorrect electronic pulse activity and create, for example, the dangerous fibrillations, which could rapidly lead to the death of the subject wearing the device. To take account of these issues, the Food and Drug Administration (FDA), for example, has made guidelines and recommendations available online.

3.2. Picture Archiving and Communication System

The *Picture Archiving and Communication System* (PACS) [2,3] is a medical device software (defined by the FDA as a Class II medical device) dedicated to the management of a diagnosis reached using the medical imaging. A PACS embeds several parts such as *elaborators, workstations, digital-databases, digital data-stores, digital-applications*. In the PACS, several software components are dedicated to the image downloading, uploading and manipulation. These actions clearly imply issues of data security and integrity, if we consider that a PACS is a deposit of patients' data with the inference of aspects related to the *data privacy and protection*. It is evident that the *cybersecurity* assumes strategic importance in the PACS in several tasks/activities of the digital radiology, in particular:

1. During the diagnostic/decision-making processes;
2. During the various phases of information manipulation ranging from image acquisition to its storage and subsequent sharing according to *client/server* type architectures.

3.3. Health Care Networks

As is well known, hospital companies today are strongly based on digital technologies. The *cyber risk* is rapidly increasing with [2,3,7]:

1. The so-called dematerialization of administrative processes;
2. The increased dependence on *computerized biomedical* and *non-biomedical technologies* (as described above);
3. The large amount of data stored in the Hospital Information Systems (HIS).

Recently, we have assisted in attacks on the HIS, both based on viruses (in minor cases) and by real complex systems, managed by increasingly capable and ingenious unlawful organizations. This means that the HIS can be attacked and breached in terms of both privacy and of activities [7]. It should be considered that the HISs have a criticality of the highest level, since the activity (based on specifically designed softwares) is linked to the health of people. With regard to the HIS, *cybersecurity* has, therefore, a leading role in the defense of IT infrastructures and in the final analysis of the citizen.

4. Conclusions

The *cybersecurity* in healthcare includes all the general actions employed both in the consumer and industrial sectors (Network Security, Application Security, Information Security, Operational Security, Disaster Recovery and Operational Continuity, End-User Training) tuned and specialized for the health-care sector. It should be considered that the criticality of the healthcare systems is of the highest level, since the activity is linked to the health of people; therefore, a correct and effective implementation of the cybersecurity assumes the utmost importance. All traditional health sectors and those emerging from eHealth and mHealth must be addressed with the utmost attention, and can and should be investigated by scholars. Training and information must be key aspects of cybersecurity in healthcare.

It will be necessary to foresee specific investigations with targeted scientific studies in each of the above-described fields. It will be also necessary to set up specific studies based on survey tools, to understand the perception and the state of the correct use of cybersecurity on the actors involved, from the medical specialist to the common people, who are disadvantaged and have a low level of instruction.

It could be also useful to understand whether it is appropriate to expand and better generalize the role of cybersecurity in new border areas of the health sector, such as, for example, (a) the sector of non-medical apps that can be confused with medical devices and whose non-compliant use could put patient safety at risk, especially during this COVID-19 pandemic period (perspective articles here are also strongly needed and welcome), and (b) the sector of the new Apps for the digital contact tracing, where discussion is increasing on the position of the citizen: with, on the one hand, his or her privacy rights and, on the other hand, the need to make every effort in order to stop the Covid-19 pandemic (reviews which analyze this issue are also welcome here) [8,9].

Conflicts of Interest: The author declares no conflict of interest.

References

1. Giansanti, D.; Monoscalco, L. The cyber-risk in cardiology: Towards an investigation on the self-perception among the cardiologists. *mHealth* **2020**. [CrossRef]
2. Giansanti, D.; Grigioni, M.; Monoscalco, L.; Gulino, R.A. Chapter: A Smartphone Based Survey to Investigate the Cyber-Risk Perception on the Health-Care Professionals. In *Mediterranean Conference on Medical and Biological Engineering and Computing, Proceedings of the XV Mediterranean Conference on Medical and Biological Engineering and Computing—MEDICON 2019, Coimbra, Portugal, 26–28 September 2019*; Henriques, J., Neves, N., de Carvalho, P., Eds.; Springer: Berlin, Germany, 2019; Volume 76, pp. 914–923. [CrossRef]
3. Giansanti, D. *Health in the Palm of Your Hand: Between Opportunities and Problems, Rapporti ISTISAN 19/15*; Istituto Superiore di Sanità: Roma, Italy, 2019; pp. 1–60.
4. Baranchuk, A.; Alexander, B.; Campbell, D.; Haseeb, S.; Redfearn, D.; Simpson, C.; Glover, B. Pacemaker Cybersecurity. *Circulation* **2018**, *138*, 1272–1273. [CrossRef] [PubMed]
5. Kramer, D.B.; Fu, K. Cybersecurity concerns and medical devices: Lessons from a pacemaker advisory. *JAMA* **2017**, *318*, 2077–2078. [CrossRef] [PubMed]
6. O'Keeffe, D.T.; Maraka, S.; Basu, A.; Keith-Hynes, P.; Kudva, Y.C. Cybersecurity in artificial pancreas experiments. *Diabetes Technol. Ther.* **2015**, *17*, 664–666. [CrossRef] [PubMed]
7. Coronado, A.J.; Wong, T.L. Healthcare cybersecurity risk management: Keys to an effective plan. *Biomed. Instrum. Technol.* **2014**, *48* (Suppl. 1), 26–30. [CrossRef] [PubMed]
8. Giansanti, D. Introduction of medical Apps in telemedicine and e-health: Problems and opportunities. *Telemed. J. E-Health* **2017**, *23*, 773–776. [CrossRef] [PubMed]
9. Censi, F.; Mattei, E.; Triventi, M.; Calcagnini, G. Regulatory frameworks for mobile medical applications. *Expert Rev. Med. Devices* **2015**, *12*, 273–278. [CrossRef] [PubMed]

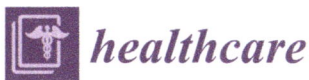

Article

A Cybersecurity Culture Survey Targeting Healthcare Critical Infrastructures

Fotios Gioulekas [1], Evangelos Stamatiadis [1], Athanasios Tzikas [1], Konstantinos Gounaris [1], Anna Georgiadou [2,*], Ariadni Michalitsi-Psarrou [2], Georgios Doukas [2], Michael Kontoulis [2], Yannis Nikoloudakis [3], Sergiu Marin [4], Ricardo Cabecinha [5] and Christos Ntanos [2]

1. 5th Regional Health Authority of Thessaly & Sterea, Mezourlo, 411 10 Larissa, Greece; fogi@dypethessaly.gr (F.G.); vstam@dypethessaly.gr (E.S.); atzi@uhl.gr (A.T.); kgounaris@ghv.gr (K.G.)
2. Decision Support Systems Laboratory, National Technical University of Athens, 15 780 Zografou, Greece; amichal@epu.ntua.gr (A.M.-P.); gdoukas@epu.ntua.gr (G.D.); mkontoulis@epu.ntua.gr (M.K.); cntanos@epu.ntua.gr (C.N.)
3. Department of Electrical & Computer Engineering, Hellenic Mediterranean University, 710 04 Heraklion, Greece; nikoloudakis@pasiphae.eu
4. Polaris Medical Clinica de Tratament si Recuperare, Str. Principală, 407062 Suceagu, Romania; sergiu.marin@polarismedical.ro
5. Hospital do Espírito Santo de Évora, EPE, Largo Senhor da Pobreza, 7000-811 Évora, Portugal; rjcabecinha@hevora.min-saude.pt
* Correspondence: ageorgiadou@epu.ntua.gr

Abstract: Recent studies report that cybersecurity breaches noticed in hospitals are associated with low levels of personnel's cybersecurity awareness. This work aims to assess the cybersecurity culture in healthcare institutions from middle- to low-income EU countries. The evaluation process was designed and performed via anonymous online surveys targeting individually ICT (internet and communication technology) departments and healthcare professionals. The study was conducted in 2019 for a health region in Greece, with a significant number of hospitals and health centers, a large hospital in Portugal, and a medical clinic in Romania, with 53.6% and 6.71% response rates for the ICT and healthcare professionals, respectively. Its findings indicate the necessity of establishing individual cybersecurity departments to monitor assets and attitudes while underlying the importance of continuous security awareness training programs. The analysis of our results assists in comprehending the countermeasures, which have been implemented in the healthcare institutions, and consequently enhancing cybersecurity defense, while reducing the risk surface.

Keywords: cybersecurity culture; awareness; security assessment; healthcare domain

1. Introduction

Cybersecurity has become one of the dominant information technologies (IT) domains in the health sector [1]. Over recent decades, various scientific attempts have been made towards identifying, classifying, and addressing vulnerabilities and weaknesses in healthcare institutions and hospitals [2–5]. However, this effort did not discourage nor limit the continuously evolving cybercrime in this domain. The European Union Agency for Cybersecurity (ENISA) stated that the healthcare sector accounted for 27% of the overall cyberattacks in Europe in 2018 [6].

The coronavirus outbreak, among its many side-effects, resulted in a significant cybercrime increase [7,8]. Critical infrastructures, as categorized based on the 2016/1148 NIS Directive [9], have major targets. Among them, EU hospitals are experiencing patient data loss [10,11], ransomware, and availability attacks. The following are two of the most troubling examples:

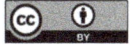

- The Brno University Hospital in the Czech Republic which, on 12 March 2020, was forced to shut down its entire IT network, impacting two of the hospital's other branches, the Children's Hospital and the Maternity Hospital [12].
- A fatality in a German hospital linked to a cyberattack [13].

Although security infrastructure is of critical importance for the defense against cybercriminals' tactics and techniques, an organization's biggest threat to privacy and security has been acknowledged to be its own personnel [14]. ENISA's report in 2018 [6] revealed that 50.6% of attacked hospitals identified insider threats as their most serious adversary.

As anticipated, a significant scientific effort has been made towards assessing healthcare personnel readiness over recent years [15–17]. Recognizing the multidisciplinary approach dictated towards this challenge, researchers soon adopted a holistic approach, and the term "cybersecurity culture" soon emerged.

Cybersecurity culture denotes the combination of attitudes, behaviors, knowledge, and awareness the organization's personnel display about common cyber risks and threats to protect the information assets [18]. Its evaluation involves the conduction of focused campaigns, which often results in the initiation of education programs, ICT infrastructure auditing, and the reassessment of current security policies to cultivate hospital personnel's culture and sense of responsibility when processing sensitive information in daily business operations, thus preventing attacks or leakages [19,20]. Several endeavors towards assessing healthcare personnel's cybersecurity culture were based on surveys. Indicatively, the surveys in Poland [21] and Finland [22] reported that medical professionals lack sufficient cybersecurity training. The analysis in [23] confirmed human error as one of the most common reasons for security incidents in hospitals. Authors in [24,25] highlighted that lack of security culture, awareness, and employee negligence or maliciousness constitute significant factors for the adoption of security policies.

Regarding the ICT resources utilization in hospitals, an analysis in 2008 [26] recorded a variation from 0.082 to 0.210 of ICT professionals (full-time job) per hospital bed in USA hospitals (0.142 in average, or equivalently, 1 ICT employee to total staff ratio of 60.7). Eurostat's general report in 2018 [27] documented an EU average value of 3.9% for the relative share of ICT specialists in total corporate employment.

This study analyses, before the COVID-19 situation, the overall disposition towards cybersecurity in healthcare institutions, which exhibit a proportion of ICT specialists in total employment below the EU average and compares the findings with relevant analyses in hospitals from Northern America and Northern Europe. We selected three different healthcare organizations from three different countries, i.e., Greece, Portugal, and Romania. In contrast to the above methods, we aimed to capture the cybersecurity awareness level of the organizations by first focusing on the ICT employees and consequently assessing the impact of this recorded level on the rest of the healthcare professionals.

The organizations under evaluation were the following: (i) a health region in Greece that comprises a significant number of reference hospitals and health centers (hereafter Institution A); (ii) a reference hospital in a large Portuguese region (henceforth Institution B); (iii) a Romanian medical clinic for impatient rehabilitation (henceforward Institution C). According to Eurostat [27], the percentage of ICT personnel to the total corporate staff for Greece was 1.8%, for Portugal it was 2.4%, and for Romania it was 2.2%. To the best of our knowledge, this is the first time that such an assessment has been conducted.

2. Methods and Materials

The Cybersecurity Culture Framework was developed in 2019 in the context of the EnergyShield [28], a European Union (EU) project targeting cybersecurity in the electrical power and energy system (EPES). It was officially introduced to the scientific community in 2020 [29] in a manuscript detailing an evaluation methodology of both individuals' and organizations' security culture indicators. Its model consists of dimensions and domains analyzed into a combination of organizational and individual security factors (Figure 1). Thus, facilitating the assessment of organizational security policies and procedures in conjunction with employees' characteristics, behaviors, attitudes, and skills. The specific framework exploits a variety of evaluation techniques, varying from surveys to more sophisticated approaches, such as simulations and serious games.

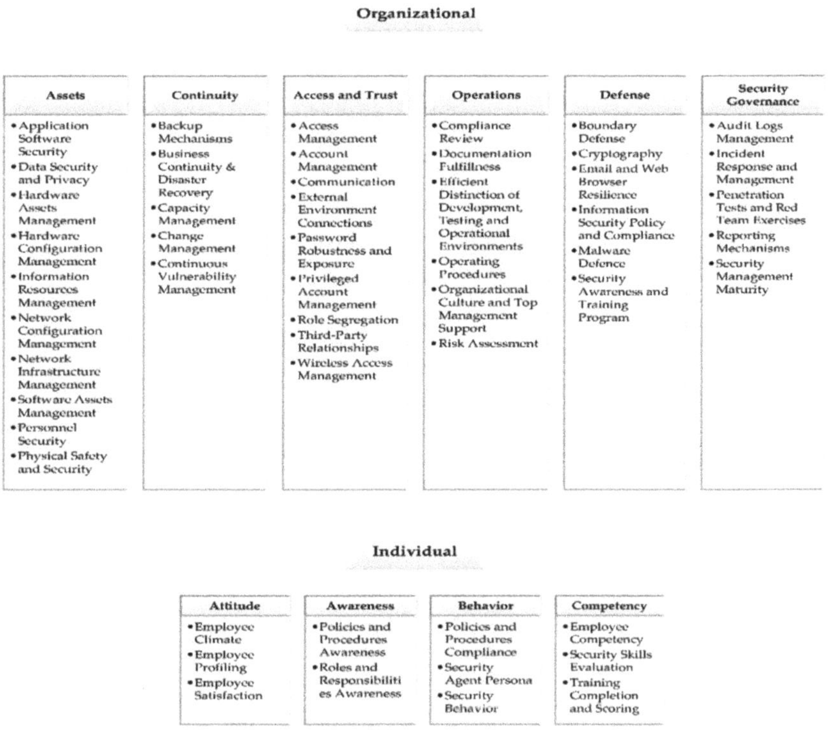

Organizational

Assets	Continuity	Access and Trust	Operations	Defense	Security Governance
• Application Software Security • Data Security and Privacy • Hardware Assets Management • Hardware Configuration Management • Information Resources Management • Network Configuration Management • Network Infrastructure Management • Software Assets Management • Personnel Security • Physical Safety and Security	• Backup Mechanisms • Business Continuity & Disaster Recovery • Capacity Management • Change Management • Continuous Vulnerability Management	• Access Management • Account Management • Communication • External Environment Connections • Password Robustness and Exposure • Privileged Account Management • Role Segregation • Third-Party Relationships • Wireless Access Management	• Compliance Review • Documentation Fulfillness • Efficient Distinction of Development, Testing and Operational Environments • Operating Procedures • Organizational Culture and Top Management Support • Risk Assessment	• Boundary Defense • Cryptography • Email and Web Browser Resilience • Information Security Policy and Compliance • Malware Defence • Security Awareness and Training Program	• Audit Logs Management • Incident Response and Management • Penetration Tests and Red Team Exercises • Reporting Mechanisms • Security Management Maturity

Individual

Attitude	Awareness	Behavior	Competency
• Employee Climate • Employee Profiling • Employee Satisfaction	• Policies and Procedures Awareness • Roles and Responsibilities Awareness	• Policies and Procedures Compliance • Security Agent Persona • Security Behavior	• Employee Competency • Security Skills Evaluation • Training Completion and Scoring

Figure 1. Cybersecurity Culture Framework.

This study, using the aforementioned cybersecurity culture framework, aims to capture the perspective and the level of personnel's cybersecurity awareness in the prior presented healthcare institutions. The percentage of the ICT staff compared to the total workforce is 0.45% for Institution A (average number among all the supervised units), 0.78% for Institution B, and 0.92% for Institution C (values lower than the Eurostat recorded statistics for these countries). The following two discrete online questionnaires were carefully designed to target two different personnel categories:

- Employees occupied in the ICT departments (ICT questionnaire);
- Non-ICT healthcare employees (non-ICT questionnaire) i.e., doctors, nurses, auxiliary, laboratory, and administrative personnel.

The survey's questionnaires are presented in Appendices A and B, while the participation was on a voluntary and anonymous basis.

The ICT questionnaire comprised the following five parts: The first part included questions about demographics, years of experience, and serving population derived from the *Employee Profiling* domain of the *Attitude* dimension (individual level). The second part focused on ICT aspects involving the number of cybersecurity trainings performed, percentages of total budget allocation to ICT, and cybersecurity deriving from the *Security Awareness and Training Program* domain of the *Defense* dimension along with the *Security Management Maturity* domain of the *Security Governance* dimension (organization level). The Section 3 targeted computer network policies and external parties' access combining indicators from different domains of the *Access and Trust* and *Assets* dimensions (organizational level). The fourth part requested individuals to answer questions about current cybersecurity methods and practices used deriving from the *Policies and Procedures Awareness* domain of the *Awareness* dimension (individual level). The last part focused on cybersecurity performance indicators (e.g., number of cyber security incidents over time and mean time for resolving an incident) deriving from the *Security Governance* dimension (organizational level).

The non-ICT questionnaire included questions for demographics, employment status, cybersecurity, or related trainings such as General Data Protection Regulation (GDPR), the ability to understand cyberattacks, cybersecurity processes' availability, and precautions taken. Security metrics were once again a combination of different indicators described in multiple layers of the cybersecurity culture framework aiming to obtain an overall evaluation of the non-ICT personnel culture. To sense if the non-ICT personnel had previously participated in cybersecurity campaigns, we used technical terminology in some questions of the questionnaire. In other words, several techniques were used to carefully trim and adjust the assessment process to the targeted audience.

The deployed numbers of computers are approximately 2800, 850, and 90 for Institutions A, B, and C, respectively. Knowing that it is generally difficult to voluntarily collect answers from the non-ICT personnel, due to the nature of their work, we sent the invitations (electronic and paper-based) to all the employees with the target to increase the response rate for the non-ICT personnel, and especially of those that have access to computers. Additionally, multiple-choice based questionnaires were translated from English to the native languages of the participants for better comprehension of their contents and to lift the language barrier and alleviate it from the equation. The collected data was translated back to English, harmonized, and checked for consistency.

The surveys were conducted from September 2019 to November 2019. There was no time limit for the completion of the questionnaires and participants were not reimbursed or offered any other incentive. Furthermore, since our analysis focused on middle- to low-income countries, we conducted an extensive literature survey on evaluations of the cybersecurity awareness status of hospitals in the USA, Canada, and Northern Europe (high- to middle-income countries) so as to comparatively analyze our findings.

3. Results

We invited 10,418 healthcare professionals (8500 from Greece, 1700 from Portugal, and 218 from Romania) and 69 ICT hospital employees (60 from Greece, 7 from Portugal, and 2 from Romania) to participate in the online survey. The participation rate is graphically presented in Figure 2. In total, 736 individuals responded to the surveys (37 for ICT and 699 for non-ICT). The overall answers to the ICT personnel were 28 (Institution A), 7 (Institution B), and 2 (Institution C), respectively, while for the non-ICT, the responses to the healthcare questionnaire were 449 (Institution A), 124 (Institution B), and 126 (Institution C). The response rate for the ICT personnel was 53.62%. The response rate for the non-ICT employees was 18.69% on the basis of the deployed computers and 6.71% on the basis of total employees, respectively.

3.1. Employed ICT Cybersecurity Procedures and Methods

The results revealed that 89%, 100%, and 50% of the ICT personnel in Institutions A, B and C, respectively, acknowledged the complete absence of dedicated cybersecurity departments in their institutions. Similar responses were given by the non-ICT personnel (86%, 63%, and 68% for Institutions A, B, and C, respectively). This deviation is due to the participants' inability to distinguish between ICT and cybersecurity departments. In total, 100% of the ICT personnel in Institutions A and B and 50% in Institution C, responded they did not follow an incident response plan form responding to a data breach in a timely and cost-effective manner.

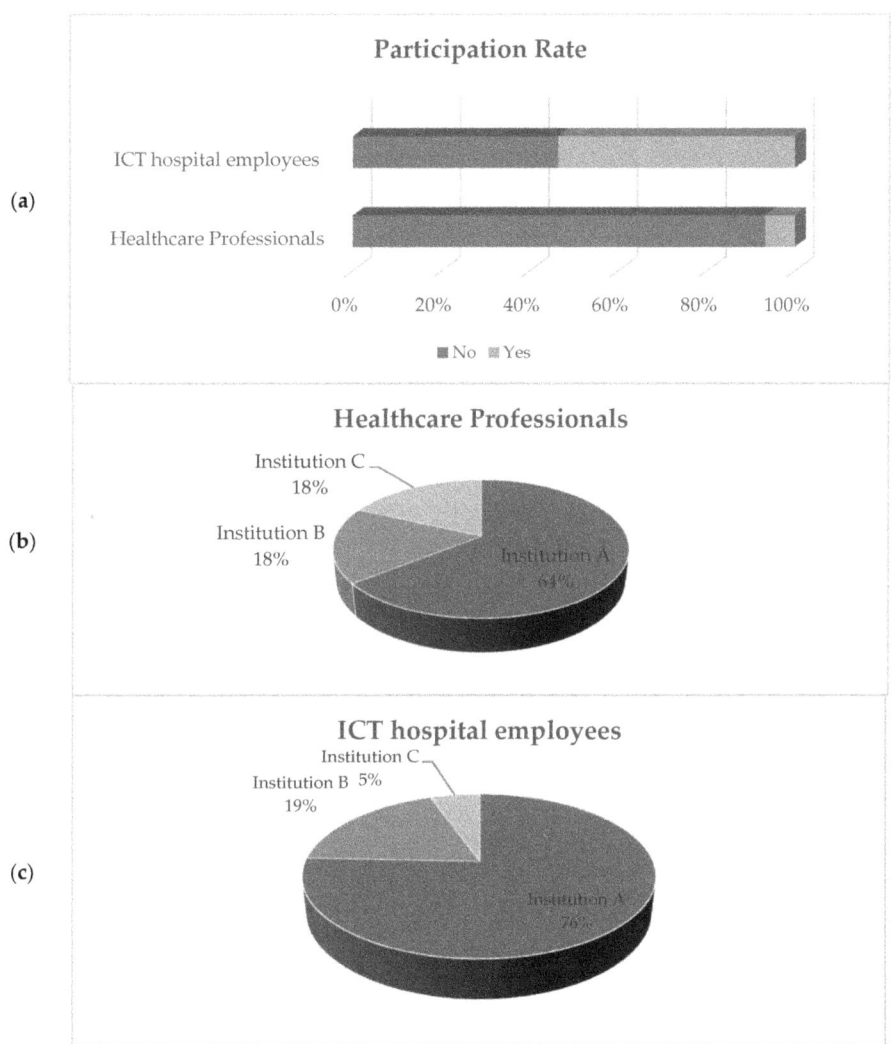

Figure 2. Campaign general participation information: (**a**) per profession, (**b**) healthcare professional per institution, and (**c**) ICT hospital employees per institution.

The ICT questionnaire responses on common vulnerabilities (Figure 3) revealed they did not adopt common policies, irrespectively of their education status, gender, or age. Although obsolete and black-boxed technologies, deployed in hospitals, play a significant role in data breaches, 40.5% of ICT personnel indicated the usage of legacy systems with known vulnerabilities in their day-to-day operations (representing more than 50% of the total equipment). Additionally, only 24.3% were aware of the existence of cybersecurity terms within the service level agreements (SLA) with vendors. The importance of setting up a unique identifier policy for users and roles for the mitigation of the impact of internal threats was acknowledged only by 48.6% of the ICT personnel. The need for secure sockets layer (SSL) certificates to be used by the web-based health information system (HIS) was identified by only 48.6%. Only 48.6% of the ICT personnel were aware that certain attacks, such as distributed denial of service (DDoS), are considered criminal actions. On the other hand, 75.7% acknowledged the usage of proactive backup measurements.

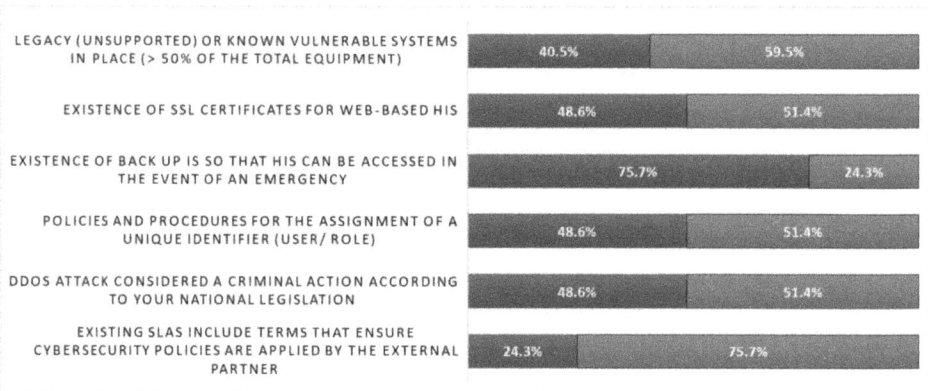

Figure 3. ICT personnel responses on common cybersecurity vulnerabilities.

Furthermore, 54% of the ICT personnel indicated that no records were kept, rendering a forensic analysis impossible and also resulting in no lessons learnt about the organizations' response. Moreover, as shown in Figure 4, the ICT personnel replied that most identified cybersecurity incidents took up to 6 h to resolve. The analysis revealed that the "Mean Downtime" was equal to the "Mean Time to Resolve the Incident", which means that parts of ICT facilities and related ICT-enabled services might have lost availability and functionality during the incident, a fact that possibly translates that no continuity plan was in place. This is in line with the finding that a small number of cybersecurity penetration tests were conducted during the last two years (affirmative answers: only 18% from A, 57% from B, and 50% from C). All the above indicate the necessity of performing regular ICT penetration tests and iterative trainings.

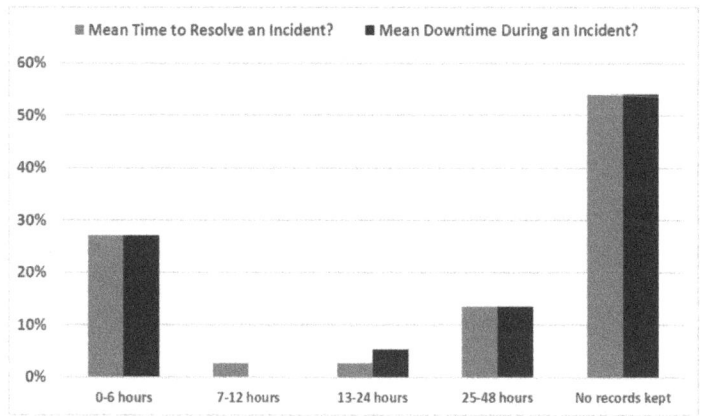

Figure 4. Cybersecurity Incident: Downtime and Time to Resolve.

3.2. Training on Cybersecurity and Data Protection

The survey exposed the lack of cybersecurity-related training across the three institutions. 70% of the ICT personnel admitted they have not received official cybersecurity training in the past 3 years, with the remaining 30% revealing a frequency of less than one training per year even on European legislation and guidance, such as Directive (EU) 2016/1148 NIS Directive and the GDPR. Nevertheless, the ICT personnel responded they were aware of those acts at 80% in A, 86% in B and 50% in C. On the other hand, 73% of non-ICT personnel replied they had access to sensitive information and were aware of GDPR (Figure 5).

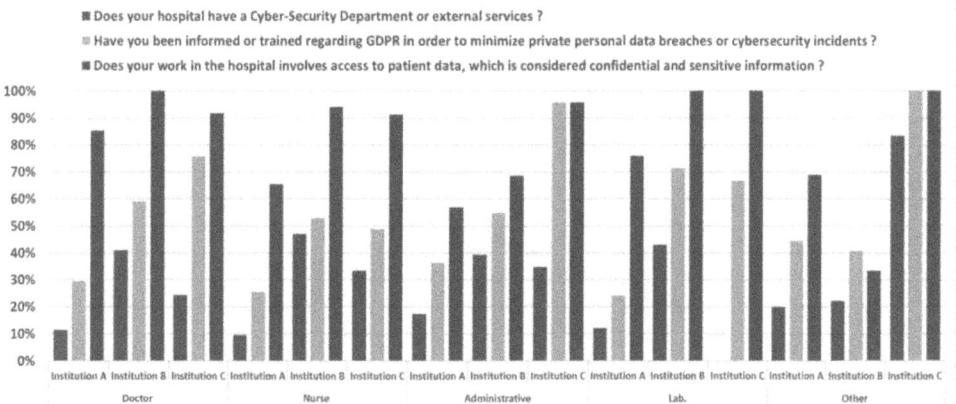

Figure 5. Awareness of Non-ICT personnel on legal aspects, privacy and cybersecurity structure.

39% of the ICT personnel in Institution A, 57% in Institution B and 100% in Institution C replied they used to perform internal cybersecurity awareness training (e.g., about phishing). The latter indicates the recorded low number of ICT staff might have played a significant role in not conducting training.

3.3. Cybersecurity Awareness Level

Figure 6 shows the positive answers of the non-ICT group to questions related to cybersecurity awareness. Only 22.7% of the non-ICT personnel felt sufficiently trained in security, while only 38.5% were confident they could recognize a security issue or incident if they encountered one. This confidence was mainly supported by personnel in Institution C, while in the other two institutions they were perceived to be low-to-moderately trained. Trying to sensor the adequacy of the personnel's awareness of cybersecurity threats such as email phishing and their reactions to them, it was found that only 26.8% of the participants knew what a social engineering attack was, while only 21.9% knew how to detect an email phishing attack. Although participants acknowledged they handled sensitive data on a daily basis, only 23.3% perceived the level of importance of their terminals' content to hackers. 40.9% answered they knew when their terminals had been compromised and whom to contact in such a case. 30.9% understood the consequences of sharing their terminal or credentials, while 37.3% knew how to handle email attachments. More than 50% of the non-ICT personnel acknowledged the existence of antivirus software and the policy of locking their terminals when they leave. Their majority also responded (76%) that following security policies would help them do their job better.

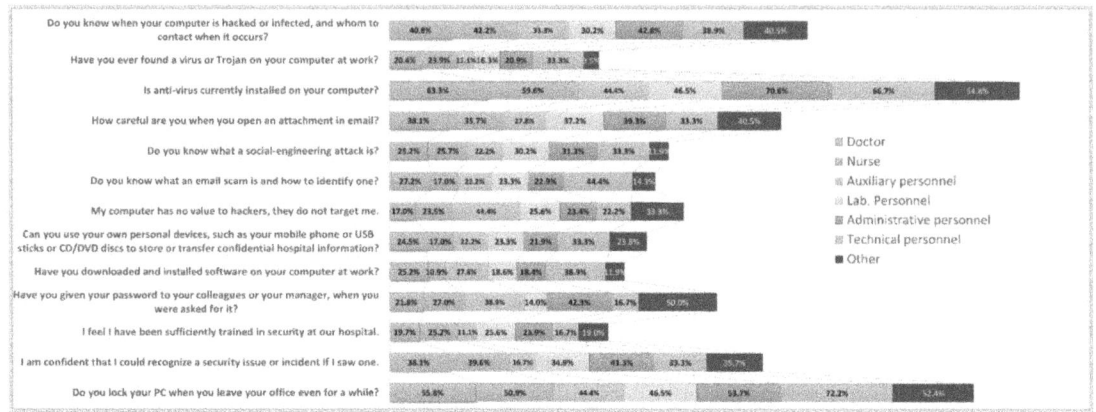

Figure 6. Digital behavior and security comprehension level of non-ICT Healthcare Employees.

4. Discussion

Our findings showed healthcare ICT personnel represented a very small percentage of the total workforce, generally below **1%**. The surveyed organizations have dedicated only a small amount of their total ICT budget (below **5%**) to cybersecurity purposes. The importance of budget allocation to cybersecurity is illustrated in the 2019 report [30] of the Healthcare Information and Management Systems Society (HIMSS) in the USA. Although our surveyed organizations reported less than **5%** in ICT budget allocation for cybersecurity, the report among **166** USA health information security specialists in [30] acknowledged a significant increase in this budget category (**10%** of the respondents acknowledged cybersecurity funding of more than **10%**, **11%** responded 7–10%, while **25%** answered 3–6%). The identified differences in the ICT investments indicate that smart hospitals have invested more in cybersecurity and in associated human resources to protect their information assets, rather than traditional hospitals [9], which are in the process of digital transformation. The ongoing application of the EU's digital convergence policies (e.g., cross-border health data exchange) is expected to bridge the aforementioned gap.

Almost all of the respondents (**96%**) in the 2019 HIMSS survey [30] indicated their respective organizations conducted risk assessments (**37%** of which were comprehensive, resulting in the adoption of new or improved security measures by **72%** of them). In our study, the lack of cybersecurity departments and that **70%** of ICT employees have not received official cybersecurity training in the past **3** years, accounted for the low adoption and lack of standard or common policies in cybersecurity incidents (**100%** for A and B and **50%** for C). Only **48.6%** of the ICT personnel (A, B, and C) acknowledged the importance of applying a unique identifier policy for users and roles, in contrast to the 2017 survey [31] among **39%** of all the USA's hospitals, where more than **90%** of them used unique identification for system users (supported by automatic logoff of system users, required use of strong passwords, etc.). Additionally, **40.5%** of the ICT personnel in our study indicated the usage of legacy systems (more than **50%** of the total equipment). The legacy-systems impediment is also acknowledged in [30] (**69%** of respondents), but in a lower percentage of the total equipment (more than **10%** for only **14%** of respondents). Moreover, in contrast to our study (see Section 3.2.), only **18%** of respondents in [30] stated their organization did not conduct phishing tests and trainings due to a lack of personnel with the appropriate cybersecurity knowledge and expertise. Furthermore, in our study, **21.9%** acknowledged they do not know how to detect an email phishing attack, which suggests that the actual percentage of a real, ongoing phishing attack might be even higher. In contrast to that, a recent study at US health care institutions [15] indicates a median click rate on phishing campaigns of **16.7%**, which is further reduced on subsequent ones, highlighting the importance of training on that matter.

Regarding the non-ICT personnel, comparing our findings (Table 1) with a 2020 study in Poland [21], a 2019 study in a health region of western Finland [22], and a 2019 study in a health organization in western Canada [19], revealed the low level of cybersecurity awareness status. In Institutions A, B, and C, the **22.7%** that felt sufficiently trained in security and the **23.3%** that perceived the importance of the terminals' content to hackers, appeared significantly lower next to the **51.31%** of the **1200** Finnish professionals reporting bring sufficiently aware of the information and the cybersecurity matters pertaining to their job. About the same percentage (**55.7%**) of **586** non-ICT professionals in the Canadian healthcare organization, declared their satisfaction with ICT security in their daily activities. **73.2%** of our non-ICT participants did not know what a social engineering attack was, which makes them a potential hazard of disclosing sensitive information (e.g., passwords). **69.1%** could not realize the consequences of sharing their terminal or credentials with other employees. The Finnish study reported a negative answer to disclosing one's password over the phone, either if requested by an authority (**96%**), or by an ICT manager (**83%**), while the Canadian one states that **93.6%** would never share login information with other employees. Only **21.9%** of the respondents in our study could detect spam emails and phishing attacks, and only **37.3%** could handle attachments, which both fell behind the Finnish awareness score (**41.54%**) and the Canadian personnel that acted correctly upon them (**55%**).

Table 1. Percentage (%) of answers related to cybersecurity awareness along with the corresponding standard deviations for non-ICT personnel.

Question	Institution A $n = 449$ (100%)	Institution B $n = 124$ (100%)	Institution C $n = 126$ (100%)
Do you have cyber-security policies at your hospital?			
Yes	11% ± 0.5	55% ± 4.9	60% ± 5.3
No	14% ± 0.7	2% ± 0.2	7% ± 0.6
Do not know	75% ± 3.5	43% ± 3.8	33% ± 2.9
Have you been informed or trained regarding General Data Protection Regulation (GDPR) in order to minimize private personal data breaches or cybersecurity incidents?			
Yes	31% ± 2.5	31% ± 0.2	31% ± 0.1
No	69% ± 0.08	69% ± 0.2	69% ± 0.1
How careful are you when you open an attachment in email?			
I always make sure it is from a person I know, and I am expecting the email	32% ± 6.7	48% ± 15.9	50% ± 18.4
As long as I know the person or company that sent me the attachment, I open it	59% ± 7.7	42% ± 15.4	45% ± 18.4
There is nothing wrong with opening attachments	9% ± 6.3	10% ± 12.3	5% ± 7.4
Have you given your password to your colleagues or your manager, when you were asked for it?			
Yes	33% ± 9.1	26% ± 14.2	30% ± 24.1
No	67% ± 9.1	74% ± 14.2	70% ± 24.1
Is anti-virus currently installed on your computer?			
Yes	60% ± 2.8	16% ± 1.4	79% ± 6.9
No	11% ± 0.5	65% ± 5.8	5% ± 0.4
Do not know	29% ± 1.3	19% ± 2.7	17% ± 1.5
I am confident that I could recognize a security issue or incident if I saw one.			
Strongly agree	4% ± 2.4	4% ± 4.6	14% ± 12.3
Agree	24% ± 8.1	39% ± 18.3	59% ± 15.3
Neither agree nor disagree	42% ± 10	34% ± 18	8% ± 7.8
Disagree	23% ± 8.3	20% ± 9.1	17% ± 10.3
Strongly disagree	7% ± 4.5	3% ± 3	2% ± 1.9

Low to moderate knowledge and awareness in the above fields pose a potential risk during daily working activities, such as processing patients' data or communicating medical information to other parties. Therefore, it is deduced that there is a high risk of security incidents triggered by non-ICT employees because the aforementioned threats and attacks and the associated impact of potential incidents have not been efficiently communicated to them by the ICT staff. All the above indicate that decreasing the endpoint complexity as proposed in [32], along with training conduction, is essential in raising awareness amongst personnel and motivating them to pay attention to cyber-threats and policies to limit human errors [33–35]. The adoption of a risk-aware attitude and associated skills by the non-ICT staff through cybersecurity trainings and a robust organizational monitoring strategy could lead to a more GDPR-compliant status. Even in New Zealand, a country where robust cybersecurity practices have long been in their agendas, the majority of internet users, as revealed by a 2019 survey [36], still take low to no security measures, while they perceive monitoring practices, such as the use of monitoring software, as highly technical. The necessity for intense cybersecurity awareness trainings, even from a young age, is highlighted.

5. Considerations and Limitations

The response rate of the non-ICT personnel was correlated with the number of the deployed computers they use daily. However, due to the variations in the clinic shift patterns, it was hard to stringently identify the non-ICT personnel that used computers. Therefore, we tried to collect responses by sending the non-ICT participation invitation mainly through their direct management, assuming it would be communicated to the total number of employees. Due to the voluntary and anonymous nature of the questionnaires, the commitment of all doctors and nurses was not totally ensured. Nevertheless, the collected answers proved to conform to the findings from the ICT questionnaire, where we managed to achieve high response rates. The availability of similar studies in the literature for the health care sector, especially recent ones, is not abundant, and comparisons were performed mainly against data from surveys conducted in hospitals in the USA, Canada, and some territories of northern Europe.

6. Conclusions

The implementation and deployment of security awareness programs in healthcare institutions along with training procedures proves to be a necessity. Furthermore, 76% of the non-ICT personnel replied that following hospitals' security policies would help them perform their job better. Consequently, the findings were communicated to the management of the institutions, and certain courses of proactive and reactive cybersecurity measures have been triggered and implemented during the COVID-19 crisis. Specifically, a certain budget was allocated to procure or upgrade cybersecurity systems and software (e.g., antivirus databases, UTM firewalls with IDS/IPS). A specialised workshop has been conducted with ENISA's support for the ICT staff, which in several cases was reinforced accordingly. Additionally, in-house awareness campaigns for non-ICT employees about anti-phishing or anti-social engineering have periodically been conducted. Moreover, those who deal daily with sensitive data and processes have participated in GDPR related seminars. In the future, we aim to revisit the updated cybersecurity measures and strategies and re-perform an extensive assessment to re-evaluate the new level of cybersecurity awareness and personnel readiness.

Author Contributions: Conceptualization, F.G., E.S., A.T., K.G., S.M. and R.C.; methodology, F.G., E.S., A.T., K.G. and C.N.; validation, F.G., E.S., A.T., K.G., A.G., A.M.-P. and Y.N.; formal analysis, F.G., E.S., A.T., K.G., G.D., A.G., A.M.-P. and C.N.; resources, A.M.-P. and C.N.; writing—original draft preparation, F.G., G.D., M.K. and C.N.; writing—review and editing, F.G., E.S., A.T., K.G., S.M., R.C., Y.N., A.G., A.M.-P. and C.N.; visualization, G.D., M.K. and F.G.; supervision, F.G., E.S. and C.N.; project administration, F.G., E.S. and C.N.; funding acquisition, E.S. and C.N. All authors have read and agreed to the published version of the manuscript.

Funding: This work was funded by the Sphinx project that has received funding from the European Union's Horizon 2020 Research and Innovation Programme under Grant Agreement No. 826183 on Digital Society, Trust and Cyber Security E-Health, Well-being and Ageing. Moreover, it was funded by the European Union's Horizon 2020 Research and Innovation Programme, Grant Number 832907. The funding body have not participated in the design of the study or in the analysis of the data and manuscript elaboration.

Institutional Review Board Statement: Not applicable.

Informed Consent Statement: Not applicable.

Data Availability Statement: The data presented in this study are available on request from the corresponding author.

Acknowledgments: This project has received funding from the European Union's Horizon 2020 Research and Innovation Programme under Grant Agreements Nos. 832907 and 826183. Moreover, authors would like to thank all the anonymous healthcare professionals that voluntarily spent part from their busy schedule to complete the surveys and their supervisors for their support.

Conflicts of Interest: The authors declare no conflict of interest.

Appendix A

ICT Personnel Questionnaire

1. General Characteristics
   a. Demographics
      i. Age:
         20–39 ☐
         40–60 ☐
         60+ ☐
      ii. Gender:
         Male ☐
         Female ☐
   b. Education:
      Secondary Education ☐
      Vocational training Institution ☐
      Bachelor's Degree ☐
      MSc ☐
      PhD ☐
   c. Position:
      ICT director ☐
      ICT manager ☐
      ICT staff ☐
   d. Years of experience
      0–5 ☐
      6–10 ☐
      more than 10 ☐
   e. Healthcare Organization:
      Hospital ☐
      Clinic ☐
      Health Authority ☐
      National ☐
      Regional ☐
      Local ☐
         Employees <100 ☐

Employees 100–300 ☐
Employees 301–600 ☐
Employees 601–1000 ☐
Employees >1000 ☐
Population <100 k ☐
Population 100 k–300 k ☐
Population >300 k ☐

2. Specific ICT

   a. Proportion of ICT employees in total employment (%)

   0–1% ☐
   1.1–2% ☐
   2.1–3% ☐
   3.1–4% ☐
   4.1–5% ☐
   5.1–6% ☐
   6.1–7% ☐

   b. Existence of a Cybersecurity Department

   Yes ☐
   No ☐

   c. Official Trainings had in ICT cybersecurity during the last 3 years (number)

   0 ☐
   1 ☐
   2 ☐
   3 ☐
   4 ☐

   d. Do you perform internal cybersecurity awareness trainings (e.g., phishing) in order to teach employees what to check in the received emails?

   Yes ☐
   No ☐

   e. Average yearly organization's budget allocated to ICT during the last 3 years (in Euros)

   0–100 K ☐
   101–200 K ☐
   201–300 K ☐
   301–400 K ☐
   401–500 K ☐
   Do not know ☐

   f. Percentage of current ICT budget allocated to cybersecurity (e.g., antivirus purchasing or license renewal, firewall purchase or firewall license renewals, etc.) during the last 3 years (%)

   0–5% ☐
   6–10% ☐
   11–15% ☐
   16–20% ☐
   21–25% ☐
   26–30% ☐
   Do not know ☐

3. Network Communication with External Partners and Collaborators

   a. Usage of secure method or other methods for third party accesses

   VPN ☐
   TeamViewer ☐

AnyDesk ☐
Remote Desktop ☐
Other secure method ☐
Other unsecure method ☐

b. Communication ports opened and monitored during daily operations (constantly or on demand)

Port TCP 22 (SSH) ☐
Port TCP 23 (Telnet) ☐
Port TCP 3389 (RDP) ☐
Port TCP 20 (FTP data) ☐
Port TCP 21 (FTP control) ☐
other ☐

c. Do existing SLAs include terms that ensure cybersecurity policies are applied by the external partner for preventing data breaches when connected remotely to hospital's information systems?

Yes ☐
No ☐
Do not know ☐

4. Cybersecurity Methods & Practices

a. Does your organization have an official cybersecurity plan?

Yes ☐
No ☐
Do not know ☐

If the previous answer is yes, which of the following plans?

Risk Assessment ☐
Incident Respond Plan ☐
Mitigation plan ☐
Report plan ☐

b. Have any cybersecurity tests been performed in your organization during the last 2 years?

Yes ☐
No ☐

If the previous answer is yes, which of the following tests?

Scanning ☐
Penetration ☐
Weak password identification ☐
Phishing ☐
Virus/malware checking ☐
Verification of latest updates/outdates ☐
Other ☐

c. Are you familiar with the Directive (EU) 2016/1148 NIS Directive and GDPR regulation?

Yes ☐
No ☐
Partially ☐

d. Is a DDoS attack considered a criminal action according to your national legislation?

Yes ☐
No ☐
Do not know ☐

e. Does your working practice have policies and procedures for the assignment of a unique identifier for each authorized user according to its role?
Yes ☐
No ☐
Do not know ☐

f. Does your working practice have back up information systems so that it can access HIS in the event of an emergency or when your practice's primary systems become unavailable i.e., in the event of a disaster?
Yes ☐
No ☐

g. Do SSL certificates exist for web-based hospital information systems?
Yes ☐
No ☐
Partially ☐

h. Which of the following tools do you use daily for information security?
Antivirus/malware ☐
Firewall(s) ☐
Data encryption (data in transit) ☐
Data encryption (data at rest) ☐
Patch & vulnerability management ☐
Intrusion detection systems (IDS) ☐
Network monitoring tools ☐
Mobile device management ☐
User access controls ☐
Intrusion prevention system ☐
Access control lists ☐
Single sign on ☐
Web security gateway ☐
Multi-factor authentication ☐
Data loss prevention (DLP application) ☐
Messaging security gateway ☐
Audit logs of each access to pt. health and financial records ☐
My duties do not include cyber-security activities ☐

5. Cybersecurity Performance Indicators

a. Percentage of legacy (unsupported) or known vulnerable systems in place (e.g., end of life operating systems in medical devices) in total equipment (%)
0–10% ☐
11–20% ☐
21–30% ☐
31–40% ☐
41–50% ☐
51–60% ☐
More than 60% ☐
Do not know ☐

b. Number of cyber security incidents during the last 3 years (e.g., phishing attacks, virus infections, etc.)?
0–5 ☐
6–10 ☐
11–15 ☐
16–20 ☐
21–25 ☐

26–30 ☐
No records kept ☐
- c. Number of unauthorized login attempts in HIS, Active Directory, RIS/PACS per month?

  0–5 ☐
  6–10 ☐
  11–15 ☐
  16–20 ☐
  21–25 ☐
  26–30 ☐
  No records kept ☐
  No records kept but it is monitored regularly ☐
- d. Mean time to resolve an incident?

  0–6 h ☐
  7–12 h ☐
  13–24 h ☐
  25–48 h ☐
  3–7 days ☐
  More than a week ☐
  No records kept ☐
- e. Mean downtime during an incident?

  0–6 h ☐
  7–12 h ☐
  13–24 h ☐
  25–48 h ☐
  3–7 days ☐
  No records kept ☐

Appendix B

Non-ICT Personnel Questionnaire

1. General Characteristics
   - a. Demographics
     - i. Age:

       21–30 ☐
       31–40 ☐
       41–50 ☐
       51–60 ☐
       61+ ☐
     - ii. Gender:

       Male ☐
       Female ☐
   - b. Education

     Secondary Education ☐
     Vocational training Institution ☐
     Bachelor's Degree ☐
     MSc ☐
     PhD ☐
   - c. Position

     Doctor ☐
     Nurse ☐

Auxiliary personnel ☐
Lab. personnel ☐
Administrative personnel ☐
Technical personnel ☐
Other ☐

2. Does your hospital have a cybersecurity department or external services?
   Yes ☐
   No ☐
   Do not know ☐

3. Does your work on the hospital involves working on a computer at any time?
   Yes ☐
   No ☐

4. Have you been informed or trained regarding General Data Protection Regulation (GDPR) in order to minimize private personal data breaches or cybersecurity incidents?
   Yes ☐
   No ☐

5. Does your work in the hospital involves access to patient data, which is considered confidential and sensitive information?
   Yes ☐
   No ☐

6. Do you have cybersecurity policies at your hospital?
   Yes ☐
   No ☐
   Do not know ☐

7. Do you know when your computer is hacked or infected, and whom to contact when it occurs?
   a. Yes, I know when my computer is hacked or infected and I know whom to contact.
   b. No, I do not know when my computer is hacked or infected and I do not know whom to contact.
   c. Yes, I know when my computer is hacked or infected, but I do not know whom to contact.
   d. No, I do not know when my computer and I know whom to contact.

8. Have you ever found a virus or trojan on your computer at work?
   a. Yes, my computer has been infected before
   b. No, my computer has never been infected
   c. I do not know what a virus or trojan is

9. Is an anti-virus currently installed on your computer?
   a. Yes
   b. No
   c. Do not know

10. How careful are you when you open an attachment in email?
    a. I always make sure it is from a person I know, and I am expecting the email
    b. As long as I know the person or company that sent me the attachment, I open it
    c. There is nothing wrong with opening attachments

11. Do you know what a social engineering attack is?
    a. Yes, I do
    b. No, I do not

12. Do you know what an email scam is and how to identify one?
    a. Yes, I know what an email scam is and how to identify one
    b. I know what an email scam is, but I do not know how to identify one
    c. No, I do not know what an email scam is or how to identify one
13. My computer has no value to hackers; they do not target me.
    a. True
    b. False
14. Can you use your own personal devices, such as your mobile phone or USB sticks or CD/DVD discs to store or transfer confidential hospital information?
    a. Yes
    b. No
    c. Do not know
15. Have you downloaded and installed software on your computer at work?
    a. Yes
    b. No
16. Have you given your password to your colleagues or your manager when you were asked for it?
    a. Yes
    b. No
17. Which of these is closer to your thinking, even if neither is exactly right?
    a. Following security policies at our hospital prevents me from doing my job
    b. Following security policies at our hospital helps me do my job better
18. I feel I have been sufficiently trained in security at our hospital.
    a. Strongly agree
    b. Agree
    c. Neither agree nor disagree
    d. Disagree
    e. Strongly disagree
19. I am confident that I could recognize a security issue or incident if I saw one.
    a. Strongly agree
    b. Agree
    c. Neither agree nor disagree
    d. Disagree
    e. Strongly disagree
20. Do you lock your PC when you leave your office even for a while?
    Yes ☐
    No ☐

References

1. Giansanti, D. Cybersecurity and the *Digital-Health*: The Challenge of This Millennium. *Healthcare* **2021**, *9*, 62. [CrossRef] [PubMed]
2. Jalali, M.S.; Russell, B.; Razak, S.; Gordon, W. EARS to cyber incidents in health care. *J. Am. Med. Inform. Assoc.* **2019**, *26*, 81–90. [CrossRef] [PubMed]
3. Razaque, A.; Amsaad, F.; Khan, M.J.; Hariri, S.; Chen, S.; Siting, C.; Ji, X. Survey: Cybersecurity Vulnerabilities, Attacks and Solutions in the Medical Domain. *IEEE Access* **2019**, *7*, 168774–168797. [CrossRef]
4. Appari, A.; Johnson, M.E. Information security and privacy in healthcare: Current state of research. *Int. J. Internet Enterp. Manag.* **2010**, *6*, 279. [CrossRef]
5. Coventry, L.; Branley, D. Cybersecurity in healthcare: A narrative review of trends, threats and ways forward. *Maturitas* **2018**, *113*, 48–52. [CrossRef] [PubMed]
6. Sfakianakis, A.; Douligeris, C.; Marinos, L.; Lourenço, M.; Raghimi, O. *ENISA Threat Landscape Report 2018—15 Top Cyberthreats and Trends*; European Union Agency for Network and Information Security (ENISA): Athens, Greece, 2019.

7. Reason Cybersecurity. *COVID-19, Info Stealer & the Map of Threats—Threat Analysis Report*; ReasonLabs: New York, NY, USA, 9 March 2020; Available online: https://blog.reasonsecurity.com/2020/03/09/covid-19-info-stealer-the-map-of-threats-threat-analysis-report/ (accessed on 26 January 2022).
8. Interpol. *Pandemic Profiteering: How Criminals Exploit the COVID-19 Crisis*; Interpol: Lyon, France, 2020.
9. European Union Agency for Network and Information Security (ENISA). *Smart Hospitals—Security and Resilience for Smart Health Service and Infrastructures*; European Union Agency for Network and Information Security (ENISA): Athens, Greece, 2016.
10. Gyles, S. Cyberattacks Hit Hospitals and Health Departments Amid COVID-19 Coronavirus Pandemic. Available online: https://vpnoverview.com/news/cyberattacks-hit-hospitals-and-health-departments-amid-covid-19-coronavirus-pandemic/ (accessed on 17 March 2020).
11. Martin , A. Coronavirus: Cyber Criminals Threaten to Hold Hospitals to Ransom-Interpol. Available online: https://news.sky.com/story/coronavirus-cyber-criminals-threaten-to-hold-hospitals-to-ransom-interpol-11968602 (accessed on 5 April 2020).
12. Porter, S. Cyberattack on Czech hospital forces tech shutdown during coronavirus outbreak. *Healthcare IT News*. 19 March 2020. Available online: https://www.healthcareitnews.com/news/emea/cyberattack-czech-hospital-forces-tech-shutdown-during-coronavirus-outbreak (accessed on 26 February 2021).
13. Howell, P. A Patient Has Died after Ransomware Hackers Hit a German Hospital. Available online: https://www.technologyreview.com/2020/09/18/1008582/a-patient-has-died-after-ransomware-hackers-hit-a-german-hospital/(accessed on 18 September 2020).
14. Doherty, N.F.; Fulford, H. Do Information Security Policies Reduce the Incidence of Security Breaches: An Exploratory Analysis. *Inf. Resour. Manag. J.* **2005**, *18*, 19. [CrossRef]
15. Gordon, W.J.; Wright, A.; Aiyagari, R.; Corbo, L.; Glynn, R.J.; Kadakia, J.; Kufahl, J.; Mazzone, C.; Noga, J.; Parkulo, M.; et al. Assessment of Employee Susceptibility to Phishing Attacks at US Health Care Institutions. *JAMA Netw. Open* **2019**, *2*, e190393. [CrossRef] [PubMed]
16. Landolt, S.; Hirsche, J.; Schlienger, T.; Businger, W.; Zbinden, A.M. Assessing and Comparing Information Security in Swiss Hospitals. *Interact. J. Med. Res.* **2012**, *1*, e11. [CrossRef] [PubMed]
17. Jalali, M.S.; Bruckes, M.; Westmattelmann, D.; Schewe, G. Why Employees (Still) Click on Phishing Links: An Investigation in Hospitals. *J. Med Internet Res.* **2020**, *22*, e16775. [CrossRef] [PubMed]
18. Yeng, P.K.; Yang, B.; Snekkenes, E.A. Framework for Healthcare Security Practice Analysis, Modeling and Incentivization. In Proceedings of the 2019 IEEE International Conference on Big Data (Big Data), Los Angeles, CA, USA, 9–12 December 2019.
19. Arain, M.A.; Tarraf, R.; Ahmad, A. Assessing staff awareness and effectiveness of educational training on IT security and privacy in a large healthcare organization. *J. Multidiscip. Heal.* **2019**, *12*, 73–81. [CrossRef] [PubMed]
20. Gardner, B.; Thomas, V. *Building an Information Security Awareness Program: Defending Against Social Engineering and Technical Threats*; Elsevier: Waltham, MA, USA, 2014.
21. Hyla, T.; Fabisiak, L. Measuring Cyber Security Awareness within Groups of Medical Professionals in Poland. In Proceedings of the 53rd Hawaii International Conference on System Sciences, Maui, HI, USA, 7–10 January 2020. [CrossRef]
22. Haukilehto, T.; Hautamäki, J. Survey of Cyber Security Awareness in Health, Social Services and Regional Government in South Ostrobothnia, Finland. In *Internet of Things, Smart Spaces, and Next Generation Networks and Systems*; Springer: Cham, Switzerland, 2019; pp. 455–466. [CrossRef]
23. Evans, M.; He, Y.; Luo, C.; Yevseyeva, I.; Janicke, H.; Maglaras, L.A. Employee Perspective on Information Security Related Human Error in Healthcare: Proactive Use of IS-CHEC in Questionnaire Form. *IEEE Access* **2019**, *7*, 102087–102101. [CrossRef]
24. Shahri, A.B.; Ismail, Z. Security effectiveness in health information system: Through improving the human factors by education and training. *Aust. J. Basic Appl. Sci.* **2012**, *6*, 226–233.
25. Ponemon Institute LLC. *The Human Factor in Data Protection*; Ponemon Institute LLC: Traverse City, MI, USA, 2012.
26. Hersh, W.; Wright, A. What workforce is needed to implement the health information technology agenda? Analysis from the HIMSS analytics database. In *AMIA Annual Symposium Proceedings*; American Medical Informatics Association: Washington, DC, USA, 2008; Volume 2008, pp. 303–307.
27. *ICT Specialists in Employment*; European Commission, Eurostat: Luxembourg, 2021.
28. Energy Shield. 2019. Available online: https://energy-shield.eu/ (accessed on 25 March 2020).
29. Georgiadou, A.; Mouzakitis, S.; Bounas, K.; Askounis, D. A Cyber-Security Culture Framework for Assessing Organization Readiness. Available online: https://www.researchgate.net/publication/347119168_A_Cyber-Security_Culture_Framework_for_Assessing_Organization_Readiness (accessed on 10 November 2020).
30. HIMSS Healthcare Cybersecurity Survey. Available online: https://www.himss.org/resources/himss-healthcare-cybersecurity-survey (accessed on 16 November 2020).
31. American Hospital Association. *Hospitals Implementing Cybersecurity Measures*; American Hospital Association: Cleveland, OH, USA, 2017.
32. Jalali, M.S.; Kaiser, J.P. Cybersecurity in Hospitals: A Systematic, Organizational Perspective. *J. Med. Internet Res.* **2018**, *20*, 1–18. [CrossRef] [PubMed]

33. Waly, N.; Tassabehji, R.; Kamala, M. Improving Organisational Information Security Management: The Impact of Training and Awareness. In Proceedings of the 2012 IEEE 14th International Conference on High Performance Computing and Communication & 2012 IEEE 9th International Conference on Embedded Software and Systems, Washington, DC, USA, 25–27 June 2012; pp. 1270–1275. [CrossRef]
34. Ghazvini, A.; Shukur, Z. Awareness Training Transfer and Information Security Content Development for Healthcare Industry. *Int. J. Adv. Comput. Sci. Appl.* **2016**, *7*, 361–370. [CrossRef]
35. *ISO/IEC 27005*; Information Technology—Security Techniques—Information Security Risk Management. International Organization for Standardization (ISO): Geneva, Switzerland, 2018.
36. Tirumala, S.S.; Valluri, M.R.; Babu, G. A survey on cybersecurity awareness concerns, practices and conceptual measures. In Proceedings of the 2019 International Conference on Computer Communication and Informatics (ICCCI), Coimbatore, India, 23–25 January 2019.

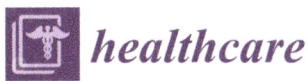

Review

Communication Requirements in 5G-Enabled Healthcare Applications: Review and Considerations

Haneya Naeem Qureshi [1,2,*], Marvin Manalastas [1,2], Aneeqa Ijaz [2], Ali Imran [2], Yongkang Liu [1] and Mohamad Omar Al Kalaa [1]

1. Center for Devices and Radiological Health, U.S. Food and Drug Administration, Silver Spring, MD 20993, USA; marvin@ou.edu (M.M.); yongkang.liu@fda.hhs.gov (Y.L.); omar.al-kalaa@fda.hhs.gov (M.O.A.K.)
2. AI4Networks Research Center, School of Electrical & Computer Engineering, University of Oklahoma, Tulsa, OK 74135, USA; aneeqa@ou.edu (A.I.); ali.imran@ou.edu (A.I.)
* Correspondence: haneya@ou.edu

Abstract: Fifth generation (5G) mobile communication technology can enable novel healthcare applications and augment existing ones. However, 5G-enabled healthcare applications demand diverse technical requirements for radio communication. Knowledge of these requirements is important for developers, network providers, and regulatory authorities in the healthcare sector to facilitate safe and effective healthcare. In this paper, we review, identify, describe, and compare the requirements for communication key performance indicators in relevant healthcare use cases, including remote robotic-assisted surgery, connected ambulance, wearable and implantable devices, and service robotics for assisted living, with a focus on quantitative requirements. We also compare 5G-healthcare requirements with the current state of 5G capabilities. Finally, we identify gaps in the existing literature and highlight considerations for this space.

Keywords: 5G networks; healthcare; key performance indicators; wireless communication

Citation: Qureshi, H.N.; Manalastas, M.; Ijaz, A.; Imran, A.; Liu, Y.; Al Kalaa, M.O. Communication Requirements in 5G-Enabled Healthcare Applications: Review and Considerations. *Healthcare* **2022**, *10*, 293. https://doi.org/10.3390/healthcare10020293

Academic Editor: Daniele Giansanti

Received: 21 October 2021
Accepted: 14 January 2022
Published: 2 February 2022

Publisher's Note: MDPI stays neutral with regard to jurisdictional claims in published maps and institutional affiliations.

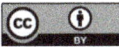

Copyright: © 2022 by the authors. Licensee MDPI, Basel, Switzerland. This article is an open access article distributed under the terms and conditions of the Creative Commons Attribution (CC BY) license (https://creativecommons.org/licenses/by/4.0/).

1. Introduction

Integrating fifth generation (5G) mobile communication technology into digital healthcare technology can facilitate healthcare delivery with expanded communication capabilities given 5G's high data speed, ultra-low latency, massive device connectivity, reliability, increased network capacity, and increased availability. These characteristics can enable novel healthcare use cases and augment existing ones [1–4]. Use cases include remote robotic-assisted surgery, remote diagnosis/teleconsultation, in-ambulance treatment by a remote physician, wearable device applications (wearable device applications are considered within the scope of the Internet of Things (IoT), narrow band IoT (NB-IoT), or Massive IoT), service robotics for assisted living, and medical big data management [1,5–9].

5G-enabled healthcare applications have diverse communication technical requirements for different use cases. Knowledge of those requirements is important for all stakeholders, including developers, network providers, and regulatory authorities in the healthcare sector, to facilitate safe and effective healthcare [6], where an understanding of the underlying communication requirements is needed to select wireless technology with features that support healthcare application design targets and expected performance [10]. 5G promises to provide the low latency and high bandwidth to enable modern healthcare applications such as remote robotic surgery and in-ambulance treatment. Accordingly, designing, deploying, and evaluating the systems needed to implement those use-cases can be informed with a clear understanding of the underlying communication requirements that can enable the intended functionality.

For instance, the expansive set of 5G configuration and optimization parameters offer network operators flexible options in setting up their networks and dynamically optimizing network performance to achieve a desired objective. Accordingly, a large set of parameters can impact the needed performance for a 5G-healthcare use case. Accordingly, quantitative key performance indicators (KPIs) can help 5G network providers assess the feasibility of a given 5G-enabled healthcare use case, provide the level of service needed for the safe and effective functioning of 5G-enabled healthcare applications, and draft service level agreements with their customers. Clearly specified KPIs can also inform regulatory authorities like the U.S. Food and Drug Administration (FDA) when evaluating whether communication service levels and quality of service are met to support the safe and effective use of a 5G-enabled medical device. Finally, end users such as healthcare facilities and patients can use this knowledge for developing, negotiating, and managing relevant service level agreements (SLAs) with the 5G network provider [6].

In this review paper, we identify, compare, and summarize the communication requirements for several healthcare use cases that can be enabled by 5G. The focus of this paper is on quantitative requirements. Furthermore, we identify gaps in the existing literature and highlight considerations in this area. Specifically, we survey the technical requirements for remote robotic-assisted surgery, mobile connected ambulance (i.e., in-ambulance treatment by remote physicians), wearable and implantable devices, and service robotics for assisted living.

This article is unique in detailing a comprehensive review of the quantitative KPI requirements of 5G-healthcare use cases. To the best of our knowledge, the closest work to our review paper on the similar topic is the recent magazine article by Cisotto et al. [11], which highlights select quantitative requirements for the use cases of telepresence and robotic-assisted telesurgery, remote pervasive monitoring, healthcare in rural areas, and mobile health (m-Health). Compared to the related work, our review paper includes references specific to the use of 5G in healthcare, in addition to those addressing the communication requirements of the healthcare applications regardless of the enabling communication technology, which can inform how applications use 5G. Our literature search results extend until 29 June 2021. Accordingly, we have significantly expanded the scope of the considered references to comprehensively capture the state-of-the-art and include a comparative study between planned and existing 5G capabilities. We have also identified gaps in this space and considerations for 5G-healthcare requirements, which were not within the scope of [11]. Moreover, after identifying literature that reported KPIs for the use of 5G in healthcare use cases, we have traced the original sources of the referenced KPIs in those papers.

The rest of the paper is organized as shown in Figure 1. In Section 2, an overview of 5G KPIs with specifications of their definitions is provided. Sections 3.1–3.4 identify four potential areas of 5G healthcare applications and review KPI requirements in individual areas, which include telesurgery (Section 3.1), connected ambulance (Section 3.2), healthcare IoT (Section 3.3), and robots for assisted living (Section 3.4). The identified 5G-healthcare requirements are then compared with the current state of 5G capabilities in Section 4, and gaps in this space are highlighted in Section 5. Finally, Section 6 concludes the paper.

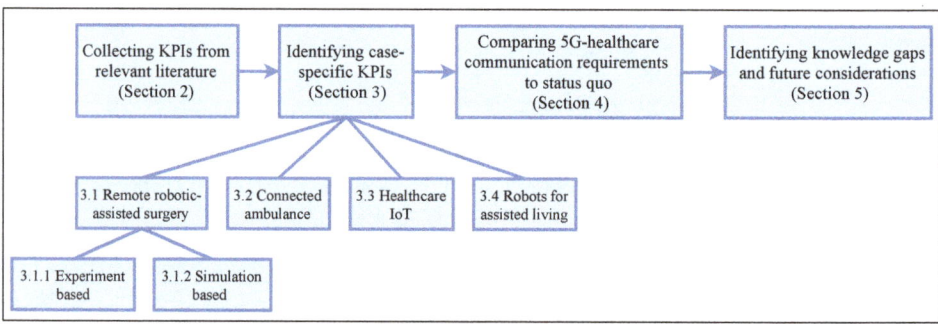

Figure 1. Methodology and organization of paper.

2. Key Performance Indicators for 5G-Healthcare

While KPIs such as data rate, accessibility, reliability, and mobility have been widely used in the performance evaluation of 4G cellular networks, the diversity and heterogeneity of 5G applications are calling for further expansion to incorporating novel sets of KPIs for measuring adequacy and efficacy of 5G-enabled services. The taxonomy shown in Figure 2 highlights the vastness of 5G network KPIs. Inspired by [12–14] and combined with domain knowledge, this taxonomy classifies 5G KPIs into four categories: network, service, application, and user. Each category also includes high-level and low-level KPIs. High-level ones measure the overall performance of the network based on metrics defined by the standardization bodies such as 3rd Generation Partnership Project (3GPP). However, most of the time, these high-level KPIs are focused on characterizing general features of the cellular system/service. In this regard, we also introduce low-level KPIs under each high-level one to further instantiate specific requirements. A certain 5G-enabled healthcare application might depend on a given set of KPIs to deliver its function while having low sensitivity to others.

The service level KPIs often discussed in 5G-enabled healthcare literature to address several aspects of the communication network, including *availability, accessibility, reliability, data rate*, and *retainability*. Availability is the fraction of time the network is available to provide the services users demand [15]. Accessibility is discussed in the context of connectivity time, which measures the time to establish a network connection, starting at the user request and ending at the beginning of the data transmission. Reliability is addressed through numerous low-level KPIs shown in Figure 2: *throughput, latency, jitter*, and *packet loss rate (PLR)*, and *bit error rate (BER)*. User throughput during active time is the size of a burst divided by the time between the arrival of the first packet and the reception of the last packet of the burst. Latency corresponds to the travel time of data packets from the source to the destination (i.e., one-way, or end-to-end latency) [16]. The round-trip latency is the time it takes a signal to be sent plus the time spent to receive an acknowledgement of that signal. Jitter is a measure of the variation in the time of arrival between packets. If uncontrolled, jitter impacts the audio and video quality, which can negatively impact applications where this type of communication is used (e.g., telesurgery, remote diagnosis, and service robotics for assisted living). PLR is the fraction of packets that failed to reach the receiver out of total number of transmitted packets. BER is the total number of bits received in error over the total number of bits sent. Like jitter, high BER/PLR negatively impacts audio and video quality. Also relevant to the service level is the data rate, which is a measure of the volume of successfully received application data, expressed in bits, within a period expressed in seconds. A high data rate is relevant in applications that transport large volumes of data. Service retainability refers to the count of radio link interruptions following the activation of that link between the user and the network. A related measure of service retainability is the number of reconnections, i.e., the count of attempts a user performs to re-establish network connection following a link failure.

The overall network characteristics are addressed in the literature with several network level KPIs such as network *bandwidth, utilization* and *spectral efficiency*. Bandwidth refers to the network maximum aggregated data transmission rate. *Connection density* and *traffic density* are measures of utilization. Connection density refers to the number of connected devices per unit area. This is relevant in connected IoT application, where the number of connected devices is large. Traffic density (or area traffic capacity) is a measure of the volume of catered data in a unit area. Spectral efficiency is the maximum number of bits the network can provide to users every second using a given bandwidth.

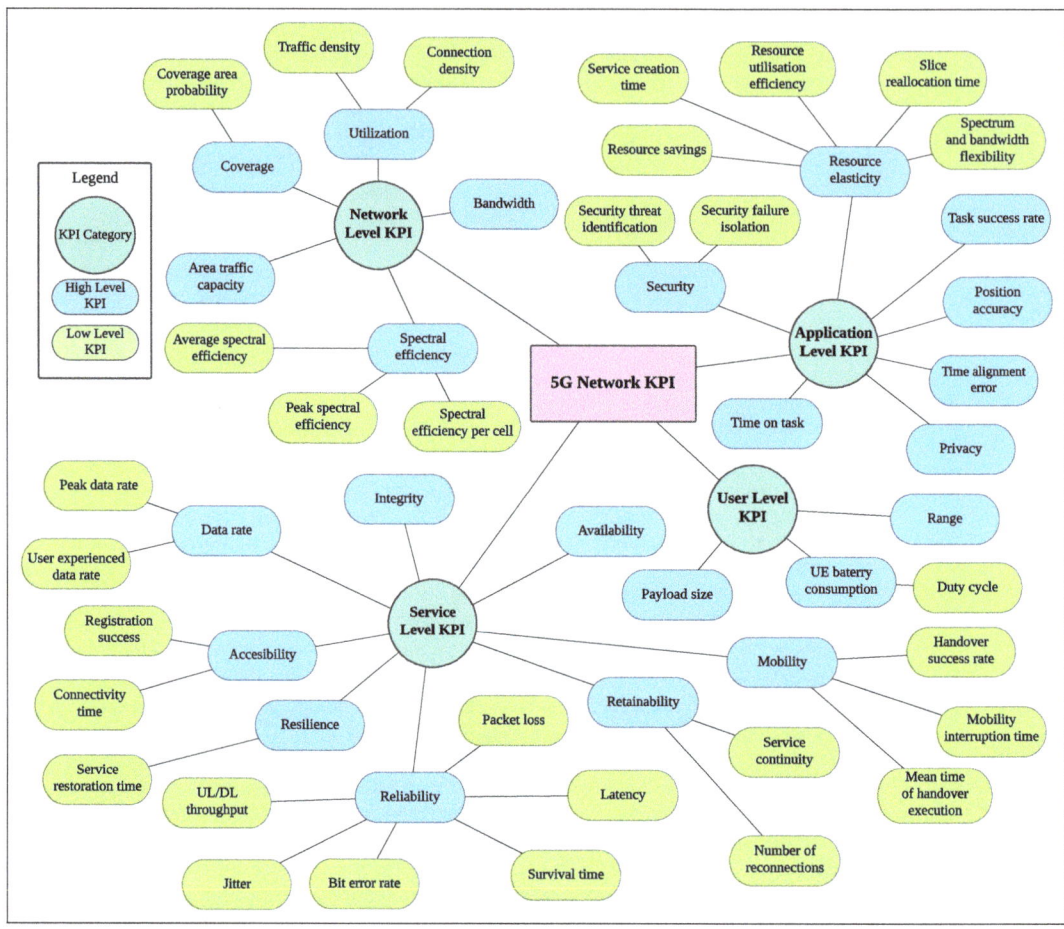

Figure 2. Taxonomy of 5G network KPIs.

On the user level, KPIs of *battery or power consumption, range,* and *payload size* are commonly reported in literature covered in this paper. User battery consumption and the its associated low-level KPI, *duty cycle*, which is the ratio between an application active (ON) and idle (OFF) times, are relevant in IoT devices where transmissions are intermittent and battery lifetime is limited. Range is the distance at which the signal transmitted is sufficient for the transmitter and receiver to communicate effectively. Another relevant KPI discussed in literature is the user payload size, which can be controlled to balance the transferred data volume with the incurred transmission overhead. This promotes efficient network resource usage while helping to meet specific application needs.

On the application level, *security* and *position accuracy* are the most commonly discussed KPIs in literature reviewed in this paper. Security refers to the network ability to identify, isolate, and eliminate threats to its infrastructure, users, and their data. Position accuracy is a measure of the difference between the estimated and actual user locations. The 3GPP (the entity that develops 5G specifications) has set different position accuracy targets for different scenarios ranging from several meters for emergency calls to a few decimeters for indoor plant operations and vehicle-to-everything (V2X) [17].

Although relevant to enabling 5G healthcare functions, some KPIs are seldom addressed in the articles reviewed in this paper. For example, the *network-coverage* is relevant to all applications using its services. While network *coverage area probability* is related to user activity range, it refers to the percentage of service area where users can receive a desired service. On the application level, *privacy* is relevant to healthcare applications because it refers to the ability of the network to keep the data that passes through it or is stored privately in it. Also on the application level, network *resource elasticity* is relevant in applications with temporary need for elevated connection capabilities such as in-ambulance treatment and other emergency related applications. Resource elasticity describes the network ability of responding to temporal and spatial fluctuations in traffic demand by redistributing available resources to seamlessly meet the demand of critical applications [18]. On the service level, *mobility* is relevant to applications that are mobile such as connected ambulance. Mobility is the maximum user speed that a network can support. It also refers to the ability of a network to support mobile users. A measure of mobility can be the *rate of successful handovers* between the coverage sites. Additional examples of KPIs related to the service level include the *service restoration time* under resilience and *survival time* under reliability. The former refers to the period in which the services are restored to normal operating status after experiencing a downtime. The latter is the tolerable packet delay in which an application can still function effectively.

Figure 3 illustrates a subjective summary of the general relevance of the high-level 5G network KPIs we investigated in Figure 2 to the following applications: remote robotic-assisted surgery, connected ambulance or in-ambulance treatment by remote physician, healthcare IoT applications, medical data management, teleconsultation and remote diagnosis, and service robotics for assisted living. These applications are only considered as generic concepts, which recognizes that realistic medical devices implementing one or more of these application concepts have unique KPI needs. Furthermore, the FDA guidance document on radio frequency wireless technology in medical devices recommends that the medical device wireless quality of service (QoS) is specific to the medical device [10]. Accordingly, this summary can help inform the KPI value specifications that should be determined for the specific intended use of a medical device and its design. Relevance is qualitatively described as high, medium, or low. Notably, remote robotic-assisted surgery needs careful provisioning of several KPIs, including reliability, where low-level KPIs such as latency, jitter, and packet loss fall under. However, when the scenario is implemented in an operating room, mobility is not as relevant as other KPIs since the connection will not move across multiple network cells. On the contrary, in-ambulance treatment by remote physician or connected ambulance needs exceptional mobility support since the data exchange occurs while the ambulance is mobile. Support for mobility in this case complements other relevant KPIs such as reliability, data rate, availability, coverage, and resource elasticity to enable the exchange of diverse data streams (e.g., video, audio, file transfer, and control commands). The number of connected wearable devices is expected to grow globally from 720 million in 2019 to more than 1 billion in 2022 [19]. Accordingly, the KPIs of utilization and UE battery consumption are highly relevant for enabling the network connectivity for such devices given their energy constraints. In the case of medical data management, security and privacy are more relevant compared to other KPIs, such as reliability. Like other services that use audio and video, remote diagnosis or teleconsultation are negatively impacted with degraded reliability. Other relevant KPIs for this use case include coverage, range, and utilization, to facilitate the service access by many users. Finally, we note that reliability, range, and position accuracy are relevant in the service robotics for assisted living use case where the robot is mobile in a limited area. The following sections will review the related literature for each of these use cases.

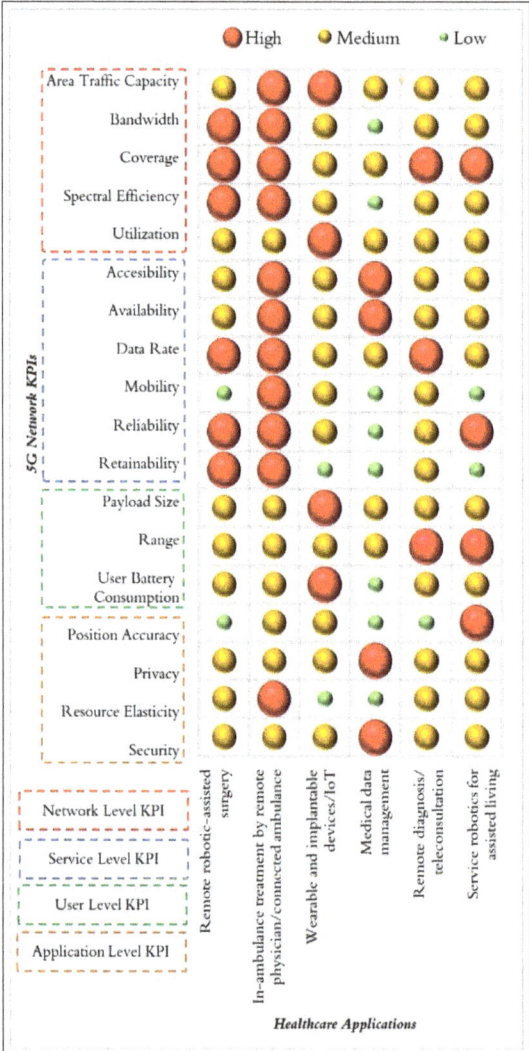

Figure 3. Examples of 5G-enabled healthcare application concepts and their projected needs for some communication KPIs.

3. KPIs for Specific 5G-Healthcare Use Cases

3.1. Remote Robotic-Assisted Surgery

Several studies have addressed quantitative KPI requirements for remote robotic-assisted surgery, which we also refer to as telesurgery for the remainder of this review. This use case involves the use of a robotic-assisted surgery platform by a surgeon located in a remote geographic location. The most commonly reported KPIs include latency, data rate, and packet loss [11,20–47]. Few studies have also reported quantitative requirements for reliability, communication service availability, payload size, traffic density, connection density, service area dimension, survival time, range, and duty cycle [11,30,34,44]. Table A1 presents the reported latency requirements for several communication streams that can be used during telesurgery such as camera flows, vital signs, and feedback for force and vibration. Latency in this context is considered end-to-end. Compared to latency, quantitative requirements for jitter have been investigated less investigated in the literature. The reported jitter requirements are detailed in Table A2. Similarly, requirements for data rate are detailed in Table A3. These requirements can be influenced by different compression techniques used. Reported packet loss and BER requirements are presented in Table A4. Reports of other KPIs, such as reliability, availability, survival time, etc., are listed in Table A5. By big payload in Table A5, we mean when the packet exceeds 10 Kb [11]. The ability of current 5G networks to meet these KPIs will be discussed in Section 4.

Notably, the reported KPI values are inconsistent across literature reports, which could be attributed to the varying type of tasks considered by the researchers during telesurgery. Additionally, the equipment used to perform telesurgery and the simulation environment also varies across studies. To detail the context of the telesurgery KPI specification, we also labeled the original source of the reported KPIs in each study as detailed in Tables A1–A5. Most KPI values were found in experiment and simulation settings of the individual studies with exceptions where the values were a consensus view of the achievable performance by wireless stakeholders [22,33], and Refs. [22,30] contain a white paper by the 5G Infrastructure Public Private Partnership (5GPPP) that highlighted use cases for 5G in healthcare and suggested quantitative requirements. A technical requirements document was compiled by the IEEE 802.15 Task Group 6 for Body Area Networks (BAN), formed in 2007 to help develop a communication standard optimized for the low power devices and operation, in or around the human body to serve a variety of applications, including medical applications. The report in [30] outlined findings from the National Science Foundation (NSF)-funded workshop on ultra-low latency wireless networks. The report addressed healthcare application requirements of the emerging applications, including telesurgery, in terms of throughput, latency, and reliability. In the following, the relevant experimental and simulation studies are summarized.

3.1.1. Experiment Based

The Aesop 1000TS robot (Computer Motion, Goleta, CA, USA) was adapted to hold a metal pin in addition to a laparoscope and camera (Stryker Instruments, San Jose, CA, USA) in [23]. Programmed incremental time delays were introduced in the audiovisual acquisition, and the number of errors made while performing tasks at various time delay intervals was noted. A remote surgeon in Baltimore, MD performed tasks 9000 miles away in Singapore and determined that a delay of <700 ms is acceptable.

A teleoperation capable ZEUSTM robotic minimally invasive surgery system was used in [24], with a dedicated communication link by Bell Canada and Telesat Canada. This link included a wired link with a roundtrip delay of 64 ms, a satellite link with a roundtrip delay of 580 ms, and a software simulated delay link through a local switch. Different tasks were performed from London, Ontario to Halifax, Nova Scotia, Canada. These included dry (typical surgical maneuvers at latencies from 0 to 1 s, in increments of 100 ms) and wet (internal mammary artery takedown on a pig) experiments. A heuristic mathematical model accompanied the task completion times and error rate results, showing acceptable delays of up to 300 ms and 800 ms for simple tasks with training. It was concluded that the effect of delay is not pronounced until the round-trip time exceeds 400 ms and the maximum tolerable delay is approximately 600 ms.

Researchers from European Institute of Telesurgery used the ZEUS system, which is transcontinental, which attempted a remote robot-assisted laparoscopic cholecystectomy on a 68-year-old woman with a history of abdominal pain and cholelithiasis. The surgeon's subsystem (Equant's point of presence, New York) and patient's subsystem (operating room in European Institute of Telesurgery, Strasbourg) were connected via a high-speed terrestrial network (i.e., ATM service), with a round-trip distance of over 14,000 km. Robot motion data had a high priority and a rate guarantee of 512 Kbps within the 10 Mbps virtual path. The operation was carried out successfully in 54 min, with a 155 ms mean time lag for transmission. The study estimated that 300 ms was the maximum time tolerable delay.

Dohler et al. [32] attempted a robot-assisted laparoscopic gall bladder removal for six pigs, with the surgeon located in Strasbourg, France and animals located in Paris, France, using the ZEUS system. The time lag was artificially increased from 20 ms up to 551.5 ms. It was concluded that no packets were lost during the surgical procedures, and the round-trip delay was 78–80 ms, with additional 70 ms for video coding and decoding and a few milliseconds for rate adaptation, summing to 155 ms [32].

To study the impact of haptic feedback in virtual environments, two experimental platforms were implemented in [40]. Platform 1 consisted of two sites at the University of Belfast separated by a few hundred meters and linked by Gigabit Ethernet connection. The configuration of the experimental platform consisted of four 100 Mbps Ethernet segments, two 1000 Mbps fiber optic segments, and four PCs. One PC was connected to a PHANToM Desktop, two generated background traffic, and one ran the remote virtual environment. In Platform 2, one of the computers is used to emulate network impairments. Haptic data, network congestion, and network-impairments were analyzed using these two platforms by introducing controlled delay (0 ms to 50 ms), jitter (1 ms to 15 ms), and packet loss (0.1% to 50%). Study participants self-scored the sense of force feedback. The haptic QoS requirements were summarized by less than 10 ms delay, less than 3 ms jitter, 1% to 5% for packet loss rate, and haptic data transmission rate of approximately 1 kHz.

The study in [29] involved both simulation and practical experiments, where multi-modal data were transmitted over a QoS-enabled Internet Protocol (IP) network. The force feedback device was the PHANToM desktop from SensAble Technologies Inc., which could provide force up to 3.3 N in 3 axis directions and generate 1000 packets/s of position and force data during the haptic collaboration actions. In the experiments, the force feedback device was used to manipulate moving virtual objects and to provide the user with feedback from the virtual environment. The end-to-end delay experienced by the haptic traffic was found to decrease from 200 ms (best effort) to 40 ms by running the haptic application in a Differentiated Services (DiffServ) network.

To understand the impact of vibration feedback latency, authors of [37] built a system consisting of a liquid crystal display (LCD), touch sensor, rod device with a vibrator, microcontroller, and a host computer. The microcontroller (NXP semiconductors, mbed NXP LPC1768) controlled the feedback latency from 0.1 to 25.6 ms, according to an adaptive staircase algorithm. Twenty-four participants first sat in front of the touchscreen and were instructed to tap the touchscreen by raising the rod as quickly as possible after the rod head made contact with the touchscreen with an approach velocity of 0.1–0.5 m/s. After the practice, they experienced a 25.6 ms delayed vibration. The participants then conducted eight staircases for further experiments involving two surface conditions (wood or metal). The results showed a 5.5 ms detection threshold of the vibration feedback latency.

Another experimental study proposed a multiplexing scheme that was evaluated using a teleoperation system consisting of a KUKA light weight robot arm (KUKA Robotics), a JR3 force/torque sensor, a force dimension Omega 6 haptic device [31], and real-time Linux-based Xenomai development software. Using the robot arm, the human operator could move toys and peg them in corresponding holes, which was considered as a representative task for the teleoperation applications. Haptic teleoperation experiments were performed, and KPIs considered were varying end-to-end signal latencies (force delay, video delay, audio delay), packet rates, peak delay, convergence time, and peak signal-to-noise ratio (PSNR) for visual quality.

In [39], researchers from Touch Lab, MIT demonstrated an experiment on haptic interaction between two users over a network with 2.4 Gbps connection. Authors used two PHANToM force-feedback devices at both sites; one was located at UCL VECG Lab, London, UK and the second was in MIT Touch Lab, Massachusetts, USA. The experimental subjects were to cooperate in lifting a virtual box together under different conditions.

A mutual tele-environment system named "HaptoClone" is proposed by researchers from the University of Tokyo in [36], which mutually copies adjacent 3D environments optically and physically using micro-mirror array plates technology. Haptic feedback was also given by using an airborne ultrasound tactile display. Different objects were touched by users, and the perceived delay of tactile feedback was measured. Simulations showed that a 100 ms delay was allowable to achieve the real-time interaction.

Other experimental studies using robot systems of SoloAssist (AKTORmed) in Germany, Panda robot (Franka Emika) in Italy, 3D-microscope (Karl Storz) and TiRobot system (Tinavi), and MicroHand (WEGO Group) in China are surveyed in [46].

3.1.2. Simulation Based

The surgical simulator dV-Trainer from Mimic technologies Inc., Seattle, WA, USA was used in [26,27]. In [26], sixteen medical students performed an energy dissection and a needle-driving exercise on the dV-Trainer, with latencies varying between 0 and 1000 ms with a 100 ms interval. These latencies were communication latencies from the time that a movement was initiated by the surgeon until the image of the movement is visible on the surgeon's monitor. The difficulty, security, precision, and fluidity of manipulation were self-scored by subjects. It was concluded that the surgical performance deteriorates in an exponential way as the latency increases. This study further concluded that latencies less than 200 ms were ideal for telesurgery; 300 ms was also suitable; 400–500 ms may be acceptable; and 600–700 ms was only acceptable for low-risk and simple procedures. Surgery was quite difficult at 800–1000 ms. The same simulator was utilized in [27]. However, in this study, instead of students, 37 surgeons were involved and performed different exercises in an easy-to-difficult order. The dV-Trainer simulator was permitted to introduce fixed latencies into the exercises between the gesture on the grips and the visual feedback on the console. Instead of a self-scoring system as in [26], the dV-trainer in [27] included a built-in scoring system, capturing instrument collisions, drops, etc. This study concluded that although the impact of delay is related to the difficulty of the procedures, overall, delays of 100 to 200 ms caused no significant impact, delays higher than 500 ms caused a noticeable increase in surgical risk, and surgery became extremely difficult and should be avoided at delays higher than 700 ms.

In [29], following experiments on a testbed (PHANToM devices), a probability density function (PDF) model of the haptic traffic from a distributed haptic virtual environments (DHVE) application was created for the use in a simulated DiffServ network using OPNET simulation tool. Subsequently, the effect of running the haptic traffic over a DiffServ IP network was obtained. Results indicated that the haptic throughput increases with the increase in the queue scheduling weight.

Another work leveraging a similar testbed used a force-feedback haptic device in the PHANToM experimental testbed [41]. The set-up involved two computers that were connected through a gigabit Ethernet fiber optic link running on the best effort IP service. The collected network traces from the test network were used to generate statistical models of each type of DVHE traffic that can be used in the standard network simulation packages such as OPNET. The measured network parameters included throughput, packet lost, delay, and jitter. Results from this simulation model showed a close match of simulation network throughputs with experimental throughputs of 850 Kbps and 630 Kbps in asynchronous and synchronous modes, respectively. DHVE effective throughput deteriorated sharply above 90% background load. End-to-end delays of more than 5 ms occurred at above 90% background load. The impact of jitter, latency, and packet loss was studied in [38] using the analytical models, OPNETWORK, and OPNET simulators. For audio, the simulated traffic behavior model was based on two-state (ON-OFF) Markov modulated rate process (MMRP) with the exponentially distributed time at each state. For video, the model was based on K-state MMRP. The QoS requirements for the audio were reported as: delay < 150 ms, jitter < 30 ms, and packet loss $< 1\%$. For video, these requirements were concluded as: delay < 400 ms, jitter < 30 ms, and packet loss $< 1\%$.

Another simulation-based study to investigate the haptic-audio-visual data communication used an interpersonal communication system, HugMe, which consisted of a haptic jacket for a remote person to simulate nurture touching, a haptic device for a local person to communicate his feelings with the remote person, and a depth camera to capture the image and depth information of the remote person and send it back [28].

Several studies citing jitter requirements for telesurgery have referred to the work in [43] that used Image Server and Haptic Handshake applications. The network emulation in [43] consisted of two endpoint computers and a third intervening computer that simulates the network using NISTNet software. The Handshake application is intended to train students remotely in surgical procedures by placing a haptic device at each endpoint and having the instructor guide the movements of the student remotely. The performance was evaluated under varying packet loss, delay, and jitter conditions. Minimum end-to-end performance requirements for throughput was 128 Kbps, packet loss was less than 10%, delay was less than 20 ms with abrupt movement and less than 80 ms with gentle movement, and jitter was less than 1 ms.

The authors investigated the effect of packet loss and latency in multimodal telepresence systems in [35]. The packet loss caused the impression of time delay and influenced the perception of the subsequent events. The simulated haptic feedback force was generated via PHANToM haptic device. The visual 3D environment was presented on a monitor, which was fixed above the haptic device and tilted 80° toward the observer. The visual space was collocated with (i.e., projected into) the haptic space by means of a mirror, and participants viewed the mirrored image through a pair of shutter glasses for the stereo image presentation. Visual-haptic event judgment was investigated under packet loss rates of 0, 0.1, 0.2, and 0.3, respectively. The minimum required latency for visual-haptic events was concluded to be 50 ms. Finally, telesurgery reports using software-defined networking (SDN), fog, and cloud infrastructures are described and compared in [48]. For more details on the use of SDN, fog, and cloud in emerging healthcare, the reader is referred to the works in [49–53].

The reported KPI values are inconsistent across literature reports due to factors such as varying types of tasks during telesurgery, varying equipment, and varying simulation environments across the studies. For example, latency ranges from as low as 1 ms for haptic feedback to as high as 700 ms for camera flow data, jitter ranges from 1 ms for haptic feedback to 55 ms for 3D camera flow, and the data rate requirements vary between 10 Kbps for vital signs transmission and 1.6 Gbps for 3D camera flow. Similarly, the BER also varies between 10^{-10} to 10^{-3} depending on the data type.

3.2. Connected Ambulance

Table 1 summarizes the literature relevant to the connected ambulance use case in terms of the investigated communication KPIs. The literature covers a wide range of applications termed connected ambulance. In essence, this involves providing medical care enroute to a healthcare facility while exchanging relevant data (e.g., imaging, vital signs, audio, and video) with healthcare providers. Requirements for 5G-enabled mobile healthcare in general are discussed in [21], where the authors propose to implement two-way connectivity between ambulances and hospitals across the UK. The KPIs discussed in the paper include the maximum allowed end-to-end latency for different data types (i.e., 150 ms for camera and audio flow, 250 ms for vital signs, and less than 10 ms for force and vibration). Data rate requirements for different data types were also specified, with the highest data rate requirement being 10 Mbps for two-way visual multimedia streaming, followed by haptic feedback, including force and vibration data types with 400 Kbps each, and then audio multimedia stream with a requirement of 200 Kbps. Depending on the required quality and bandwidth constraints, the data rate requirements for audio data can vary between 22 and 200 Kbps. Moreover, different types of vital signs were assigned different data rates, with EEG having the highest requirement of up to 86.4 Kbps [21].

Table 1. Summary of literature for relevant connected ambulance KPIs.

Use Case	KPIs	Data Type	Tools	Study Year
Ambulance transporting stroke patients to hospital	Throughput, number of reconnections	Audio, video, and vital signs	TeleBAT system in ambulance	[54] 2000
Ambulance transporting cardiac patients to hospital	Retainability, PLR	12-lead ECGs	Rhythm-surveillance and defibrillation equipment	[55] 2002
Ambulance transporting cardiac patients to hospital	Latency, PLR	12-Lead ECG	Philips standard (basic device model without advanced features such as computer-assisted ECG interpretations), embedded, and integrated ECG device	[56] 2010
Ambulance transporting stroke patients to hospital	Retainability	Audio, video	VIMED CAR, head and body cameras, and specialized microphones	[57] 2012
Ambulance transporting stroke patients to hospital	Retainability, bandwidth (mean and maximal upload and download speeds for data transfer), accessibility	Audio-video, blood pressure, heart rate, blood oxygen saturation, glycemia, and electronic patient identification	PreSSUB 3.0 system in ambulance	[58] 2014
Ambulance transporting stroke patients to hospital	Reliability, retainability	Audio, video	In-Touch RP-Xpress telemedicine device, Verizon Jetpack 4G LTE mobile hotspot (4620LE) for 4G LTE	[59] 2014
Ambulance transporting stroke patients to hospital	Bandwidth (median maximal and average upload download speed)	Audio-video, blood pressure, heart rate, blood oxygen saturation, glycemia, temperature, cardiac rhythm, Glasgow Coma Scale (GCS), and electronic patient identification	PreSSUB 3.0 system in ambulance	[60] 2016
Mobile stroke treatment units for patients with acute onset of stroke-like symptoms	Service restoration time, PLR, and latency	CT, audio-video, and vital signs	MSTUs with CT system, camera (RP-Xpress; InTouch Health)	[61] 2016
Testing of video encoding framework on ultrasound videos of carotid artery in connected ambulance scenario	Bitrate, data rate, time-varying bandwidth availability	Ultrasound videos of the common carotid artery	Multi-objective optimization, Philips ATL 5000 ultrasound machine, x265 open source software, and Ubuntu 14.04.4 LTS/Linux 64-bit platform	[62] 2017
A mobile small cell-based ambulance in the uplink direction in a heterogeneous network	Latency, data rate, PLR, retainability, and spectral efficiency	Ultrasound video	LTE Sim system level simulator	[63] 2018
Project proposal aiming to capture more than 6000 ambulances across the UK provided by 200 different vendors	Latency, data rate, PLR	Ultrasound video, in-ambulance video vital signs, EEG, ECG, force, vibration	Sonography and vital-signs-measuring equipment in ambulances	[21] 2019
Connected ambulance prototype study with QoS control in network slicing environment	Uplink/downlink throughput, latency (average per-hop)	Video slices (eHealth, conferencing, surveillance and entertainment)	MEC-based TeleStroke service by SliceNet, NetFPGA cards, SimpleSumeSwitch architecture, LTE eNodeBs, OpenFlow-enabled switches, Software Development Kit (SDK), Dell Edge Gateway, and P4 NetFPGA	[64] 2019
Connected Ambulance prototype study in network slicing environment	Average packet loss, latency (round trip time), throughput (frames per second)	Audio, video	eHealth infrastructure at Dell, Ireland, pfSense security, OpenVPN, Dell Edge Gateway series 3003, LTE SIMS, OpenMANO OSM, and MEC by SliceNET	[65] 2019

Table 1. Cont.

Use Case	KPIs	Data Type	Tools	Study Year
Prediction of ambulances' future locations to overcome mobility-based challanges	Position accuracy	GPS data	Apache Spark, Spark SQL, and algorithms	[66] 2020
Proposition of an architecture for connected ambulance	Uplink/downlink rate, number of device connections, latency, speed, reliability, and jitter	Ultrasound image, vital signs, and video	Vital signs monitor, ultrasound equipment, and video cameras	[67] 2020
Report compiled by industry experts and academic researchers based on their studies	Latency, jitter, survival time, communication service availability, reliability, and data rate	4K video, audio	Reference given to [22]	[11] 2020
Simulation of mobile ambulance using emulated biosensor data	Latency, average throughput, and PLR	Body temperature, blood pressure, and heart rate	Data Distribution Service (DDS) middleware, and biosensor emulator	[68–70] 2015, 2020
Ambulance transporting stroke patients in rural area to hospital	Retainability, reliability	Audio, video,	iPad, Jabber video app, University of Virginia Health System firewall, COR IBR600 LE-VZ; CradlePoint router, 4G Verizon Wireless sim, and AP-CW-M-S22-RP2-BL and AP-CG-S22-BL antennas	[71,72] 2016, 2020
Connected ambulance evaluation in network slicing environment using a test platform	Downlink/uplink data rate, and uplink latency	Video, CT image, vital signals, and medical record	5G customer-premises equipment (CPE) signal transceiver, 5G user plane function (UPF) gateway service flow forwarding device, and medical data acquisition device, MEC cloud computing node	[73] 2021
Stroke patients in mobile stroke units en route to hospital	Reliability, retainability	Audio, video, ECG, and vital signs	MEYTEC GmbH telemedicine systems of Vimed car and Vimed Doc for videoconferencing and teleradiology	[74,75] 2019, 2021

The studies in [11,22] also highlighted some general requirements for this use case, including 10 ms latency, 2 ms jitter, <2 ms survival time, $1 - 10^{-5}$ service availability, $1 - 10^{-7}$ reliability, and 0.05 Mbps data rate.

The project "improving treatment with rapid evaluation of acute stroke via mobile telemedicine" (iTREAT) in [71] reported that 93% of connected ambulance cases achieved a minimum 9 min of continuous, and live video transmission with a mean mobile connectivity time of 18 min, and 87.5% of tests achieved bidirectional audio video quality with ratings of 4 out of 5 or higher, excluding one route with poor transmission quality. The transport routes were 20 min to the University of Virginia Medical Center, and 30 test runs were performed. Limitations of this study include manual ratings of the service quality, not explicitly incorporating patient while testing, exclusion of one route with poor coverage conditions, small size of study, and being limited to one region.

Another e-ambulance study used biosensor emulators in a laboratory to mimic biosensor communication behavior and studied KPIs with the varying number of biosensors and payload sizes [68–70]. Reported outcomes include an upper bound of 250 ms on latency, and 0.4 Mbps for average overall throughput, and the success ratio of transmitted samples varied between 97.7% and 99.9%.

A connected ambulance use case was investigated in [62] in the context of proposing a video encoding configuration that jointly optimizes the clinical video quality, time-varying bandwidth availability, and heterogeneous device's performance capabilities. The proposed model estimated structural similarity quality with a median accuracy error of less than 1%, bitrate demands with the deviation error of 10% or less, and encoding frame rate within a 6% margin.

The study in [67] proposed measurement-based requirements for high-definition ultrasound images (uplink rate > 20 Mbps, downlink rate > 5 Mbps, network delay < 80 ms, jitter < 30 ms), 4K video (uplink rate > 20 Mbps, downlink rate > 20 Mbps, network delay < 50 ms, jitter < 20 ms). Reliability was set to 99.99%, and mobility was 0–120 km/h. The measured download rate inside the ambulance, which is a user of a 5G private network, reached 1361.21 Mbps, and upload rate reached 257.52 Mbps.

Handling specific patient conditions was also addressed in the context of connected ambulance, e.g., prehospital stroke evaluation and treatment [76]. A Prehospital Stroke Study at the Universitair Ziekenhuis Brussel investigated the safety, technical feasibility, and reliability of in-ambulance telemedicine [58]. A total of 43 attempts were made to perform a prehospital teleconsultation of neurological and non-neurological conditions (e.g., strokes, trauma, respiratory, gastro-intestinal, acute pain, intoxication, labor, dysglycemia, and vascular disease). The authors concluded that 30 teleconsultations were performed, with success rate of 73.2%. Transient signal loss occurred during 6 teleconsultation sessions (14.6%). The time before the connection was re-established varied from 38 seconds to 5 minutes and 47 seconds. Permanent signal losses occurred in five teleconsultations (12.2%). The success rates for the communication of blood pressure, heart rate, blood oxygen saturation, glycemia, and electronic patient identification were 78.7%, 84.8%, 80.6%, 64.0%, and 84.2%, respectively. Communication of a prehospital report to the in-hospital team had a 94.7% success rate and prenotification of the in-hospital team 90.2%. Most problems were caused by unstable bandwidth of the 3G/4G mobile network; limited high speed broadband access; and software, hardware, or human error. The study's main limitations include the small sample size, short study duration, and complex observational design. A continuation of this study was carried out in [60], which addressed patients with suspected acute stroke and reported median maximal and average upload speeds as 196 Kbps and 40 Kbps, respectively. The download median maximal speed is reported as 407 Kbps, and average speed is reported 12 Kbps, using 4G. An experimental study evaluated the use of mobile stroke treatment units (MSTUs) to diagnose and treat 100 residents of Cleveland who had an acute onset of stroke-like symptoms [61]. It was concluded that there were six instances of video disconnection, of which five were because of an area of poor wireless reception, and one was due to the compatibility issue of the devices. No video disconnections lasted longer than 60 s. One limitation pointed out by the authors is the small sample size of this study.

TeleBAT system in [54] used an integrated mobile telecommunications system while transporting patients to the University of Maryland hospital via an ambulance. Results showed feasibility of the case, with number of disconnections resulting from coverage holes, or network switching.

Another case study on mobile stroke units (MSU), a11, consisted of a combination of two studies: PrioLTE2 (Reliability of Telemedically Guided Pre-hospital Acute Stroke Care With Prioritized 4G Mobile Network Long-Term Evolution) study and TeDir (TeleDiagnostics in Prehospital Emergency Medicine [Tele-Diagnostik im Rettungsdienst]) study. A remote neurologist rated the audiovisual quality. The authors in [74] reported high interrater reliabilities between the onboard and remote neurologists, and 16 out of 18 treatment decisions agreed. Limitations of this study included 12.6% of the teleconsultations not being completed due to the failure of video connection, higher rate of aborted attempts than the previous studies (1% in [61] and 2% in [77]), small number of patients, and inclusion of the data from two separate studies with different assessment metrics.

A prehospital utility of rapid stroke evaluation using in-ambulance telemedicine (PURSUIT) pilot feasibility study was conducted in [59]. Actors performing pre-scripted stroke scenarios of varying stroke severity were used in live acute stroke assessments. It is concluded that 80% of the sessions were conducted without major technological limitations. Reliability of video interpretation was defined by a 90% concordance between the data derived during the real-time sessions and those from the scripted scenarios. A previous pilot study, StrokeNET in Berlin, could not conclude assessments because the audio video was lost in 18 out of 30 scenarios [57].

As for cardiac patients, a study published in 2010 [56] demonstrated the transmission of 12-lead electrocardiography (ECG) in an ambulance driving at 50–100 km/h to the cell phone of the attendant emergency medical technician and then to the hospital and to the cell phones of off-site cardiologists using a 3G network, after going through the hospital ECG-processing server. It was concluded that the ECG can be transmitted successfully at the first attempt in all five trials, except in one remote, mountainous ambulance service area. The average transmission time of an ECG report ranged from 91 to 165 s. Interruption of ambulance ECG transmission occurred in up to 27% of transmissions. Rehman et al. in [55] reported a 1 year study included data from 17 ambulances enroute to Silkeborg Central Hospital (distance ranging from 20–75 km) transmitting 12-lead ECGs and involving 250 patients with the suspected diagnosis of acute myocardial infarction. Results indicated that 86% of prehospital diagnoses were successful. Geographically related transmission problems were the primary reason for failure. Limitations of this study included patient history taking by direct communication between the physician and patient and the lack of a randomized setup.

Mobility is one of the unique features of the connected ambulance use cases and this raises the connectivity issues that can be observed in high-speed moving vehicles (e.g., poor signal quality, multiple handovers, greater occurrences of connection drops, and penetration loss from metallic walls of vehicle). To address these challenges, authors in [63] evaluated data streaming between one ambulance and hospital nodes on the uplink with a small cell inside the ambulance traveling at a speed of 120 km/h. In the simulation scenario, a transceiver was installed on the roof of the ambulance to transmit/receive data to/from the backhaul macrocell network. The small cell installed inside the ambulance made a wireless connection between the paramedics and the small cell access point (SAP). The SAP and the transceiver were connected through a wired network. The PLR value when using the small cell was reduced to 4.8% compared to 14% in case of 10 users trying to connect to the outside macrocell base station. All 10 users were located in the same ambulance. Throughput also improved by a small amount with the small cell. Authors concluded that using small cell inside the ambulance could be particularly useful in high bandwidth congestion scenarios. Another way to help address mobility challenges can be to predict the future location of the ambulance based on its previous locations as reported in [66]. The authors proposed an algorithm, NextSTMove, which is 300% faster than traditional algorithms and achieved accuracies of 75% to 100%.

Among the 5G features that can enable connected ambulances is network slicing, where logical network resources can be provisioned to accommodate specific application demands. A study conducted in network slicing environment using facilities at the 5G Prototyping Lab at Dell EMC facilities Ireland and SliceNet reported an average round trip latency of 296.91 ms from client to core, an average round trip time of 50.68 ms from client to edge, and an average packet loss of 7.2% for the core and 0.1% at the edge [65]. Another study was carried out in [64] using the same experimental tools with the added features like QoS control based on the data plane programmability and low-latency cloud-based mobile edge computing (MEC) platform. Throughput was evaluated for the coordinated and uncoordinated network slicing strategies and ranged from 0 to 18 Mbps. In QoS-aware slicing, average delay of less than 0.05 ms was observed. However, in non-QoS aware slicing, no guarantee of low latency was given for any network transmission.

Another network-slicing system architecture for 5G-enabled ambulance service was tested in the experimental settings with ambulance speed of 30 km/h. Two types of data were considered in this study: video data for remote consultation and uploading of 4.5 GB of computed tomography (CT) image data from an ambulance to a destination hospital affiliated with the Zhengzhou University [73]. For video data, the average downlink speed of 1080 p 30 Hz HD video in the 5G network environment was 4.6 Mbps, compared to 3.5 Mbps with unstable network and packet loss in 4G. For CT data, the upload time was shortened by 33 percent in 5G as compared to 4G and the average latency for 5G was 12.88 ms, compared to 76.85 ms for 4G which was 6 times that of 5G.

Other relevant studies are ongoing by the groups such as PRE-hospital Stroke Treatment Organization's (PRESTO) [75,78] and EU 5G PPP Trials working group by SliceNET [79,80].

The reported KPI values for connected ambulance use case vary across literature reports with the variation in considered ambulance mobility, which has a range of 0–120 km/h across reports. Accordingly, latency ranges from around 10 ms for haptic feedback to around 250 ms for vital signs transmission. However, one study also reports latency of as low as 0.05 ms using a QoS-aware slicing scheme. Jitter ranges from 2 ms to 30 ms, depending on the data type and survival time remains less than 2 ms. The maximum data rate requirement reported in literature is around 1360 Mbps and the minimum is 22 Kbps, depending on the communication quality and bandwidth constraints. The average packet loss is reported to be in the 0.1% to 7.2% range.

3.3. Healthcare IoT

Based on the American Society of Engineers, medical internet of things refers to the amalgamation of the medical devices and applications that connect to healthcare information technology systems by leveraging the networking technologies [81]. Healthcare IoT systems encompass diverse applications and computational capabilities and target diverse populations. Notably, many healthcare IoT systems predate 5G and are being used with 4G and local area wireless technologies such as Wi-Fi and Bluetooth. However, 5G can enable an expanded use of healthcare IoT and facilitate the development of novel applications [53]. Accordingly, we dedicate this section to highlighting the wide range of healthcare IoT applications and summarizing their reported communication KPIs. We broadly categorize healthcare IoT systems, which include, medical, and non-medical devices, into five types as shown in Figure 4: (1) fitness tracking and health improvement, (2) chronic disease monitoring, (3) aid for the physically impaired, (4) tracking of life threatening events, and (5) embedded/implantable medical devices.

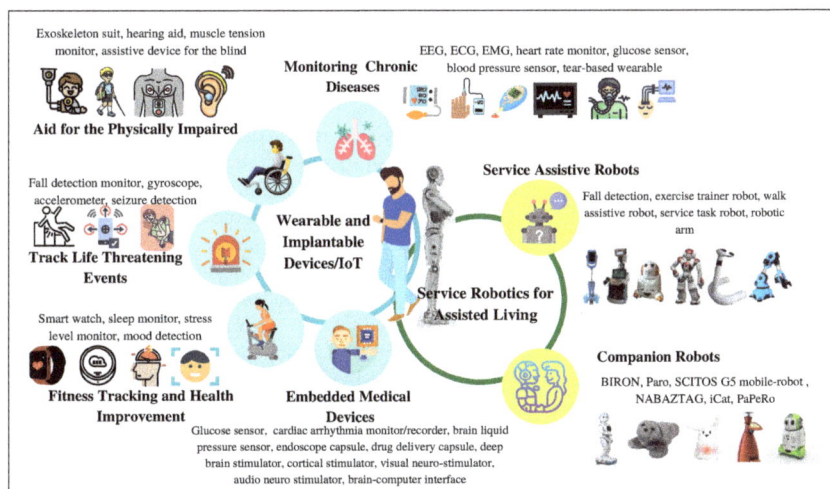

Figure 4. Types of healthcare IoT devices and service assistive robots.

Applications targeted for healthy individuals can be used for a wide range of purposes, including routine monitoring, lifestyle improvement, or disease prevention, where they act as early warning systems [82]. Examples include smart watches [83,84] that can monitor heart rate, blood glucose level, blood pressure, and breathing rate. Other fitness and health improvement wearables include temperature sensors [85,86]; pulse oximeter SpO$_2$ [87–89];

sleep trackers [90]; fertility and pregnancy trackers [91]; and monitors for respiration [92], blood pressure [93–96], pH [97,98], stress [99], mood [100], and sleep [101].

Patients with underlying conditions or those who need assisted living in chronic scenarios can benefit from applications for measuring and reporting electroencephalogram (EEG) [102,103], ECG [93,104,105], electromyography (EMG) [106,107] heart rate [108–110] for cardiac patients, glucose [111,112], insulin for diabetic patients [113–115], and continuous respiratory rate for chronic respiratory patients [116]. For assisting the physically impaired, there are numerous wearable devices to help improve quality of life, such as hearing aids (ear-to-ear communication) [117,118]; devices for disability assistance, e.g., muscle tension monitor [119]; muscle tension stimulation [120]; wearable assistive devices for the blind [121–124]; devices for speech impairment [125,126]; artificial/wearable limbs [127–129]; and exoskeleton suits [130]. Other examples that can be used by the elderly, or by Alzheimer's or epilepsy patients, include wearables for fall detection [131–133] and seizure detection [134,135], and gyroscopes [136] and accelerometers [137] for localization monitoring. Examples of implantable devices include pacemakers [138] and implantable cardioverter defibrillators (ICD) [139], and implanted actuator [140,141].

Despite the diversity of healthcare IoT applications, the underlying KPIs requirements are shared by most. However, KPI levels vary for different applications. Following are some of the KPI requirements for this category.

Energy efficiency is vital for battery-operated devices, where the needed battery lifetime can range from a few days to a few years. Accordingly, battery lifetime can be >1 week (the life-time numbers are expected/calculated based on normal use conditions for continuous monitoring) for non-implantable devices, and for monitoring ECG, EEG, EMG, glucose, etc. [142]. For implantable devices, this figure can grow to several years (e.g., >3 years for deep brain stimulator) or remain within the range of hours for some applications such as >24 h for capsule endoscopes [34]. The importance of battery lifetime increases in implanted devices given the risks associated with the device replacement because of depleted battery. In an attempt to overcome constraints on the battery form factor to accommodate specific implant application, solutions for energy harvesting were considered in the literature that can benefit from the energy present in the environment, human body, and wireless signals [143]. Duty cycle is also relevant in this context, where a lower duty cycle contributes to longer battery lifetime. It captures the tradeoff between the need to timely communicate data and the cost of battery power to do so. The work in [34] reports on duty cycle requirements ranging from <1% (e.g., temperature sensors, fall detection devices, and respiration monitors) to <50% (e.g., implantable endoscope capsules).

The efficiency of data transmission during the device ON time is described by the data rate, with varying requirements according to the application and the used transmission protocol. Literature reports offer a wide array of data rate requirements. For example, the researchers in, patel2010applications report that monitoring devices for temperature, heart rate, breathing, blood pressure, blood sugar, and oxygenation require <10 Kbps data rate, 72 Kbps for ECG, 86.4 Kbps for EEG, 1 Mbps for deep brain stimulation and capsule endoscopy, and 1–1.5 Mbps for EMG and location tracking devices [34,144]. Other references [142,145–147] listed different values, including 128–320 Kbps for deep brain stimulators, 3 Kbps per ECG channel per link, and 16 bps for the wearable temperature sensors. Data rate can be influenced by device processing capabilities, the data use model (i.e., real-time processing by an external processor is associated with demand for a high data rate, while applications suitable for post-processing can use a low data rate), and the capabilities of the wireless technology being considered. With the advancement of 5G, literature reports now point to a higher data rate to be supported by wearables (e.g., 10 Mbps [148], 0.1–5 Mbps [11].) Requirements for BER also varied by application and were reported in [149], generally ranging from 10^{-10} to 10^{-5}. Specific examples included an ultrasonic wearable device prototype designed to be used as heart rate monitor, and ECG respiratory rate monitor, and step counter reported a BER requirement of lower than 10^{-5} using a transmission power of 13 dBm [150]. BER for vital sign monitoring devices such as ECG, pulse oximeters, and implantable devices such as hearing aids are reported as $<10^{-10}$ [34]. To facilitate the diverse healthcare IoT applications, the overall reliability and service availability should be $1 - 10^{-3}$ [11].

Latency requirements also varied across the applications and by the source. The authors in [144] report <50 ms latency for monitors of chronic disease and emergency event detection. Vital signs monitors were assigned a latency of <1 s, while fitness tracking devices increased latency tolerance to a few seconds. A blanket latency requirement for wearables was set at 250 ms in [11,34], while survival time was set at 10 ms in [11,22] and jitter <25 ms in [11]. Other reported latency values include <50 ms for deep brain stimulators and <100 ms for hearing aids [142]. In [151], LTE-based data transmission experiments using a real-time video wearable device (i.e., BlueEye) under impaired channel loss and propagation loss were performed. The purpose of the study was to test whether mHealth services could be used in the locations with poor coverage conditions. For different mobility scenarios, the jitter values obtained were 0.473 ms for the static users, 2.05 ms for the pedestrian users, and 3.54 ms for the vehicular users. In an attempt to reduce latency in healthcare IoT applications, significant research was dedicated to data processing and analytics at the edge side of the system to circumvent delays caused by the processing lag and cross network data transfer [53,152]. In this context, latency of transmitting various raw ECG captures from a gateway to a remote cloud was compared with the total latency of processing on fog computing service and transmitting preprocessed ECG data in [153]. At the data rate of 9 Mbps there was 48.5% latency reduction by leveraging fog computing in this case. This comes at the cost of addressing data security and privacy while in transport between the device and the cloud. To help manage medical device risks, including security, a risk management process is specified in the international organization for standardization (ISO) 14,971 standard for the application of risk management to the medical devices [154]. Moreover, the FDA published a draft guidance on the content of premarket submissions for the management of cybersecurity in medical devices [155], which provides recommendations to industry regarding cybersecurity aspects of the medical device cybersecurity management, such as risk assessment. Security KPIs in the context of 5G-enabled healthcare applications are summarized in [6], including authenticity, confidentiality, integrity, agility, vulnerability, resilience, mitigation/recovery time, and proactiveness.

Network-level KPIs were addressed in the context of healthcare IoT, including a connection density of 20,000 devices/km^2 in remote pervasive monitoring settings such as in smart home wearables and 10, 000 devices/km^2 for general mHealth wearables [11,22]. Other reported KPIs include 50 Gbps/km^2 traffic density and 50 km user activity range [11].

Given that the healthcare IoT includes diverse applications that can be used in diverse environments, their enabling KPIs can be influenced by practical deployment factors such as number of nodes, topology, operating frequencies, transmit power restrictions height of device [156], interference, and co-existence [156,157], and others. Finally, we note that one of the emerging 5G-enabled healthcare applications is medical augmented reality/virtual reality (AR/VR). According to a study by Qualcomm [158], the requirements for AR/VR can go to as high as 10–50 Mbps for 360° 4 K video, 50–200 Mbps for 360° 8 K video, and up to 5000 Mbps (or 5 Gbps) for 6 degree-of-freedom (DoF) video. Moreover, a study by Facebook indicates a real-time playback rate of 4 Gbps (or 32 Gbps) for 6 DoF video, indicating there might be some use cases where individual sustained per-user rates of >1 Gbps might be needed [159]. The varying applications and diverse IoT device categories contributed to the reported KPI covering a broad range of values. For instance, the battery lifetime ranges from 24 h for capsule endoscopes to several years for other implantable devices. The data transmission rate for wearable devices varies from as low as <10 Kbps to 10 Mbps. Similarly, the BER also varies between 10^{-10} and 10^{-3} depending on the data type. The latency ranges from 0.473 ms for wearable devices for vital signs monitoring to a few seconds for fitness tracking devices, while the network-level KPIs include a connection density of 10,000–20,000 devices/km^2.

3.4. Robots for Assisted Living

Robots in assisted living environments have been widely studied in literature [11,20–47]. An assistive robot can be defined as an aiding device that has the ability to process the sensory information for helping the physically/mentally impaired or elderly persons to perform tasks of daily living without the need of attendants, in hospital or at home [160]. Assistive robots can be broadly classified into two categories, i.e., services assistive robots and companion robots as shown in Figure 4. In this section, our focus is on the communication KPIs for this application with a summary provided in Table 2 of the reported cellular network KPIs.

Table 2. Summary of literature for relevant assistive robots KPIs.

KPI	Service Robot	Assigned Tasks	Target Population	Study
UE battery	Mobile robot BENDER with telepresence capabilities	Assistance in routine tasks and user localization	Elderly	[161]
Latency, PLR	Companion robot	User finding and medication reminder	Elderly	[162]
Latency, data rate	Cloud robot	Monitoring of vital signs	Elderly	[163]
Accessibility, position accuracy	Domestic health assistant Max	Assistance in routine tasks, user searching and following	Healthy elderly	[164]
Throughput (packets per seconds)	Domestic robot DoRo	Video streaming through robot cameras	Elderly and children	[165]
Latency, PLR, position accuracy (mean localization error)	Service robot	Recognition and localization of users	Healthy elderly	[166]
Latency (round trip time), retainability (total service time)	Mobile robot DoRo	Personalized medical support and pre-set reminder event	Elderly people with chronic diseases (multimorbidity)	[167]
Latency, reliability	Nao, Qbo and Hanson robots	Streaming of teleoperation website	Elderly and children	[168]
Position accuracy	ASTRO robot	Assistance in routine tasks, health related reminders	Healthy elderly	[169]
Position accuracy	Assistive robotic arm	Tablet placement infront of patient	Patients with limited or no mobility	[170]
Position accuracy	Mobile humanoid robot GARMI	Support for household tasks and emergency assistance	Elderly and patients	[171]

Position accuracy is pertinent to robots used for fall detection and real-time assistance. The authors in [172] demonstrated that by exploiting the information from the reflected multipath components, increased accuracy and robustness in localization can be achieved. Moreover, they proposed 5G mmWave as one of the promising solutions for indoor accurate localization for assistive living.

According to the EU Horizon 2020 project "Robots in Assisted Living Environments" [173], assisted living considerations include reliability, connectivity, low battery discharge profile, low latency, high communication success rate, and minimum localization error, with appropriate feedback to support people with limited mobility, who require assistance and companionship.

To provide personalized medical support to the elderly in the presence of several chronic diseases, the authors in [167] designed a hybrid robot–cloud approach. The robot autonomously reached the user with the pre-set reminder events acting as a physical reminder. This case study in DomoCasa Lab (Italy) evaluated the robot (DoRo) based on KPIs such as latency (i.e., round trip time), retainability (i.e, in terms of total service time), robot processing time (RPT), average travel time, and mean velocity. Latency over the 20 experimental trials was reported as 56 ms and RPT as 0.012 ms. For the use case where DoRo had to travel 12.6 m to deliver the services with a mean velocity of 0.31 m/s, the total service time was 40.08 s.

The ASTROMOBILE system was evaluated in [169]. The mean path length for the simplest use case (moving in the kitchen) was 9.6 m with a mean velocity of 0.51 m/s, path jerk of 0.023×10^6, and a mean position accuracy error is 0.98 m.

Under the German research project SERROGA, which lasted from 2012 to mid 2015, a companion robot for domestic health assistance was developed [164]. Its services include communication, emergency assistant, physical activity motivator, navigation services, pulse rate monitoring, and fall detection. The robot was evaluated in different apartments and labs for a minimum of 29 min and a maximum duration of 255 min, with a velocity range of 0.25–0.27 m/s for distance covered of 355–2600 m. The robot was able to complete the user following tasks with a positioning accuracy of 95%.

A cloud-robotic system for the provisioning of assistive services for the promotion of active and healthy ageing in Italy and Sweden was assessed in [166] on the basis of latency (i.e, round trip time), PLR (i.e, data loss rate), position accuracy (i.e, mean localization error), and localization root mean square error (RMSE) KPIs. The reliability and responsiveness of the cloud Database Management Service (DBMS) was evaluated based on latency as the time a robot waits for the user position, after a request to the server. The study took place in two sites: smart home in Italy (Domocasa lab) and residential condominium in Sweden (Angen). The mean latency in Domocasa lab was 40 ms, while for the Swedish site it was 134.57 ms. The local host latency acquired during the experimentation was 7.46 ms and was used as a benchmark. The rate of service failures was less than 0.5% in Italy, and 0.002% for the Angen site. In Domocasa and Angen, the mean absolute localization errors were 0.98 m and 0.79 m, respectively, while the RMSE were 1.22 m and 0.89 m, respectively. On average, the absolute localization error considering the two setups was 0.89 m, and the RMSE was 1.1 m. The use of the presence sensors increased the localization accuracy in the selected positions by an average of 35%.

Assistive living robots domain can suffer from errors caused by the communication connection issues, latency, and spatiotemporal dynamic environment changes. To improve the autonomy and efficiency of robots in smart environment, the authors in [174] proposed a framework for the improvement of the assistive robot performance through a context acquisition method, an activity recognition process, and a dynamic hierarchical task planner. Additionally, authors in [175] proposed to use full duplex 5G communication for reliable and low-latency robot-based assistive living.

In a trend similar to the other investigated use-cases, the reported communication KPI values for assistive robots varied across reports, with latency varying from 7.46 ms to 134.57 ms and velocity varying from 0.25 m/s to 0.51 m/s. The localization error has a narrow range from 0.89 m–0.98 m, while the distance covered by the assistive robots has a broad range from 12.6 m–2600 m, and service time varies from 0.08 s–255 min.

4. 5G-Healthcare Requirements vs. Status of 5G Capabilities

5G technology was developed to meet the use cases specified by the International Telecommunication Union (ITU) International Mobile Telecommunications-2020 (IMT-2020). These are enhanced mobile broadband (eMBB), ultra-reliable, and low-latency communications (URLLC), and massive machine type communications (mMTC). As detailed in the previous sections, many healthcare applications can benefit from the communication capabilities of these 5G use cases. A study based on simulation confirmed that the 3GPP

5G system complies with the ITU IMT-2020 performance requirements [176]. 5G trials and commercial deployments are accelerating throughout the world [177–179]. These show varying levels of performance toward theoretical goals. For example, 2 Gbps throughput and 3 ms latency were achieved in Austria using spectrum in the 3.7 GHz band [177]. In another 5G trial in Belgium, 2.94 Gbps throughput and 1.81 ms latency were achieved. The peak throughputs of 15 Gbps, 5 Gbps, and 4.3 Gbps in 5G trials were also reported by European network operators Telia, Elisa, and Tele2 Lithuania, respectively [177]. In the U.S., AT&T reported on 5G use cases such as video streaming, downloading, and conferencing and achieved upload and download speeds around 1 Gbps [177]. Sprint tested streaming 5G virtual reality systems and 4K video and achieved peak download speeds of more than 2 Gbps using the 73 GHz mmWave spectrum [178]. Verizon achieved 4.3 Gbps speeds by aggregating C-band spectrum with mmWave spectrum in a lab trial [179].

Although commercial 5G coverage is still limited [180–182], 5G tests by OpenSignal in 2020 compared services offered by Verizon (mmWave), T-Mobile (mmWave, 600 MHz), Sprint (2.5 GHz), and AT&T (850 MHz) [183]. The report concluded that users should not automatically expect speeds of several hundred Mbps on 5G because in the tests they observed an average 5G download speeds ranging from 47.5 Mbps to 722.9 Mbps. They also noted that the U.S. carrier's 5G services are held back by 5G spectrum availability and some services are fast; however, they are limited by the coverage. Those with greater coverage offer slow speeds due to the limited spectrum. They also highlighted the need for the U.S. carriers to repurpose large portions of the mid-band spectrum for 5G in the U.S. to facilitate the 5G performance goals.

Comparing the realistic performance reports with the most stringent data rate requirement for telesurgery (i.e., 1.6 Gbps for 3D camera flow as listed in Table A3), we note that the throughput requirements of many healthcare use cases might be possible to meet with existing 5G capabilities. However, use cases requiring 6 DoF content such as AR/VR might be challenging those current capabilities. Furthermore, our review highlights that the latency for the haptic feedback can go as low as 1 ms, and for connected ambulance, the lower limit is 10 ms. However, realistic latency figures are expected to remain in the 10–12 ms range [184,185], rather than 1–2 ms. Notably, the 1 ms latency is specified in next-generation radio access network (NG-RAN) domain, which is defined as the link between the end user and base station (including MEC). This latency increases when the communication needs to be transmitted to the core network. Therefore, the end-to-end latency target could be around 5 ms [186]. The additional delay can impact the applications that utilize the core network (e.g., remote expert for collaboration in surgery, video analytics for behavioral recognition, and remote patient monitoring). 5G mmWave frequencies—also known as frequency range 2 (FR2)—can support large subcarrier spacing, resulting in smaller transmission time interval and thus improving latency. This indicates a favorable latency requirement support for healthcare use cases when using the mmWave spectrum. However, this comes at the expense of limited coverage due to the wave propagation properties in the mmWave spectrum, which can impact applications that need mobility support such as the connected ambulance. Moreover, the realistic deployments and trials are limited by the specific used configurations and the small set of reported KPIs like downlink throughput and latency. Accordingly, enabling a specific healthcare application using 5G requires a collaboration between the application developer, 5G network service provider, and the application user to ensure that the service meets the application requirements for communication and that the application can be used safely.

5. Gaps in Literature and Future Considerations

A considerable part of the existing literature addresses the communication requirements for the healthcare applications qualitatively, for example, using descriptors such as "big", "small", and "extremely low". Where quantitative requirements are mentioned, the focus is on high-level KPIs, which leaves a gap in describing how a given application can be supported in certain scenarios. For example, when addressing throughput, uplink and downlink throughput are commonly discussed; however, cell edge throughput is not considered. Similarly, mobility is commonly mentioned in terms of speed in the case of connected ambulance, but other mobility-related KPIs, such as handover success/failure rates or handover execution time, are not specified.

Although some reports describe individual KPIs in detail, the trade-offs between multiple KPIs and their interactions with configuration and optimization parameters (COPs) in a healthcare applications are often omitted. For example, one trade-off between throughput and latency for next-generation video content is described in [158], which states that achieving 5–20 ms latency requires 400–600 Mbps throughput, while achieving 1–5 ms latency requires 100–200 Mbps throughput. Another example of trade-offs is between coverage, capacity, and load balancing [187], or the trade-off between coverage, height of BS, and antenna parameters [188]. Such trade-offs are rarely considered in the literature on 5G-enabled healthcare use cases, which can complicate applications with conflicting requirements such as achieving high throughput with high mobility or low battery consumption. One way to study these trade-offs might be to combine several KPIs into a new one. For example, Samsung developed representative KPIs to describe the performance of multi-objective optimization involving more than two KPIs, such as sum of log of data rate, considering both throughput and fairness. It can be used as a joint KPI of wearable devices applications to represent both energy efficiency and throughput, energy efficiency, and delay, or energy efficiency and reliability [189].

Another gap in the literature is the limited 5G network scenarios that are assessed. Limitations include the small number of network trials, small number of infrastructure configurations, small coverage area, and the lack of spatiotemporal variability for trials being conducted in the laboratory settings. A critical analysis of 5G network failure modes that can impact 5G-enabled healthcare use cases is an open question not addressed in the literature. For example, only the success of the connected ambulance use case is discussed in the literature. However, this use case might be negatively impacted in situations with extremely high mobility, high user density, a disaster scenario where a large number of ambulances rush to the same point, a cell outage, or the presence of multiple critical traffic flows in the network.

Moreover, network KPIs are commonly vendor-specific, where each network equipment vendor specifies the performance metrics using its own set of counters and naming conventions. This may give rise to the challenge of managing non-standardized KPIs. The large number of technical counters in the heterogeneous 5G deployments, the use of vendor-specific monitoring tools by the network operators, and the lack of unified data format for collecting and reporting the performance data also pose a challenge for managing the service level agreements between the 5G network operators and the end users of the 5G-enabled healthcare systems [6]. For further reflection on avenues for addressing the highlighted considerations in practice and research, the reader is referred to [6,190].

Finally, we note that real-time systems and time-sensitive networks (TSNs) can benefit several of the discussed healthcare applications such as remote robotic-assisted surgery and in-ambulance treatment. This can be supported by 5G's technical features such as the near-instantaneous data transmission. For instance, the telerobotic spinal surgeries conducted using 5G-enabled robots have been enabled by a minimal lag between the robot and the remote physician [191]. Similarly, authors in [192] presented a survey on application requiring near real-time response, including healthcare applications such as AR, VR, tele-diagnosis, tele-surgery, and telerehabilitation. Accordingly, future considerations for 5G-enabled healthcare include the investigation and analysis of real-time systems and TSNs and their role in supporting healthcare applications. 5G can also contribute to enabling connected healthcare applications in small-scale healthcare facilities like those in rural areas [193,194].

6. Conclusions

5G communication features promise to enable novel healthcare applications and expand network access in the existing connected medical devices. Understanding the communication KPI requirements for 5G-enabled healthcare use cases can help healthcare application developers, 5G network providers, and regulatory authorities in the healthcare sector to promote safe and effective healthcare. In this paper, we have surveyed quantitative and qualitative KPI requirements for different use cases, including remote robotic-assisted surgery, mobile-connected ambulances, wearable and implantable devices in the healthcare IoT, and service robotics for assisted living. A comparison of 5G-healthcare requirements with the status of 5G capabilities reveals that some healthcare applications can be supported by the existing 5G services while others might be challenging, especially those with stringent latency requirement. This calls for a collaboration between the healthcare application developers and the network service providers to explore, document, and manage the possible connectivity support for a given application throughout its lifecycle.

We have also identified gaps in the existing literature and highlight considerations in this space, including the lack of focus on quantitative requirements, omitting relevant KPIs, overlooking the trade-offs between multiple KPIs and COPs, the lack of unified KPI specifications across different network operators and equipment vendors, and (lastly) the limitations 5G scenarios conducted in the existing trials. The gaps in this space and considerations highlighted in this paper can help direct future 5G-enabled medical device studies and facilitate the safe, effective, and efficient implementation of 5G technology in healthcare. Medical devices must integrate 5G technology safely and effectively to facilitate patient access to 5G-enabled medical device applications. As a part of the overall medical device risk management process, documenting and meeting the communication requirements for diverse 5G-healthcare use cases comes under service level agreements. Therefore, knowledge of requirements for 5G-enabled medical use cases highlighted in this paper can also help network service providers, users, and regulatory authorities in developing, managing, monitoring, and evaluating service-level agreements in 5G-enabled medical systems.

Author Contributions: Conceptualization, A.I. (Ali Imran) and M.O.A.K.; methodology, H.N.Q., M.O.A.K. and A.I. (Ali Imran); validation, H.N.Q., A.I. (Aneeqa Ijaz), M.M. and Y.L.; formal analysis, H.N.Q., M.O.A.K. and A.I. (Ali Imran); investigation, H.N.Q., A.I. (Aneeqa Ijaz) and M.M.; resources, A.I. (Ali Imran) and M.O.A.K.; writing—original draft preparation, H.N.Q., A.I. (Aneeqa Ijaz) and M.M.; writing—review and editing, M.O.A.K. and Y.L.; visualization, M.M. and H.N.Q.; supervision, M.O.A.K., A.I. (Ali Imran) and Y.L.; project administration, M.O.A.K., A.I. (Ali Imran) and Y.L.; funding acquisition, M.O.A.K. and A.I. (Ali Imran). All authors have read and agreed to the published version of the manuscript.

Funding: This research received no external funding.

Institutional Review Board Statement: Not applicable.

Informed Consent Statement: Not applicable.

Data Availability Statement: Not applicable.

Acknowledgments: This project was supported in part by an appointment to the Research Participation Program at the U.S. Food and Drug Administration, administered by the Oak Ridge Institute for Science and Education through an interagency agreement between the U.S. Department of Energy and the U.S. Food and Drug Administration.

Conflicts of Interest: The mention of commercial products, their sources, or their use in connection with material reported herein is not to be construed as either an actual or implied endorsement of such products by the Department of Health and Human Services.

Appendix A. Telesurgery KPIs

Table A1. Latency requirements for telesurgery.

Data Type	Reported Latency	Source	Distance
2D camera flow	<150 ms [20,21] <200 ms [11,22] <700 ms [23] <600 ms [24] <300 ms [25]	Experiment [32] Other [22] Experiment [23] Experiment [24] Experiment [25]	14,000 km ≈1000 m 9000 miles 14,000 km 14,000 km
3D camera flow	<150 ms [20,21] <300 ms [26] <500 ms [27] <400 ms [28,29] 280 ms [195] 20–50 ms [30] 2–60 ms [46] 146–202 ms [197] 28 ms [191] 258–278 ms [198] 0.25–5 ms [48]	Experiment [32] Experiment [26] Experiment [27] Simulation [38] Experiment [195] Other [30] Experiment [196] Experiment [197] Experiment [191] Experiment [198] Simulation [48]	14,000 km - - - 15 km 200 km - 4 km, 6.1 km ≈740 km, 1260 km, 144 km, 190 km, 3160 km 3000 km -
Audio flow	<150 ms [20,21,28,31] 100 ms [30]	Experiment [32] Other [30]	14,000 km 200 km
Temperature	<250 ms [11,20,21,33,34]	Other [33]	-
Blood pressure	<250 ms [11,20,21,33,34]	Other [33]	-
Heart rate	<250 ms [11,20,21,33,34]	Other [33]	-
Respiration rate	<250 ms [11,20,21,33,34]	Other [33]	-
ECG	<250 ms [11,20,21,33,34]	Other [33]	-
EEG	<250 ms [11,20,21,33,34]	Other [33]	-
EMG	<250 ms [11,20,21,33,34]	Other [33]	-
Force	3–10 ms [20,21] 1–10 ms [30] 3–60 ms [28] <50 ms [29,35] 40 ms [29] <100 ms [36]	Experiment [37] Other [30] Experiment [39] Experiment [40] & Simulation [35] Experiment & Simulation [29] Experiment [36]	- 200 km ≈3200 miles few hundred meters - -
Vibration	<5.5 ms [20,21,28,31] <50 ms [29] 1–10 ms [30]	Experiment [37] Experiment [40] Other [30]	- few hundred meters 200 km

Table A2. Jitter requirements for telesurgery.

Data Type	Reported Jitter	Source
2D camera flow	3–30 ms [11,20]	Simulation [41] Simulation [38]
3D camera flow	3–30 ms [11,20] 3–55 ms [48] <30 ms [28–30,34,38,41]	Simulation [41] Simulation [38] Simulation [48] Other [30]
Audio flow	<30 ms [11,20,28,29,34] 50 ms [30] 3–55 ms [48]	Simulation [41] Simulation [38] Other [30] Simulation [48]
Force	<2 ms [11,20,29,34] 10 ms [30] 1–10 ms [28]	Experiment [40] Simulation [41] Other [30] Experiment [42]
Vibration	<2 ms [11,20,29,34] 10 ms [30] 1–10 ms [28]	Experiment [40] Simulation [41] Other [30] Experiment [42]

Table A3. Data rate requirements for telesurgery.

Data Type	Reported Data Rate	Source
2D camera flow	<10 Mbps [20,21]	Simulation [41] Experiment [40]
3D camera flow	137 Mbps–1.6 Gbps [20,21] ≈8 Mbps [196] 95–106 Mbps [197] 2.5–5 Mbps [28,29] 1 Gbps [30] >1 Gbps [11]	Simulation [28] Experiment [196] Experiment [197] Simulation [41] Experiment [40] Other [30] Simulation [28]
Audio flow	22–200 Kbps [20,21,28,29]	Experiment [31]
Temperature	<10 Kbps [20,21,34]	Other [33]
Blood pressure	<10 Kbps [20,21,34]	Other [33]
Heart rate	<10 Kbps [20,21,34]	Other [33]
Respiration rate	<10 Kbps [20,21,34]	Other [33]
ECG	72 Kbps [20,21,34]	Other [33]
EEG	84.6 Kbps [20,21,34]	Other [33]
EMG	1.536 Mbps [20,21,34]	Other [33]
Force	128–400 Kbps [20,21] 500 Kbps–1 Mbps [29] 128 Kbps [28]	Experiment [28,31] Simulation [41] Experiment [43]
Vibration	128–400 Kbps [20] 500 Kbps–1 Mbps [29] 128 Kbps [28]	Experiment [28,31] Simulation [41] Experiment [43]

Table A4. Packet loss or bit error rate for telesurgery.

Data Type	Reported Loss	Source
2D camera flow	$<10^{-3}$ [20,21]	Experiment [40,41]
3D camera flow	$<10^{-3}$ [20,21]	Experiments [40,41]
	$<1\%$ [28,29]	Experiments [40,41] & Simulation [38]
	0.01–0.06% [48]	Simulations [48]
Audio flow	$<10^{-2}$ [20,21]	Experiments [40,41]
	0.01–0.06% [48]	Simulations [48]
	$<1\%$ [28,29]	Experiments [40,41], Simulation [38]
	10^{-5} [30]	Other [30]
Temperature	$<10^{-3}$ [20,21]	Other [33]
	$<10^{-10}$ [34] (BER)	Other [33]
Blood pressure	$<10^{-3}$ [20,21]	Other [33]
	$<10^{-10}$ [34] (BER)	Other [33]
Heart rate	$<10^{-3}$ [20,21]	Other [33]
	$<10^{-10}$ [34] (BER)	Other [33]
Respiration rate	$<10^{-3}$ [20,21]	Other [33]
	$<10^{-10}$ [34] (BER)	Other [33]
ECG	$<10^{-3}$ [20,21]	Other [33]
	$<10^{-10}$ [34] (BER)	Other [33]
EEG	$<10^{-3}$ [20,21]	Other [33]
	$<10^{-10}$ [34] (BER)	Other [33]
EMG	$<10^{-3}$ [20,21]	Other [33]
	$<10^{-10}$ [34] (BER)	Other [33]
Force	$<10\%$ [29]	Experiments [40,41]
	$<10^{-4}$ [20] [21]	Experiments [40,41]
	0.01–10% [28]	Experiments [40,41]
	<0.1 [35]	Experiments [35]
Vibration	$<10\%$ [29]	Experiments [40,41,43]
	$<10^{-4}$ [20] [21]	Experiments [40,41,43]
	0.01–10% [28]	Experiments [40,41,43]

Table A5. Other requirements for telesurgery.

KPI	Reported Requirement	Source
Reliability	$1-10^{-7}$	[11,44]
Availability	$1-10^{-5}$	[11]
Payload size	Big	[11]
Traffic density	Low [Gbps/km^2]	[11]
Connection density	Low [/km^2]	[11]
Service area dimension	10 m × 10 m × 5 m	[11]
Survival time	0 ms	[11]
Range	Up to 200 km	[30]
	300 km	[11]
Duty cycle for vital signal monitoring	<1–10%	[34]

References

1. Li, D. 5G and intelligence medicine—How the next generation of wireless technology will reconstruct healthcare? *Precis. Clin. Med.* **2019**, *2*, 205–208. [CrossRef]
2. Liu, E.; Effiok, E.; Hitchcock, J. Survey on health care applications in 5G networks. *IET Commun.* **2020**, *14*, 1073–1080. [CrossRef]
3. Hamm, S.; Schleser, A.C.; Hartig, J.; Thomas, P.; Zoesch, S.; Bulitta, C. 5G as enabler for Digital Healthcare. *Curr. Dir. Biomed. Eng.* **2020**, *6*, 1–4. [CrossRef]
4. Padmashree, T.; Nayak, S.S. 5G Technology for E-Health. In Proceedings of the 2020 Fourth International Conference on I-SMAC (IoT in Social, Mobile, Analytics and Cloud)(I-SMAC), Palladam, India, 7–9 October 2020; pp. 211–216.
5. Gupta, P.; Ghosh, M. Revolutionizing Healthcare with 5G. *Telecom Bus. Rev.* **2019**, *12*, 41.
6. Qureshi, H.N.; Manalastas, M.; Zaidi, S.M.A.; Imran, A.; Al Kalaa, M.O. Service Level Agreements for 5G and beyond: Overview, Challenges and Enablers of 5G-Healthcare Systems. *IEEE Access* **2020**, *9*, 1044–1061. [CrossRef]
7. Ullah, H.; Nair, N.G.; Moore, A.; Nugent, C.; Muschamp, P.; Cuevas, M. 5G communication: An overview of vehicle-to-everything, drones, and healthcare use-cases. *IEEE Access* **2019**, *7*, 37251–37268. [CrossRef]
8. Muzammil, S. Telehealth: Is It Only for the Rural Areas? A Review of Its Wider Use. *Telehealth Med. Today* **2020**, *5*, 30938–30953. [CrossRef]
9. Qadri, Y.A.; Nauman, A.; Zikria, Y.B.; Vasilakos, A.V.; Kim, S.W. The future of healthcare internet of things: A survey of emerging technologies. *IEEE Commun. Surv. Tutor.* **2020**, *22*, 1121–1167. [CrossRef]
10. FDA. Radio Frequency Wireless Technology in Medical Devices, Guidance for Industry and Food and Drug Administration Staff. Available online: https://www.fda.gov/media/71975/download (accessed on 29 October 2020).
11. Cisotto, G.; Casarin, E.; Tomasin, S. Requirements and Enablers of Advanced Healthcare Services over Future Cellular Systems. *IEEE Commun. Mag.* **2020**, *58*, 76–81. [CrossRef]
12. Schaich, F.; Hamon, M.H.; Hunukumbure, M.; Lorca, J.; Pedersen, K.; Schubert, M.; Kosmatos, E.; Wunder, G.; Reaz, K. The ONE5G Approach Towards the Challenges of Multi-Service Operation in 5G Systems. In Proceedings of the 2018 IEEE 87th Vehicular Technology Conference (VTC Spring), Porto, Portugal, 3–6 June 2018; pp. 1–6. [CrossRef]
13. 5GPPP. White Paper on Service Performance Measurement Methods over 5G Experimental Networks from TMV WG. Available online: https://5g-ppp.eu/white-paper-on-service-performance-measurement-methods-over-5g-experimental-networks/ (accessed on 30 June 2021).
14. 5G-Monarch. Documentation of Requirements and KPIs and Definition of Suitable Evaluation Criteria. Available online: https://5g-monarch.eu/wp-content/uploads/2017/10/5G-MoNArch_761445_D6.1_Documentation_of_Requirements_and_KPIs_and_Definition_of_Suitable_Evaluation_Criteria_v1.0.pdf (accessed on 30 June 2021).
15. Krasniqi, F.; Gavrilovska, L.; Maraj, A. The Analysis of Key Performance Indicators (KPI) in 4G/LTE Networks. In *Future Access Enablers for Ubiquitous and Intelligent Infrastructures*; Poulkov, V., Ed.; Springer International Publishing: Cham, Switzerland, 2019; pp. 285–296.
16. 3GPP. 3GPP TR 38.913, "Study on Scenarios and Requirements for Next Generation Access Technologies". V14.2.0. March 2017. Available online: http://www.3gpp.org (accessed on 30 June 2021).
17. Dwivedi, S.; Shreevastav, R.; Munier, F.; Nygren, J.; Siomina, I.; Lyazidi, Y.; Shrestha, D.; Lindmark, G.; Ernström, P.; Stare, E.; et al. Positioning in 5G networks. *arXiv* **2021**, arXiv:2102.03361.
18. Gutierrez-Estevez, D.M.; Gramaglia, M.; De Domenico, A.; Di Pietro, N.; Khatibi, S.; Shah, K.; Tsolkas, D.; Arnold, P.; Serrano, P. The path towards resource elasticity for 5G network architecture. In Proceedings of the 2018 IEEE Wireless Communications and Networking Conference Workshops (WCNCW), Barcelona, Spain, 15–18 April 2018; pp. 214–219.
19. Global Connected Wearable Devices. Available online: https://www.statista.com/statistics/487291/global-connected-wearable-devices/ (accessed on 27 June 2021).
20. Zhang, Q.; Liu, J.; Zhao, G. Towards 5G enabled tactile robotic telesurgery. *arXiv* **2018**, arXiv:1803.03586.
21. Usman, M.A.; Philip, N.Y.; Politis, C. 5G enabled mobile healthcare for ambulances. In Proceedings of the 2019 IEEE Globecom Workshops (GC Wkshps), Waikoloa, HI, USA, 9–13 December 2019; pp. 1–6.
22. Thuemmler, C.; Gavrasm, A.; Jumelle, A.; Paulin, A.; Sadique, A.; Schneider, A.; Fedell, C.; Abraham, D.; Trossen, D. 5G and e-Health; 5G-PPP White Paper. 2015; pp. 1–24. Available online: https://5g-ppp.eu/euro-5g/ (accessed on 20 July 2021).
23. Fabrlzio, M.D.; Lee, B.R.; Chan, D.Y.; Stoianovici, D.; Jarrett, T.W.; Yang, C.; Kavoussi, L.R. Effect of time delay on surgical performance during telesurgical manipulation. *J. Endourol.* **2000**, *14*, 133–138. [CrossRef] [PubMed]
24. Rayman, R.; Primak, S.; Patel, R.; Moallem, M.; Morady, R.; Tavakoli, M.; Subotic, V.; Galbraith, N.; Van Wynsberghe, A.; Croome, K. Effects of latency on telesurgery: An experimental study. In *Lecture Notes in Computer Science, Proceedings of the International Conference on Medical Image Computing and Computer-Assisted Intervention*, Palm Springs, CA, USA, 26–29 October 2005; Springer: Berlin/Heidelberg, Germany, 2005; pp. 57–64.
25. Marescaux, J.; Leroy, J.; Rubino, F.; Smith, M.; Vix, M.; Simone, M.; Mutter, D. Transcontinental robot-assisted remote telesurgery: Feasibility and potential applications. *Ann. Surg.* **2002**, *235*, 487. [CrossRef] [PubMed]
26. Xu, S.; Perez, M.; Yang, K.; Perrenot, C.; Felblinger, J.; Hubert, J. Determination of the latency effects on surgical performance and the acceptable latency levels in telesurgery using the dV-Trainer® simulator. *Surg. Endosc.* **2014**, *28*, 2569–2576. [CrossRef] [PubMed]

27. Perez, M.; Xu, S.; Chauhan, S.; Tanaka, A.; Simpson, K.; Abdul-Muhsin, H.; Smith, R. Impact of delay on telesurgical performance: Study on the robotic simulator dV-Trainer. *Int. J. Comput. Assist. Radiol. Surg.* **2016**, *11*, 581–587. [CrossRef]
28. Eid, M.; Cha, J.; El Saddik, A. Admux: An adaptive multiplexer for haptic-audio-visual data communication. *IEEE Trans. Instrum. Meas.* **2010**, *60*, 21–31. [CrossRef]
29. Marshall, A.; Yap, K.M.; Yu, W. Providing QoS for networked peers in distributed haptic virtual environments. *Adv. Multimed.* **2008**, *2008*, 841590. [CrossRef]
30. NSF. NSF Follow-on Workshop on Ultra-Low Latency Wireless Networks. In *NSF Workshop on Ultra Low-Latency Wireless Networks*; NSF: Arlington, VA, USA, 2016.
31. Cizmeci, B.; Xu, X.; Chaudhari, R.; Bachhuber, C.; Alt, N.; Steinbach, E. A multiplexing scheme for multimodal teleoperation. *ACM Trans. Multimed. Comput. Commun. Appl. (TOMM)* **2017**, *13*, 1–28. [CrossRef]
32. Marescaux, J.; Leroy, J.; Gagner, M.; Rubino, F.; Mutter, D.; Vix, M.; Butner, S.E.; Smith, M.K. Transatlantic robot-assisted telesurgery. *Nature* **2001**, *413*, 379–380. [CrossRef]
33. Zhen, B.; Patel, M.; Lee, S.; Won, E.; Astrin, A. TG6 technical requirements document (TRD). *IEEE P802* **2008**, *15*, 8.
34. Patel, M.; Wang, J. Applications, challenges, and prospective in emerging body area networking technologies. *IEEE Wirel. Commun.* **2010**, *17*, 80–88. [CrossRef]
35. Shi, Z.; Zou, H.; Rank, M.; Chen, L.; Hirche, S.; Muller, H.J. Effects of packet loss and latency on the temporal discrimination of visual-haptic events. *IEEE Trans. Haptics* **2009**, *3*, 28–36.
36. Makino, Y.; Furuyama, Y.; Inoue, S.; Shinoda, H. HaptoClone (Haptic-Optical Clone) for Mutual Tele-Environment by Real-time 3D Image Transfer with Midair Force Feedback. In Proceedings of the CHI, San Jose, China, 7 May 2016; pp. 1980–1990.
37. Hachisu, T.; Kajimoto, H. Vibration feedback latency affects material perception during rod tapping interactions. *IEEE Trans. Haptics* **2016**, *10*, 288–295. [CrossRef]
38. Bertsekas, D.P. Traffic Behavior and Queuing in a QoS Environment. OPNETWORK 2005, Session 1813; 2005. Available online: https://www.cpe.ku.ac.th/~anan/myhomepage/wp-content/uploads/2015/01/1-opnet_full_presentation.pdf (accessed on 20 October 2021).
39. Kim, J.; Kim, H.; Tay, B.K.; Muniyandi, M.; Srinivasan, M.A.; Jordan, J.; Mortensen, J.; Oliveira, M.; Slater, M. Transatlantic touch: A study of haptic collaboration over long distance. *Presence Teleoperators Virtual Environ.* **2004**, *13*, 328–337. [CrossRef]
40. Souayed, R.T.; Gaiti, D.; Yu, W.; Dodds, G.; Marshall, A. Experimental study of haptic interaction in distributed virtual environments. In Proceedings of the EuroHaptics, Munich, Germany, 5–7 June 2004; pp. 260–266.
41. Yap, K.M.; Marshall, A.; Yu, W.; Dodds, G.; Gu, Q.; Souayed, R.T. Characterising distributed haptic virtual environment network traffic flows. In *IFIP—The International Federation for Information Processing, Proceedings of the International Conference on Network Control and Engineering for QoS, Security and Mobility, Lannion, France, 14–18 November 2005*; Springer: Boston, MA, USA, 2005; pp. 297–310.
42. Park, K.S.; Kenyon, R.V. Effects of network characteristics on human performance in a collaborative virtual environment. In Proceedings of the IEEE Virtual Reality (Cat. No. 99CB36316), Houston, TX, USA, 13–17 March 1999; pp. 104–111.
43. Dev, P.; Harris, D.; Gutierrez, D.; Shah, A.; Senger, S. End-to-end performance measurement of Internet based medical applications. In Proceedings of the AMIA Symposium, San Antonio, AZ, USA, 9–13 November 2002; American Medical Informatics Association: San Antonio, AZ, USA, 2002; pp. 205–209.
44. Soldani, D.; Fadini, F.; Rasanen, H.; Duran, J.; Niemela, T.; Chandramouli, D.; Hoglund, T.; Doppler, K.; Himanen, T.; Laiho, J.; et al. 5G mobile systems for healthcare. In Proceedings of the 2017 IEEE 85th Vehicular Technology Conference (VTC Spring), Sydney, NSW, Australia, 4–7 June 2017; pp. 1–5.
45. Xia, S.B.; Lu, Q.S. Development status of telesurgery robotic system. *Chin. J. Traumatol.* **2021**, *24*, 144–147. [CrossRef] [PubMed]
46. Valdez, L.B.; Datta, R.R.; Babic, B.; Müller, D.T.; Bruns, C.J.; Fuchs, H.F. 5G mobile communication applications for surgery: An overview of the latest literature. *Artif. Intell. Gastrointest. Endosc.* **2021**, *2*, 1–11. [CrossRef]
47. Dohler, M. The Internet of Skills: How 5G-Synchronized Reality Is Transforming Robotic Surgery. In *Robotic Surgery*; Springer: Berlin/Heidelberg, Germany, 2021; pp. 207–215._20. [CrossRef]
48. Sedaghat, S.; Jahangir, A.H. RT-TelSurg: Real Time Telesurgery Using SDN, Fog, and Cloud as Infrastructures. *IEEE Access* **2021**, *9*, 52238–52251.
49. Ahvar, E.; Ahvar, S.; Raza, S.M.; Manuel Sanchez Vilchez, J.; Lee, G.M. Next generation of SDN in cloud-fog for 5G and beyond-enabled applications: Opportunities and challenges. *Network* **2021**, *1*, 28–49. [CrossRef]
50. Aggarwal, S.; Kumar, N. Fog computing for 5G-enabled tactile Internet: Research issues, challenges, and future research directions. *Mob. Netw. Appl.* **2019**, 1–28.%2Fs11036-019-01430-4. [CrossRef]
51. Hartmann, M.; Hashmi, U.S.; Imran, A. Edge computing in smart health care systems: Review, challenges, and research directions. *Trans. Emerg. Telecommun. Technol.* **2019**, e3710. [CrossRef]
52. Akrivopoulos, O.; Chatzigiannakis, I.; Tselios, C.; Antoniou, A. On the deployment of healthcare applications over fog computing infrastructure. In Proceedings of the 2017 IEEE 41st Annual Computer Software and Applications Conference (COMPSAC), Turin, Italy, 4–8 July 2017; Volume 2, pp. 288–293.
53. Mutlag, A.A.; Abd Ghani, M.K.; Arunkumar, N.A.; Mohammed, M.A.; Mohd, O. Enabling technologies for fog computing in healthcare IoT systems. *Future Gener. Comput. Syst.* **2019**, *90*, 62–78. [CrossRef]

54. LaMonte, M.P.; Cullen, J.; Gagliano, D.M.; Gunawardane, R.; Hu, P.; Mackenzie, C.; Xiao, Y. TeleBAT: Mobile telemedicine for the Brain Attack Team. *J. Stroke Cerebrovasc. Dis.* **2000**, *9*, 128–135. [CrossRef] [PubMed]
55. Terkelsen, C.; Nørgaard, B.; Lassen, J.; Gerdes, J.; Ankersen, J.; Rømer, F.; Nielsen, T.; Andersen, H. Telemedicine used for remote prehospital diagnosing in patients suspected of acute myocardial infarction. *J. Intern. Med.* **2002**, *252*, 412–420. [CrossRef]
56. Hsieh, J.C.; Lin, B.X.; Wu, F.R.; Chang, P.C.; Tsuei, Y.W.; Yang, C.C. Ambulance 12-lead electrocardiography transmission via cell phone technology to cardiologists. *Telemed. E-Health* **2010**, *16*, 910–915. [CrossRef] [PubMed]
57. Liman, T.G.; Winter, B.; Waldschmidt, C.; Zerbe, N.; Hufnagl, P.; Audebert, H.J.; Endres, M. Telestroke ambulances in prehospital stroke management: Concept and pilot feasibility study. *Stroke* **2012**, *43*, 2086–2090. [CrossRef]
58. Yperzeele, L.; Van Hooff, R.J.; De Smedt, A.; Espinoza, A.V.; Van Dyck, R.; Van de Casseye, R.; Convents, A.; Hubloue, I.; Lauwaert, D.; De Keyser, J.; et al. Feasibility of AmbulanCe-Based Telemedicine (FACT) study: Safety, feasibility and reliability of third generation in-ambulance telemedicine. *PLoS ONE* **2014**, *9*, e110043. [CrossRef] [PubMed]
59. Wu, T.C.; Nguyen, C.; Ankrom, C.; Yang, J.; Persse, D.; Vahidy, F.; Grotta, J.C.; Savitz, S.I. Prehospital utility of rapid stroke evaluation using in-ambulance telemedicine: A pilot feasibility study. *Stroke* **2014**, *45*, 2342–2347. [CrossRef]
60. Espinoza, A.V.; Van Hooff, R.J.; De Smedt, A.; Moens, M.; Yperzeele, L.; Nieboer, K.; Hubloue, I.; de Keyser, J.; Convents, A.; Tellez, H.F.; et al. Development and pilot testing of 24/7 in-ambulance telemedicine for acute stroke: Prehospital stroke study at the Universitair Ziekenhuis Brussel-Project. *Cerebrovasc. Dis.* **2016**, *42*, 15–22. [CrossRef]
61. Itrat, A.; Taqui, A.; Cerejo, R.; Briggs, F.; Cho, S.M.; Organek, N.; Reimer, A.P.; Winners, S.; Rasmussen, P.; Hussain, M.S.; et al. Telemedicine in prehospital stroke evaluation and thrombolysis: Taking stroke treatment to the doorstep. *JAMA Neurol.* **2016**, *73*, 162–168. [CrossRef]
62. Antoniou, Z.C.; Panayides, A.S.; Pantzaris, M.; Constantinides, A.G.; Pattichis, C.S.; Pattichis, M.S. Real-time adaptation to time-varying constraints for medical video communications. *IEEE J. Biomed. Health Inform.* **2017**, *22*, 1177–1188. [CrossRef]
63. Rehman, I.U.; Nasralla, M.M.; Ali, A.; Philip, N. Small cell-based ambulance scenario for medical video streaming: A 5G-health use case. In Proceedings of the 2018 15th International Conference on Smart Cities: Improving Quality of Life Using ICT & IoT (HONET-ICT), Islamabad, Pakistan, 8–10 October 2018; pp. 29–32.
64. Wang, Q.; Alcaraz-Calero, J.; Ricart-Sanchez, R.; Weiss, M.B.; Gavras, A.; Nikaein, N.; Vasilakos, X.; Giacomo, B.; Pietro, G.; Roddy, M.; et al. Enable advanced QoS-aware network slicing in 5G networks for slice-based media use cases. *IEEE Trans. Broadcast.* **2019**, *65*, 444–453. [CrossRef]
65. Roddy, M.; Truong, T.; Walsh, P.; Al Bado, M.; Wu, Y.; Healy, M.; Ahearne, S. 5G Network Slicing for Mission-critical use cases. In Proceedings of the 2019 IEEE 2nd 5G World Forum (5GWF), Dresden, Germany, 30 September–2 October 2019; pp. 409–414.
66. Kamal, M.D.; Tahir, A.; Kamal, M.B.; Naeem, M.A. Future Location Prediction for Emergency Vehicles Using Big Data: A Case Study of Healthcare Engineering. *J. Healthc. Eng.* **2020**, *2020*, 6641571. [CrossRef] [PubMed]
67. Yu, S.; Yi, F.; Qiulin, X.; Liya, S. A Framework of 5G Mobile-health Services for Ambulances. In Proceedings of the 2020 IEEE 20th International Conference on Communication Technology (ICCT), Nanning, China, 28–31 October 2020; pp. 528–532.
68. Bin-Yahya, M.A.R. E-AMBULANCE: A Real-Time Integration Platform for Heterogeneous Medical Telemetry System of Smart Ambulances. Ph.D. Thesis, King Fahd University of Petroleum and Minerals, Dhahran, Saudi Arabia, 2015.
69. Ehrler, F.; Siebert, J.N. PedAMINES: A disruptive mHealth app to tackle paediatric medication errors. *Swiss Med. Wkly.* **2020**, *150*, w20335. [CrossRef]
70. Almadani, B.; Bin-Yahya, M.; Shakshuki, E.M. E-AMBULANCE: Real-time integration platform for heterogeneous medical telemetry system. *Procedia Comput. Sci.* **2015**, *63*, 400–407. [CrossRef]
71. Lippman, J.M.; Smith, S.N.C.; McMurry, T.L.; Sutton, Z.G.; Gunnell, B.S.; Cote, J.; Perina, D.G.; Cattell-Gordon, D.C.; Rheuban, K.S.; Solenski, N.J.; et al. Mobile telestroke during ambulance transport is feasible in a rural EMS setting: The iTREAT Study. *Telemed. e-Health* **2016**, *22*, 507–513. [CrossRef] [PubMed]
72. Kim, H.; Kim, S.W.; Park, E.; Kim, J.H.; Chang, H. The role of fifth-generation mobile technology in prehospital emergency care: An opportunity to support paramedics. *Health Policy Technol.* **2020**, *9*, 109–114. [CrossRef]
73. Zhai, Y.; Xu, X.; Chen, B.; Lu, H.; Wang, Y.; Li, S.; Shi, X.; Wang, W.; Shang, L.; Zhao, J. 5G-Network-Enabled Smart Ambulance: Architecture, Application, and Evaluation. *IEEE Netw.* **2021**, *35*, 190–196. [CrossRef]
74. Geisler, F.; Kunz, A.; Winter, B.; Rozanski, M.; Waldschmidt, C.; Weber, J.E.; Wendt, M.; Zieschang, K.; Ebinger, M.; Audebert, H.J.; et al. Telemedicine in prehospital acute stroke care. *J. Am. Heart Assoc.* **2019**, *8*, e011729. [CrossRef]
75. Kandimalla, J.; Vellipuram, A.R.; Rodriguez, G.; Maud, A.; Cruz-Flores, S.; Khatri, R. Role of Telemedicine in Prehospital Stroke Care. *Curr. Cardiol. Rep.* **2021**, *23*, 1–5. [CrossRef]
76. Rajan, S.S.; Baraniuk, S.; Parker, S.; Wu, T.C.; Bowry, R.; Grotta, J.C. Implementing a mobile stroke unit program in the United States: Why, how, and how much? *JAMA Neurol.* **2015**, *72*, 229–234.
77. Wu, T.C.; Parker, S.A.; Jagolino, A.; Yamal, J.M.; Bowry, R.; Thomas, A.; Yu, A.; Grotta, J.C. Telemedicine can replace the neurologist on a mobile stroke unit. *Stroke* **2017**, *48*, 493–496. [CrossRef] [PubMed]
78. Audebert, H.; Fassbender, K.; Hussain, M.S.; Ebinger, M.; Turc, G.; Uchino, K.; Davis, S.; Alexandrov, A.; Grotta, J. The PRE-hospital stroke treatment organization. *Int. J. Stroke* **2017**, *12*, 932–940. [CrossRef] [PubMed]
79. EU 5G PPP Trials Working Group (Including J. Alcaraz Calero and Q. Wang). The 5G PPP Infrastructure-Trials and Pilots Brochure. Available online: https://5g-ppp.eu/wp-content/uploads/2019/09/5GInfraPPP_10TPs_Brochure_FINAL_low_singlepages.pdf (accessed on 24 June 2021).

80. Martinez-Alpiste, I.; Jose, M.; Alcaraz, C.; Qi, W.; Gelayol, G.; Chirivella-Perez, E.; Salva-Garcia, P. 5G Can Shape Mission-Critical Healthcare Services. Available online: https://https://www.comsoc.org/publications/ctn/5g-can-shape-mission-critical-healthcare-services (accessed on 24 June 2021).
81. MIoT. Internet of Medical Things Revolutionizing Healthcare. Available online: https://aabme.asme.org/posts/internet-of-medical-things-revolutionizing-healthcare (accessed on 26 June 2021).
82. Lukowicz, P.; Anliker, U.; Ward, J.; Troster, G.; Hirt, E.; Neufelt, C. AMON: A wearable medical computer for high risk patients. In Proceedings of the Sixth International Symposium on Wearable Computers, Seattle, WA, USA, 10 October 2002; pp. 133–134.
83. Diaz, K.M.; Krupka, D.J.; Chang, M.J.; Peacock, J.; Ma, Y.; Goldsmith, J.; Schwartz, J.E.; Davidson, K.W. Fitbit®: An accurate and reliable device for wireless physical activity tracking. *Int. J. Cardiol.* **2015**, *185*, 138. [CrossRef] [PubMed]
84. Reeder, B.; David, A. Health at hand: A systematic review of smart watch uses for health and wellness. *J. Biomed. Inform.* **2016**, *63*, 269–276. [CrossRef]
85. Trung, T.Q.; Ramasundaram, S.; Hwang, B.U.; Lee, N.E. An all-elastomeric transparent and stretchable temperature sensor for body-attachable wearable electronics. *Adv. Mater.* **2016**, *28*, 502–509. [CrossRef]
86. Yamamoto, Y.; Yamamoto, D.; Takada, M.; Naito, H.; Arie, T.; Akita, S.; Takei, K. Efficient skin temperature sensor and stable gel-less sticky ECG sensor for a wearable flexible healthcare patch. *Adv. Healthc. Mater.* **2017**, *6*, 1700495. [CrossRef]
87. Adiputra, R.; Hadiyoso, S.; Hariyani, Y.S. Internet of things: Low cost and wearable SpO2 device for health monitoring. *Int. J. Electr. Comput. Eng.* **2018**, *8*, 939. [CrossRef]
88. Azhari, A.; Yoshimoto, S.; Nezu, T.; Iida, H.; Ota, H.; Noda, Y.; Araki, T.; Uemura, T.; Sekitani, T.; Morii, K. A patch-type wireless forehead pulse oximeter for SpO_2 measurement. In Proceedings of the 2017 IEEE Biomedical Circuits and Systems Conference (BioCAS), Turin, Italy, 19–21 October 2017; pp. 1–4.
89. Chacon, P.J.; Pu, L.; da Costa, T.H.; Shin, Y.H.; Ghomian, T.; Shamkhalichenar, H.; Wu, H.C.; Irving, B.A.; Choi, J.W. A wearable pulse oximeter with wireless communication and motion artifact tailoring for continuous use. *IEEE Trans. Biomed. Eng.* **2018**, *66*, 1505–1513. [CrossRef]
90. Surrel, G.; Rincón, F.; Murali, S.; Atienza, D. Low-power wearable system for real-time screening of obstructive sleep apnea. In Proceedings of the 2016 IEEE Computer Society Annual Symposium on VLSI (ISVLSI), Pittsburgh, PA, USA, 11–13 July 2016; pp. 230–235.
91. Shilaih, M.; Goodale, B.M.; Falco, L.; Kübler, F.; De Clerck, V.; Leeners, B. Modern fertility awareness methods: Wrist wearables capture the changes in temperature associated with the menstrual cycle. *Biosci. Rep.* **2018**, *38*, BSR20171279. [CrossRef]
92. Xie, R.; Du, Q.; Zou, B.; Chen, Y.; Zhang, K.; Liu, Y.; Liang, J.; Zheng, B.; Li, S.; Zhang, W.; et al. Wearable leather-based electronics for respiration monitoring. *ACS Appl. Bio Mater.* **2019**, *2*, 1427–1431. [CrossRef]
93. Mizuno, A.; Changolkar, S.; Patel, M.S. Wearable Devices to Monitor and Reduce the Risk of Cardiovascular Disease: Evidence and Opportunities. *Annu. Rev. Med.* **2020**, *72*, 459–471. [CrossRef] [PubMed]
94. Holz, C.; Wang, E.J. Glabella: Continuously sensing blood pressure behavior using an unobtrusive wearable device. *Proc. ACM Interactive Mobile Wearable Ubiquitous Technol.* **2017**, *1*, 1–23. [CrossRef]
95. Kuwabara, M.; Harada, K.; Hishiki, Y.; Kario, K. Validation of two watch-type wearable blood pressure monitors according to the ANSI/AAMI/ISO81060-2: 2013 guidelines: Omron HEM-6410T-ZM and HEM-6410T-ZL. *J. Clin. Hypertens.* **2019**, *21*, 853–858. [CrossRef] [PubMed]
96. Arakawa, T. Recent research and developing trends of wearable sensors for detecting blood pressure. *Sensors* **2018**, *18*, 2772. [CrossRef] [PubMed]
97. Escobedo, P.; Ramos-Lorente, C.E.; Martínez-Olmos, A.; Carvajal, M.A.; Ortega-Munoz, M.; de Orbe-Paya, I.; Hernández-Mateo, F.; Santoyo-González, F.; Capitán-Vallvey, L.F.; Palma, A.J.; et al. Wireless wearable wristband for continuous sweat pH monitoring. *Sens. Actuators B Chem.* **2021**, *327*, 128948. [CrossRef]
98. Nakata, S.; Shiomi, M.; Fujita, Y.; Arie, T.; Akita, S.; Takei, K. A wearable pH sensor with high sensitivity based on a flexible charge-coupled device. *Nat. Electron.* **2018**, *1*, 596–603. [CrossRef]
99. Wijsman, J.; Grundlehner, B.; Liu, H.; Hermens, H.; Penders, J. Towards mental stress detection using wearable physiological sensors. In Proceedings of the 2011 Annual International Conference of the IEEE Engineering in Medicine and Biology Society, Boston, MA, USA, 30 August—3 September 2011; pp. 1798–1801.
100. Valenza, G.; Nardelli, M.; Lanata, A.; Gentili, C.; Bertschy, G.; Paradiso, R.; Scilingo, E.P. Wearable monitoring for mood recognition in bipolar disorder based on history-dependent long-term heart rate variability analysis. *IEEE J. Biomed. Health Inform.* **2013**, *18*, 1625–1635. [CrossRef]
101. Gruwez, A.; Bruyneel, A.V.; Bruyneel, M. The validity of two commercially-available sleep trackers and actigraphy for assessment of sleep parameters in obstructive sleep apnea patients. *PLoS ONE* **2019**, *14*, e0210569. [CrossRef]
102. Lin, C.T.; Ko, L.W.; Chang, M.H.; Duann, J.R.; Chen, J.Y.; Su, T.P.; Jung, T.P. Review of wireless and wearable electroencephalogram systems and brain-computer interfaces–a mini-review. *Gerontology* **2010**, *56*, 112–119. [CrossRef]
103. Casson, A.J.; Yates, D.C.; Smith, S.J.; Duncan, J.S.; Rodriguez-Villegas, E. Wearable electroencephalography. *IEEE Eng. Med. Biol. Mag.* **2010**, *29*, 44–56. [CrossRef]
104. Ip, J.E. Wearable devices for cardiac rhythm diagnosis and management. *JAMA* **2019**, *321*, 337–338. [CrossRef] [PubMed]
105. Jeon, B.; Lee, J.; Choi, J. Design and implementation of a wearable ECG system. *Int. J. Smart Home* **2013**, *7*, 61–69.

106. Beniczky, S.; Conradsen, I.; Henning, O.; Fabricius, M.; Wolf, P. Automated real-time detection of tonic-clonic seizures using a wearable EMG device. *Neurology* **2018**, *90*, e428–e434. [CrossRef]
107. Tsubouchi, Y.; Suzuki, K. BioTones: A wearable device for EMG auditory biofeedback. In Proceedings of the 2010 Annual International Conference of the IEEE Engineering in Medicine and Biology, Buenos Aires, Argentina, 31 August–4 September 2010; pp. 6543–6546.
108. Nathan, V.; Jafari, R. Particle filtering and sensor fusion for robust heart rate monitoring using wearable sensors. *IEEE J. Biomed. Health Inform.* **2017**, *22*, 1834–1846. [CrossRef] [PubMed]
109. Park, J.H.; Jang, D.G.; Park, J.W.; Youm, S.K. Wearable sensing of in-ear pressure for heart rate monitoring with a piezoelectric sensor. *Sensors* **2015**, *15*, 23402–23417. [CrossRef]
110. El-Amrawy, F.; Nounou, M.I. Are currently available wearable devices for activity tracking and heart rate monitoring accurate, precise, and medically beneficial? *Healthc. Inform. Res.* **2015**, *21*, 315. [CrossRef]
111. Tsai, C.W.; Li, C.H.; Lam, R.W.K.; Li, C.K.; Ho, S. Diabetes care in motion: Blood glucose estimation using wearable devices. *IEEE Consum. Electron. Mag.* **2019**, *9*, 30–34. [CrossRef]
112. Cappon, G.; Acciaroli, G.; Vettoretti, M.; Facchinetti, A.; Sparacino, G. Wearable continuous glucose monitoring sensors: A revolution in diabetes treatment. *Electronics* **2017**, *6*, 65. [CrossRef]
113. Pickup, J.C. Insulin-pump therapy for type 1 diabetes mellitus. *N. Engl. J. Med.* **2012**, *366*, 1616–1624. [CrossRef]
114. Weissberg-Benchell, J.; Antisdel-Lomaglio, J.; Seshadri, R. Insulin pump therapy: A meta-analysis. *Diabetes Care* **2003**, *26*, 1079–1087. [CrossRef]
115. Gadaleta, M.; Facchinetti, A.; Grisan, E.; Rossi, M. Prediction of adverse glycemic events from continuous glucose monitoring signal. *IEEE J. Biomed. Health Inform.* **2018**, *23*, 650–659. [CrossRef] [PubMed]
116. Angelucci, A.; Kuller, D.; Aliverti, A. A home telemedicine system for continuous respiratory monitoring. *IEEE J. Biomed. Health Inform.* **2020**, *25*, 1247–1256. [CrossRef]
117. Scherer, M.; Menachery, K.; Magno, M. SmartAid: A Low-Power Smart Hearing Aid For Stutterers. In Proceedings of the 2019 IEEE Sensors Applications Symposium (SAS), Sophia Antipolis, France, 11–13 March 2019; pp. 1–6.
118. Sudharsan, B.; Chockalingam, M. A microphone array and voice algorithm based smart hearing aid. *arXiv* **2019**, arXiv:1908.07324.
119. DJordjevic, S.; Stancin, S.; Meglc, M.; Milutinovic, V.; Tomazic, S. Mc sensor—A novel method for measurement of muscle tension. *Sensors* **2011**, *11*, 9411–9425.
120. Mansuri, B.; Torabinejhad, F.; Jamshidi, A.A.; Dabirmoghaddam, P.; Vasaghi-Gharamaleki, B.; Ghelichi, L. Transcutaneous electrical nerve stimulation combined with voice therapy in women with muscle tension dysphonia. *J. Voice* **2020**, *34*, 490.e11–490.e21. [CrossRef]
121. Velázquez, R. Wearable assistive devices for the blind. In *Wearable and Autonomous Biomedical Devices and Systems for Smart Environment*; Springer: Berlin/Heidelberg, Germany, 2010; pp. 331–349.
122. Garcia-Macias, J.A.; Ramos, A.G.; Hasimoto-Beltran, R.; Hernandez, S.E.P. Uasisi: A modular and adaptable wearable system to assist the visually impaired. *Procedia Comput. Sci.* **2019**, *151*, 425–430. [CrossRef]
123. Savindu, H.P.; Iroshan, K.; Panangala, C.D.; Perera, W.; De Silva, A.C. BrailleBand: Blind support haptic wearable band for communication using braille language. In Proceedings of the 2017 IEEE International Conference on Systems, Man, and Cybernetics (SMC), Banff, AB, Canada, 5–8 October 2017; pp. 1381–1386.
124. Sun, M.; Burke, L.E.; Mao, Z.H.; Chen, Y.; Chen, H.C.; Bai, Y.; Li, Y.; Li, C.; Jia, W. eButton: A wearable computer for health monitoring and personal assistance. In Proceedings of the 51st Annual Design Automation Conference, San Francisco, CA, USA, 1–5 June 2014; pp. 1–6.
125. Kapur, A.; Kapur, S.; Maes, P. Alterego: A personalized wearable silent speech interface. In Proceedings of the 23rd International Conference on Intelligent User Interfaces, Tokyo, Japan, 7–11 March 2018; pp. 43–53.
126. Marjanovic, N.; Piccinini, G.; Kerr, K.; Esmailbeigi, H. TongueToSpeech (TTS): Wearable wireless assistive device for augmented speech. In Proceedings of the 2017 39th Annual International Conference of the IEEE Engineering in Medicine and Biology Society (EMBC), Jeju, Korea, 11–15 July 2017; pp. 3561–3563.
127. Huo, W.; Mohammed, S.; Moreno, J.C.; Amirat, Y. Lower limb wearable robots for assistance and rehabilitation: A state of the art. *IEEE Syst. J.* **2014**, *10*, 1068–1081. [CrossRef]
128. Hadi, A.; Alipour, K.; Kazeminasab, S.; Elahinia, M. ASR glove: A wearable glove for hand assistance and rehabilitation using shape memory alloys. *J. Intell. Mater. Syst. Struct.* **2018**, *29*, 1575–1585. [CrossRef]
129. Gandolla, M.; Antonietti, A.; Longatelli, V.; Pedrocchi, A. The effectiveness of wearable upper limb assistive devices in degenerative neuromuscular diseases: A systematic review and meta-analysis. *Front. Bioeng. Biotechnol.* **2020**, *7*, 450. [CrossRef]
130. Chen, B.; Zhong, C.H.; Zhao, X.; Ma, H.; Guan, X.; Li, X.; Liang, F.Y.; Cheng, J.C.Y.; Qin, L.; Law, S.W.; et al. A wearable exoskeleton suit for motion assistance to paralysed patients. *J. Orthop. Transl.* **2017**, *11*, 7–18. [CrossRef]
131. Delahoz, Y.S.; Labrador, M.A. Survey on fall detection and fall prevention using wearable and external sensors. *Sensors* **2014**, *14*, 19806–19842. [CrossRef] [PubMed]
132. Chen, D.; Feng, W.; Zhang, Y.; Li, X.; Wang, T. A wearable wireless fall detection system with accelerators. In Proceedings of the 2011 IEEE International Conference on Robotics and Biomimetics, Karon Beach, Thailand, 7–11 December 2011; pp. 2259–2263.
133. Yi, W.J.; Saniie, J. Design flow of a wearable system for body posture assessment and fall detection with android smartphone. In Proceedings of the 2014 IEEE International Technology Management Conference, Chicago, IL, USA, 12–15 June 2014; pp. 1–4.

134. Bruno, E.; Biondi, A.; Thorpe, S.; Richardson, M.; Consortium, R.C. Patients self-mastery of wearable devices for seizure detection: A direct user-experience. *Seizure* **2020**, *81*, 236–240. [CrossRef]
135. Jeppesen, J.; Fuglsang-Frederiksen, A.; Johansen, P.; Christensen, J.; Wüstenhagen, S.; Tankisi, H.; Qerama, E.; Hess, A.; Beniczky, S. Seizure detection based on heart rate variability using a wearable electrocardiography device. *Epilepsia* **2019**, *60*, 2105–2113. [CrossRef]
136. Pierleoni, P.; Belli, A.; Palma, L.; Pellegrini, M.; Pernini, L.; Valenti, S. A high reliability wearable device for elderly fall detection. *IEEE Sens. J.* **2015**, *15*, 4544–4553. [CrossRef]
137. Atallah, L.; Lo, B.; King, R.; Yang, G.Z. Sensor positioning for activity recognition using wearable accelerometers. *IEEE Trans. Biomed. Circuits Syst.* **2011**, *5*, 320–329. [CrossRef]
138. Ouyang, H.; Liu, Z.; Li, N.; Shi, B.; Zou, Y.; Xie, F.; Ma, Y.; Li, Z.; Li, H.; Zheng, Q.; et al. Symbiotic cardiac pacemaker. *Nat. Commun.* **2019**, *10*, 1–10. [CrossRef]
139. Eicken, A.; Kolb, C.; Lange, S.; Brodherr-Heberlein, S.; Zrenner, B.; Schreiber, C.; Hess, J. Implantable cardioverter defibrillator (ICD) in children. *Int. J. Cardiol.* **2006**, *107*, 30–35. [CrossRef] [PubMed]
140. Van der Kroft, S. Design and Validation of an Implantable Actuator for Use in a Novel Dynamic Arteriovenous Shunt System. Master's Thesis, Delft University of Technology, Delft, The Netherlands, 2021.
141. Shiba, K.; Tsuji, T.; Koshiji, K. Direct drive of an implantable actuator using a transcutaneous energy transmission system. *J. Life Support Eng.* **2006**, *18*, 17–24. [CrossRef]
142. BAN Applications Matrix, Document 15-07-0735-08-0. 2008. Available online: https://www.ieee802.org/15/pub/default_page.html (accessed on 15 June 2021).
143. Rong, G.; Zheng, Y.; Sawan, M. Energy Solutions for Wearable Sensors: A Review. *Sensors* **2021**, *21*, 3806. [CrossRef]
144. Kos, A.; Milutinović, V.; Umek, A. Challenges in wireless communication for connected sensors and wearable devices used in sport biofeedback applications. *Future Gener. Comput. Syst.* **2019**, *92*, 582–592. [CrossRef]
145. Ullah, S.; Khan, P.; Ullah, N.; Saleem, S.; Higgins, H.; Kwak, K.S. A review of wireless body area networks for medical applications. *arXiv* **2010**, arXiv:1001.0831.
146. Movassaghi, S.; Abolhasan, M.; Lipman, J.; Smith, D.; Jamalipour, A. Wireless body area networks: A survey. *IEEE Commun. Surv. Tutor.* **2014**, *16*, 1658–1686. [CrossRef]
147. TG6 Applications Matrix, Document 15-08-0406-00-0006, IEEE P802. 2008. Available online: https://view.officeapps.live.com/op/view.aspx?src=https%3A%2F%2Fmentor.ieee.org%2F802.15%2Fdcn%2F08%2F15-08-0644-09-0006-tg6-technical-requirements-document.doc (accessed on 7 June 2021).
148. Jones, R.W.; Katzis, K. 5G and wireless body area networks. In Proceedings of the 2018 IEEE Wireless Communications and Networking Conference Workshops (WCNCW), Barcelona, Spain, 15–18 April 2018; pp. 373–378.
149. Soh, P.J.; Vandenbosch, G.A.; Mercuri, M.; Schreurs, D.M.P. Wearable wireless health monitoring: Current developments, challenges, and future trends. *IEEE Microw. Mag.* **2015**, *16*, 55–70. [CrossRef]
150. Santagati, G.E.; Melodia, T. A software-defined ultrasonic networking framework for wearable devices. *IEEE/ACM Trans. Netw.* **2016**, *25*, 960–973. [CrossRef]
151. Garcia-Perez, C.; Diaz-Zayas, A.; Rios, A.; Merino, P.; Katsalis, K.; Chang, C.Y.; Shariat, S.; Nikaein, N.; Rodriguez, P.; Morris, D. Improving the efficiency and reliability of wearable based mobile eHealth applications. *Pervasive Mob. Comput.* **2017**, *40*, 674–691. [CrossRef]
152. Sahni, Y.; Cao, J.; Zhang, S.; Yang, L. Edge mesh: A new paradigm to enable distributed intelligence in internet of things. *IEEE Access* **2017**, *5*, 16441–16458. [CrossRef]
153. Gia, T.N.; Jiang, M.; Rahmani, A.M.; Westerlund, T.; Liljeberg, P.; Tenhunen, H. Fog computing in healthcare internet of things: A case study on ecg feature extraction. In Proceedings of the 2015 IEEE International Conference on Computer and INFORMATION technology; Ubiquitous Computing and Communications; Dependable, Autonomic and Secure Computing; Pervasive Intelligence and Computing, Liverpool, UK, 26–28 October 2015; pp. 356–363.
154. ISO standard. ANSI/AAMI/ISO 14971:2019-Medical Devices-Application of Risk Management to Medical Devices. Available online: https://www.iso.org/standard/72704.html (accessed on 20 June 2021).
155. FDA. Content of Premarket Submissions for Management of Cybersecurity in Medical Devices: Draft Guidance for Industry and Food and Drug Administration Staff. Available online: https://www.fda.gov/media/119933/download (accessed on 25 September 2021).
156. Motani, M.; Yap, K.K.; Natarajan, A.; de Silva, B.; Hu, S.; Chua, K.C. Network characteristics of urban environments for wireless BAN. In Proceedings of the 2007 IEEE Biomedical Circuits and Systems Conference, Montreal, QC, Canada, 27–30 November 2007; pp. 179–182.
157. Al Kalaa, M.O.; Balid, W.; Refai, H.H.; LaSorte, N.J.; Seidman, S.J.; Bassen, H.I.; Silberberg, J.L.; Witters, D. Characterizing the 2.4 GHz spectrum in a hospital environment: Modeling and applicability to coexistence testing of medical devices. *IEEE Trans. Electromagn. Compat.* **2016**, *59*, 58–66. [CrossRef]
158. Qualcomm Technologies, Inc. VR and AR Pushing Connectivity Limits. Available online: https://www.qualcomm.com/media/documents/files/vr-and-ar-pushing-connectivity-limits.pdf (accessed on 25 June 2021).
159. Pozo, A.P.; Toksvig, M.; Schrager, T.F.; Hsu, J.; Mathur, U.; Sorkine-Hornung, A.; Szeliski, R.; Cabral, B. An integrated 6DoF video camera and system design. *ACM Trans. Graph. (TOG)* **2019**, *38*, 1–16. [CrossRef]

160. Feil-Seifer, D.; Mataric, M.J. Defining socially assistive robotics. In Proceedings of the 9th International Conference on Rehabilitation Robotics, 2005, ICORR 2005, Chicago, IL, USA, 28 June–1 July 2005; pp. 465–468.
161. Pavón-Pulido, N.; López-Riquelme, J.A.; Ferruz-Melero, J.; Vega-Rodríguez, M.Á.; Barrios-León, A.J. A service robot for monitoring elderly people in the context of ambient assisted living. *J. Ambient Intell. Smart Environ.* **2014**, *6*, 595–621. [CrossRef]
162. Bonaccorsi, M.; Fiorini, L.; Cavallo, F.; Esposito, R.; Dario, P. Design of cloud robotic services for senior citizens to improve independent living and personal health management. In *Ambient Assisted Living*; Springer: Berlin/Heidelberg, Germany, 2015; pp. 465–475.
163. Ma, Y.; Zhang, Y.; Wan, J.; Zhang, D.; Pan, N. Robot and cloud-assisted multi-modal healthcare system. *Clust. Comput.* **2015**, *18*, 1295–1306. [CrossRef]
164. Gross, H.M.; Mueller, S.; Schroeter, C.; Volkhardt, M.; Scheidig, A.; Debes, K.; Richter, K.; Doering, N. Robot companion for domestic health assistance: Implementation, test and case study under everyday conditions in private apartments. In Proceedings of the 2015 IEEE/RSJ International Conference on Intelligent Robots and Systems (IROS), Hamburg, Germany, 28 September–2 October 2015; pp. 5992–5999.
165. Manzi, A.; Fiorini, L.; Limosani, R.; Sincak, P.; Dario, P.; Cavallo, F. Use case evaluation of a cloud robotics teleoperation system (short paper). In Proceedings of the 2016 5th IEEE International Conference on Cloud Networking (Cloudnet), Pisa, Italy, 3–5 October 2016; pp. 208–211.
166. Bonaccorsi, M.; Fiorini, L.; Cavallo, F.; Saffiotti, A.; Dario, P. A cloud robotics solution to improve social assistive robots for active and healthy aging. *Int. J. Soc. Robot.* **2016**, *8*, 393–408. [CrossRef]
167. Fiorini, L.; Esposito, R.; Bonaccorsi, M.; Petrazzuolo, C.; Saponara, F.; Giannantonio, R.; De Petris, G.; Dario, P.; Cavallo, F. Enabling personalised medical support for chronic disease management through a hybrid robot-cloud approach. *Auton. Robot.* **2017**, *41*, 1263–1276. [CrossRef]
168. Cádrik, T.; Takáč, P.; Ondo, J.; Sinčák, P.; Mach, M.; Jakab, F.; Cavallo, F.; Bonaccorsi, M. Cloud-based robots and intelligent space teleoperation tools. In *Robot Intelligence Technology and Applications 4*; Springer: Berlin/Heidelberg, Germany, 2017; pp. 599–610.
169. Cavallo, F.; Limosani, R.; Fiorini, L.; Esposito, R.; Furferi, R.; Governi, L.; Carfagni, M. Design impact of acceptability and dependability in assisted living robotic applications. *Int. J. Interact. Des. Manuf. (IJIDeM)* **2018**, *12*, 1167–1178. [CrossRef]
170. Brunete, A.; Gambao, E.; Hernando, M.; Cedazo, R. Smart Assistive Architecture for the Integration of IoT Devices, Robotic Systems, and Multimodal Interfaces in Healthcare Environments. *Sensors* **2021**, *21*, 2212. [CrossRef]
171. Tröbinger, M.; Jähne, C.; Qu, Z.; Elsner, J.; Reindl, A.; Getz, S.; Goll, T.; Loinger, B.; Loibl, T.; Kugler, C.; et al. Introducing GARMI-A Service Robotics Platform to Support the Elderly at Home: Design Philosophy, System Overview and First Results. *IEEE Robot. Autom. Lett.* **2021**, *6*, 5857–5864. [CrossRef]
172. Witrisal, K.; Meissner, P.; Leitinger, E.; Shen, Y.; Gustafson, C.; Tufvesson, F.; Haneda, K.; Dardari, D.; Molisch, A.F.; Conti, A.; et al. High-accuracy localization for assisted living: 5G systems will turn multipath channels from foe to friend. *IEEE Signal Process. Mag.* **2016**, *33*, 59–70. [CrossRef]
173. RADIO Project. Unobtrusive, Efficient, Reliable and Modular Solutions for Independent Ageing. Available online: http://www.radio-project.eu/ (accessed on 24 June 2021).
174. Ramoly, N.; Bouzeghoub, A.; Finance, B. A framework for service robots in smart home: An efficient solution for domestic healthcare. *IRBM* **2018**, *39*, 413–420. [CrossRef]
175. Kaneriya, S.; Vora, J.; Tanwar, S.; Tyagi, S. Standardising the use of duplex channels in 5G-WiFi networking for ambient assisted living. In Proceedings of the 2019 IEEE International Conference on Communications Workshops (ICC Workshops), Shanghai, China, 20–24 May 2019; pp. 1–6.
176. Henry, S.; Alsohaily, A.; Sousa, E.S. 5G is real: Evaluating the compliance of the 3GPP 5G new radio system with the ITU IMT-2020 requirements. *IEEE Access* **2020**, *8*, 42828–42840. [CrossRef]
177. European 5G Observatory. 5G Trials That Have Been Publicly Announced in EU27, UK, Norway, Russia, Switzerland and Turkey. Available online: https://5gobservatory.eu/5g-trial/major-european-5g-trials-and-pilots/ (accessed on 25 June 2021).
178. sdx Central. 5G Trials in the United States—Steps Toward Standardization. Available online: https://www.sdxcentral.com/5g/definitions/5g-trials/ (accessed on 25 June 2021).
179. Verizon. Verizon Will Rapidly Integrate C-Band Spectrum with mmWave for Customers. Available online: https://www.verizon.com/about/news/verizon-c-band-spectrum-mmwave (accessed on 25 June 2021).
180. Verizon. Explore 4G LTE and 5G Network Coverage in Your Area. Available online: https://www.verizon.com/coverage-map/ (accessed on 26 June 2021).
181. AT&T. Wireless Coverage. Available online: https://www.att.com/maps/wireless-coverage.html (accessed on 26 June 2021).
182. T-Mobile. Coverage Maps. Available online: https://www.t-mobile.com/coverage/coverage-map (accessed on 26 June 2021).
183. Opensignal. How AT&T, Sprint, T-Mobile and Verizon Differ in Their Early 5G Approach. Available online: https://www.opensignal.com/2020/02/20/how-att-sprint-t-mobile-and-verizon-differ-in-their-early-5g-approach (accessed on 25 June 2021).
184. Digital Trends. 5G vs. 4G: How Will the Newest Network Improve on the Last? Available online: https://www.digitaltrends.com/mobile/5g-vs-4g/ (accessed on 25 June 2021).
185. Forbes. 5G Latency Improvements Are Still Lagging. Available online: https://www.forbes.com/sites/bobodonnell/2020/02/18/5g-latency-improvements-are-still-lagging/?sh=6d74337548f1 (accessed on 25 June 2021).

186. Carrozzo, G.; Siddiqui, M.S.; Du, K.; Sayadi, B.; Carrasco, O.; Lazarakis, F.; Sterle, J.; Bruschi, R. Definition and Evaluation of Latency in 5G with Heterogeneous Use Cases and Architectures. Available online: https://www.5gcity.eu/wp-content/uploads/2020/05/Definition-and-Evaluation-of-Latency-in-5G-with-Heterogeneous-Use-Cases-and-Architectures.pdf (accessed on 20 October 2021).
187. Asghar, A.; Farooq, H.; Imran, A. Concurrent CCO and LB optimization in emerging HetNets: A novel solution and comparative analysis. In Proceedings of the 2018 IEEE 29th Annual International Symposium on Personal, Indoor and Mobile Radio Communications (PIMRC), Bologna, Italy, 9–12 September 2018; pp. 1–6.
188. Qureshi, H.N.; Imran, A. On the tradeoffs between coverage radius, altitude, and beamwidth for practical UAV deployments. *IEEE Trans. Aerosp. Electron. Syst.* **2019**, *55*, 2805–2821. [CrossRef]
189. Park, S.H.; Kang, N.G.; Cho, C.; Won, E.T.; Patro, R.K.; Goyal, G.; Bhatia, A.; Bynam, K.; Naniyat, A. System Simulation Metrics for BAN—Samsung. Project: IEEE P802.15 Working Group for Wireless Personal Area Networks (WPANs). 2008. Available online: https://mentor.ieee.org/802.15/file/08/15-08-0630-00-0006-system-simulation-metrics-for-ban.ppt (accessed on 20 October 2021).
190. Qureshi, H.N.; Manalastas, M.; Imran, A.; Kalaa, M.O.A. Service Level Agreements for 5G-Enabled Healthcare Systems: Challenges and Considerations. *IEEE Netw.* **2021**, 1–8. [CrossRef]
191. Tian, W.; Fan, M.; Zeng, C.; Liu, Y.; He, D.; Zhang, Q. Telerobotic spinal surgery based on 5G network: The first 12 cases. *Neurospine* **2020**, *17*, 114. [CrossRef]
192. Parvez, I.; Rahmati, A.; Guvenc, I.; Sarwat, A.I.; Dai, H. A survey on low latency towards 5G: RAN, core network and caching solutions. *IEEE Commun. Surv. Tutor.* **2018**, *20*, 3098–3130. [CrossRef]
193. Ron Malenfant, Cisco. Industry Voices—5G Has the Potential to Transform Healthcare for Rural Communities. Available online: https://www.fiercehealthcare.com/tech/industry-voices-5g-has-potential-to-transform-healthcare-for-rural-communities (accessed on 20 October 2021).
194. OTH Amberg-Weiden. 5G4Healthcare. Available online: https://www.oth-aw.de/en/research-and-cooperation/latest-news-in-research/5g4healthcare/homepage/ (accessed on 12 January 2020).
195. Acemoglu, A.; Peretti, G.; Trimarchi, M.; Hysenbelli, J.; Krieglstein, J.; Geraldes, A.; Deshpande, N.; Ceysens, P.M.V.; Caldwell, D.G.; Delsanto, M.; et al. Operating from a distance: Robotic vocal cord 5G telesurgery on a cadaver. *Ann. Intern. Med.* **2020**, *173*, 940–941. [CrossRef] [PubMed]
196. Jell, A.; Vogel, T.; Ostler, D.; Marahrens, N.; Wilhelm, D.; Samm, N.; Eichinger, J.; Weigel, W.; Feussner, H.; Friess, H.; et al. 5th-Generation Mobile Communication: Data Highway for Surgery 4.0. *Surg. Technol. Int.* **2019**, *35*, 36–42. [PubMed]
197. Lacy, A.; Bravo, R.; Otero-Piñeiro, A.; Pena, R.; De Lacy, F.; Menchaca, R.; Balibrea, J. 5G-assisted telementored surgery. *Br. J. Surg.* **2019**, *106*, 1576–1579. [CrossRef]
198. Zheng, J.; Wang, Y.; Zhang, J.; Guo, W.; Yang, X.; Luo, L.; Jiao, W.; Hu, X.; Yu, Z.; Wang, C.; et al. 5G ultra-remote robot-assisted laparoscopic surgery in China. *Surg. Endosc.* **2020**, *34*, 5172–5180. [CrossRef]

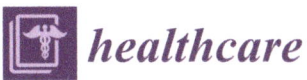

Review

Pathway of Trends and Technologies in Fall Detection: A Systematic Review

Rohit Tanwar [1,*], Neha Nandal [2], Mazdak Zamani [3,*] and Azizah Abdul Manaf [4]

1. School of Computer Science, University of Petroleum & Energy Studies, Dehradun 248007, India
2. Department of Computer Science and Engineering, Gokaraju Rangaraju Institute of Engineering and Technology, Hyderabad 500090, India; neha28nandal@gmail.com
3. Department of Computer Science, New York University, New York, NY 10012, USA
4. Independent Researcher, Kuala Lumpur 54100, Malaysia; azizahmanaf18@gmail.com
* Correspondence: r.tanwar@ddn.upes.ac.in (R.T.); mazdak.zamani@nyu.edu (M.Z.)

Abstract: Falling is one of the most serious health risk problems throughout the world for elderly people. Considerable expenses are allocated for the treatment of after-fall injuries and emergency services after a fall. Fall risks and their effects would be substantially reduced if a fall is predicted or detected accurately on time and prevented by providing timely help. Various methods have been proposed to prevent or predict falls in elderly people. This paper systematically reviews all the publications, projects, and patents around the world in the field of fall prediction, fall detection, and fall prevention. The related works are categorized based on the methodology which they used, their types, and their achievements.

Keywords: fall detection; fall prediction; fall prevention; fall risk factors; gait assessment

1. Introduction

According to the World Health Organization [1], approximately 28–35% of people with an age of 65 fall every year. The count further increases to 32–42% for people of age 70. With the rapid rise in the number of elderly people, the demand for supportive healthcare systems has also increased. The advancement in the fields of sensors, cameras, and communication makes it feasible to develop more efficient and optimized healthcare systems. Moreover, financial support from the respective governments motivates researchers to help elderly people through their valuable research [2]. Research in the medical field shows that a human being's process of aging leads towards a decreased walkability in elderly persons along with bringing down the physiological and nervous system function. Therefore, the probability of being injured during a walk becomes greater, which can cause several anile diseases. The prediction and evaluation of fall risks are very important given the surging number of aged people [3]. The impact of falls in the elderly is extensive and occurs across the world [4,5]. The process of fall prevention includes knowing and assessing the parameters responsible for a fall, predicting the possibility of a fall, and then not letting the fall happen. The process may include medical and paramedical treatment to fine-tune the fall parameters, the use of some aids, and some similar methods. It is very difficult to prevent a fall; however, long-term treatment may help in achieving fall prevention. Fall intervention is a set of techniques that help prevent future falls. Techniques that include exercise, home modification, and medication are carried out under clinical or self-administration with the aim of fall prevention in elderly persons [6].

1.1. Fall Risk Factors

Understanding the possible risk factors responsible for falls in elderly persons is required. A better understanding of these risk factors will help in developing a better fall prevention system. Numerous factors related to biology, behavior, demographics, and

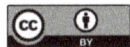

environment are there that can be a cause of falls for an elderly person [7]. A list of risk factors has been identified through the study of relevant and published literature, as shown in Figure 1. Numerous causes are responsible for the fall of an elderly person or patient. Physiological conditions and falls from the bed are the most common cause of the fall [8–10]. The authors in [11] designed a reliable and flexible method for the classification of falls in the elderly. Along with that, the operational definitions for types of falls were also provided. In the proposed three-level hierarchical classification scheme, the first level consists of four major classifications. Each major classification has further subcategories which are further divided into other subcategories of level three. The detailed categorization is shown in Figure 1.

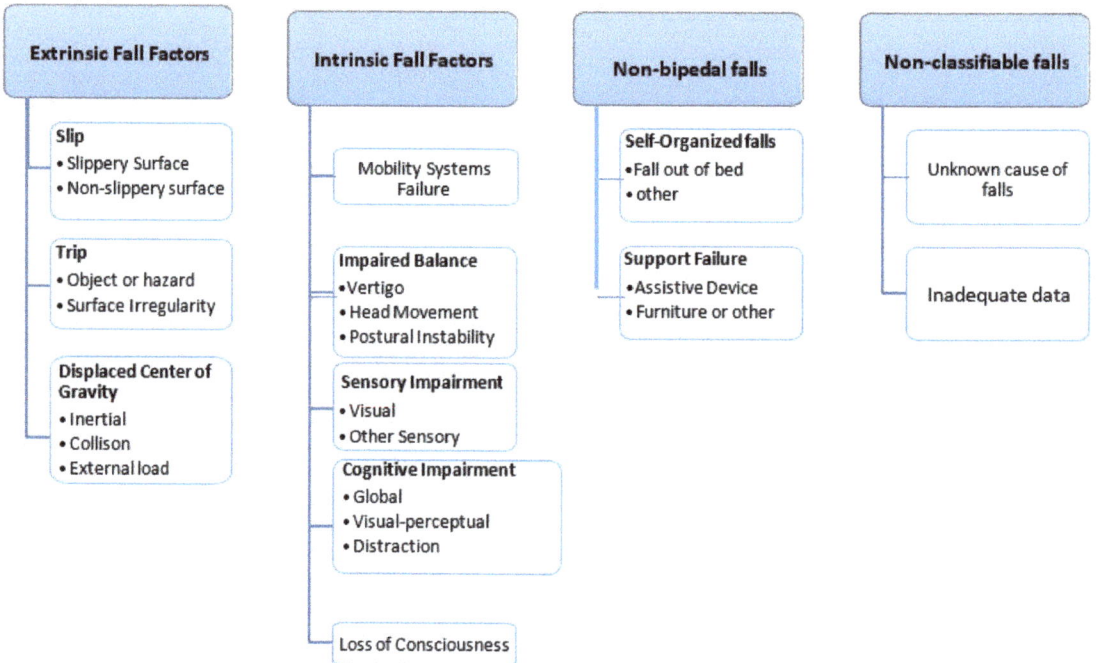

Figure 1. Fall risk factors [11].

1.2. Types of Fall

Categorizing falls used to be a great issue until the 1990s. A lack of consensus among researchers was the biggest hurdle. Most of the categorization then was based upon the factors responsible for falls. Depending on the position before a fall, a fall was considered to be of three general types, as described in Figure 2.

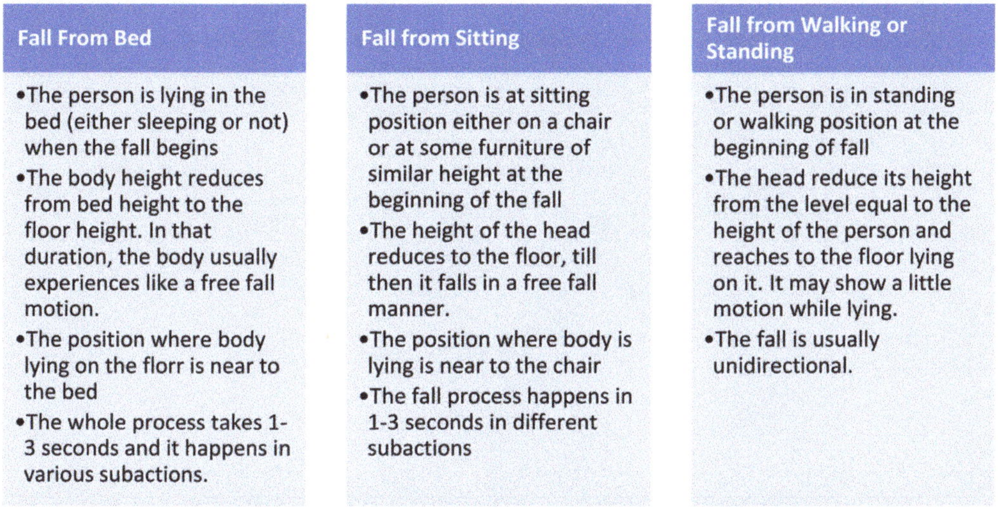

Fall From Bed	Fall from Sitting	Fall from Walking or Standing
• The person is lying in the bed (either sleeping or not) when the fall begins • The body height reduces from bed height to the floor height. In that duration, the body usually experiences like a free fall motion. • The position where body lying on the florr is near to the bed • The whole process takes 1-3 seconds and it happens in various subactions.	• The person is at sitting position either on a chair or at some furniture of similar height at the beginning of the fall • The height of the head reduces to the floor, till then it falls in a free fall manner. • The position where body is lying is near to the chair • The fall process happens in 1-3 seconds in different subactions	• The person is in standing or walking position at the beginning of fall • The head reduce its height from the level equal to the height of the person and reaches to the floor lying on it. It may show a little motion while lying. • The fall is usually unidirectional.

Figure 2. Types of falls [8–10].

1.3. Fall Detection/Prevention Approaches

A list of technologies has been developed by researchers to detect and prevent the occurrence of falls in elderly people. Numerous techniques have been used to handle the problem of falls among elderly people. These approaches are based on the integration of machine learning, IoT (Internet of things) devices, imaging techniques [12], etc. The continuous monitoring of the elderly person using either wearable or non-wearable devices and finding the probability of their fall in advance is known as fall prediction [13]; however, fall prediction is more concerned with the detection of fall risk factors. It requires a highly accurate prediction mechanism that could respond instantly in no time. However, it is not easy to achieve, but an accurate prediction will significantly contribute to preventing elderly persons from the after effects of falls. Fall detection is the process of finding out that an elderly person has experienced a fall and then sending some alarm signal to let medical professionals know about the incident. Various incidents might give an illusion of a fall, such as sitting on a chair from a standing position, bending on knees to pick something up, etc. The process is expected to differentiate actual falls from false falls and then send an alarm to pre-specified people or locations instantly. The intention is to send help to the elderly people after the fall as soon as possible so that after effects can be minimized.

Fall detection: fall detection techniques can be classified into three basic categories: (i) wearable devices, (ii) camera-based devices, and (iii) ambience devices. The categorization of fall detection is presented in Figure 3. In the wearable devices approach, some wearable gadgets or garments need to be worn by the people at risk of a fall. These devices sense the information regarding the body posture or the movement and then some algorithm processing this information decides whether it is a fall or not. The decision is then communicated to the pre-specified caregivers. However, the use of wearable devices seems to be very intrusive and an extra overhead to some users. They do not want to bother to keep on wearing any device all the time. Moreover, there is an issue regarding the placement of the device. Some activities, such as sleeping and walking, might displace the device from its original location and may result in less accurate results.

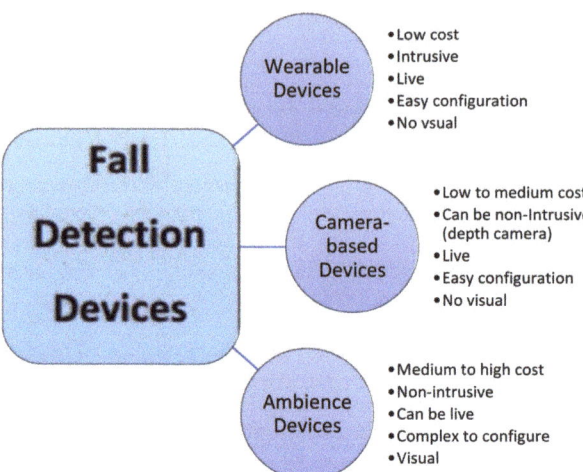

Figure 3. Fall detection approaches [2].

The camera-based approach seems to overcome some of these issues. The cameras are placed at selected locations so that continuous monitoring of the elderly people can be performed passively. Unlike sensors, it is possible to assess and analyze more than one feature using the camera. These types of systems were less preferable initially when the cost of the camera used to be very high. Additionally, the data captured through these devices can be stored for later analysis and reference. In the ambience device approach, a series of sensors are installed in the vicinity of the related persons, such as a wall, floor, bed, etc. The data are gathered from these sensors and, using that input, an algorithm decides whether there is a fall or not. Consequently, the incident is reported to the caregivers. Since there is no need to wear any sensor, the related person is not concerned about any type of overhead.

A variety of devices from different manufacturers are available in the market that send alerts when a fall occurs. According to a survey, the number of automatic systems for detecting falls will cover 60% of the fall detection systems market by 2019–20. The compound annual growth rate (CAGR) is expected to be approx. 4% from 2019 to 2029 [14]. Governments are investing more in research related to fall detection devices so that the major portion of their budget that is used in medical care and treatment of after-fall injuries could be minimized. These devices differ in their location of the mount, response time, size, etc. Some of the devices are listed [10–13] below:

1. MobileHelp
2. Medical Guardian
3. LifeFone
4. Bay Alarm Medical
5. GreatCall Lively Mobile Plus
6. Apple Watch

Fall prevention: preventing falls in elderly people is something that cannot be guaranteed and achieved 100%. It can be used as an activity for ensuring that the targeted person is in a minimal risk zone. It is performed through continuous monitoring and periodically assessing the status of identified fall risk factors. If the observed values for those parameters lie in the acceptable range, then the targeted people might be assumed to be in the safe zone. The list of activities [15,16] that can be performed for fall prevention can be listed as:

- Notice if they are holding onto walls, or something else, when walking, or if they appear to have difficulty when walking or arising from a chair.

- Talk about their medication.
- Complete a walk-through safety assessment of their home.
- Enlist their support in taking simple steps to stay safe.
- Discuss their current health conditions.
- Perform regular checkups of the eyes and spectacles.

2. Methodology

This section discusses the methodology followed for carrying out this work. The literature studied comprises the work completed as publications, patents, and funded projects or surveys in this domain in the specified time duration, as shown in Figure 4. The query used for searching is a Boolean "OR" combination of the terms "Fall Detection", "Fall Prediction", and "Fall Prevention", and it should appear in the title of the publication. A number of projects/surveys and patents completed in a window of two years starting from the year 1991–92 was sought out. The process was repeated for the subsequent two-year periods until 2020. Similarly, the number of publications was identified using Google Scholar. Additionally, the publications were also categorized according to the different publishers, including Springer, Elsevier, IEEE, etc. The publications were further grouped based on the technology used to detect/predict/prevent falls. The articles that were purely concerned with clinical research were excluded. Additionally, the articles where falls were a secondary concern, and the primary concern was some pre-existing disease, were not included. The non-availability of full text and indexing in some inappropriate databases were also considered as part of the criteria for exclusion.

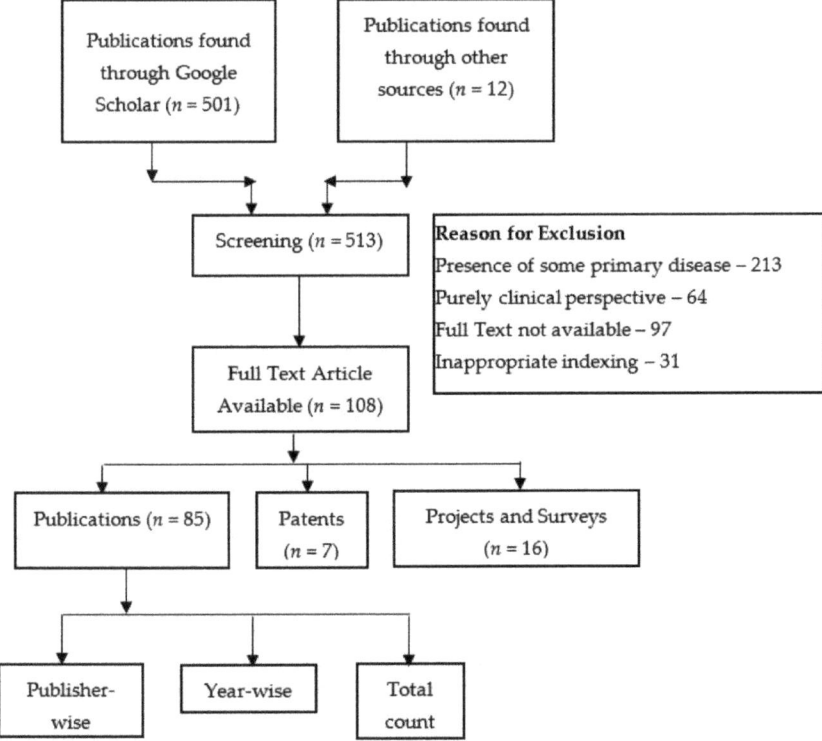

Figure 4. Review methodology.

3. Research Publications

To make the review process more systematic, the research publications that have been studied are placed in various categories depending upon the underlying technology they are focused upon. Before discussing the research publications in various categories, it is better to describe the parameters used for the evaluation of an algorithm used for fall detection or prevention.

3.1. Evaluation Parameters

A fall detection or prediction model needs to be tested for its effectiveness at analysis. The following four parameters [15,16] are used to evaluate a given model:

(i) Sensitivity: the system can detect falls correctly. It is defined as the ratio of the number of falls correctly classified and the total number of falls as follows:

$$\text{Sensitivity} = \frac{TP}{TP + FN} \quad (1)$$

where, TP = Falls correctly identified, and FN = Fall not detected by the model.

(ii) Specificity: the system can avoid false alarms (detecting an event similar to a fall, which is not a fall in actuality). It is calculated using ADL (activities of daily living) as follows:

$$\text{Sensitivity} = \frac{TN}{TN + FP} \quad (2)$$

where, TN = Number of ADL coorectly classified, FP = Number of False Falls

(iii) Accuracy: accuracy is the capability of a model to correctly identify actual falls and to recognize falls false as well. It is calculated through a balanced calculation of sensitivity and specificity:

$$\text{Accuracy} = \frac{\text{Specificity} + \text{Sensitivity}}{2} \quad (3)$$

(iv) False positive rate: this is the number of false falls identified as actual falls per hour. It is calculated as a ratio of the number of false falls to the total time of recording:

$$\text{False Positive Rate} = \frac{FP}{ADL\ time\ (in\ hrs)} \quad (4)$$

3.2. Cell Phone-Based Approaches

A simple system for fall risk prediction is developed in [3] using a cell phone along with a three-dimensional accelerometer. Practically, it is less expensive to use the accelerometer to monitor a human walking as an object. Along with the proposed work, the authors defined gait symmetry and stability under the data conditions of acceleration. The proposed gait assessment model was capable of analyzing and evaluating the stability and symmetry of an individual's gait. The proposed gait assessment model could predict the fall risk of a walking object correctly. The improved results for the performance and efficiency were obtained, justifying the effectiveness of the work. The problem of fall prediction is a manifold one, whose solution demands balanced coordination of behavioral, physiological, and environmental parameters.

Fortina and Gravina [12] designed a system comprising a smartphone and wearable accelerometer that sends an alarm when a fall is detected in real time. The system was capable of triggering fall incidents using different alerting modalities, providing emergency services with a notification in no time. The approach was tested on 20 subjects and the results reported an 83% specificity, 97% sensitivity, and 90% precision. The fall detection system in the future would be improved in terms of design and evaluation and become better because of this work. Research on the invention of modest wearable devices for blood pressure checking to detect orthostatic hypotension and the associated fall risk is almost nullified, however, although the research on using smartphones as devices to detect falls is in transit, and certain limitations are still challenges that need to be resolved, as listed below:

- It is doubtful whether the quality of the built-in sensors of cell phones [17] is good enough to properly identify falls. The accelerometer sensor of smartphones have dynamic ranges of up to ±2 g, but the level required for a fall detection device to produce an appropriate result is ±4 g to ±6 g (1 g = 9.8 m/s^2).
- The limited battery life (only a few hours) of smartphones on heavy usage is a major concern [17]. Past studies show that battery consumption rises to more than double when three sensors are used simultaneously. Using power-saver mode appears to be a genuine solution, but the performance would be affected considerably.
- Smartphones are not designed and developed purposefully for detecting falls [1]. The various compatibility and operational issues result in a compromise with accuracy when used in real time.
- The positioning of mobility sensors significantly impacts the behavior of fall detectors. The accuracy of the smartphone-based fall detection systems demands its mounting or placement at some particular and unnatural position, usually the chest or wrist [15]. However, this mandate of positioning either produces discomfort to the user or compromise with the accuracy achieved. Moreover, an additional device is needed to carry and position the smartphone at the desired point. It makes the product less attractive overall.

3.3. Sensor-Based Approaches

The use of accelerometer and gyroscope sensors either alone or in pairs has been the preferred choice of researchers to detect falls. In some research, the existing sensors of the devices are being exploited for fall detection, while in others, the desired sensor(s) is/are connected externally. Figure 5 shows the use of the different types of sensors in fall detection and prediction. The accelerometer sensor was used in 86% of the research works related to fall detection or prediction. Only 5% of the researchers used a barometer and magnetometer for fall detection.

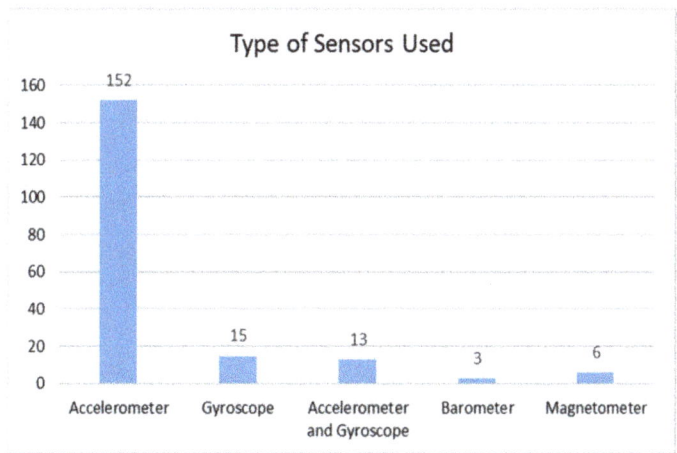

Figure 5. Types of sensors used in fall detection.

The problem of falls in the elderly is renowned and hazardous throughout the world. A delay in fall assistance may result in practical damage to the elderly person along with a decrease in movement and ease of living. The authors of [18] suggested a novel system to detect falls in aged people using the IoT. Their approach was based on utilizing energy-efficient wireless sensor networks, cloud computing, and smart devices. The wearable device was designed by embedding a 3D-axis accelerometer into a 6LoWPAN (low-power wireless personal area networks) device. The real-time data were collected from the movement of elderly people. To detect falls with improved efficiency, a decision tree-based big data model, along with a smart IoT gateway, is used for processing and analyzing sensor data. The moment a fall is detected, the system reacts by sending an alert message to the caregivers or emergency services chosen for providing care. The data are managed and stored in the cloud. The medical professionals can use that data for further analysis. Additionally, there is a system service that generates another machine learning model based on these data to adapt to future falls. The experimental consequences were improved fall detection success rates, measured using accuracy, gain, and precision.

Gait analysis and the monitoring of mobility are usually performed using accelerometers and gyroscopes in wearable systems. Most of the researchers recently have worked on obtaining and analyzing the data from accelerometers and gyroscope sensors for the assessment of fall risks [17,19]. Bourke et al. [20] analyzed different permutations of the magnitude of acceleration, sensor velocity, and body posture and, based on that, a fall detection system was developed. They observed that the maximum value of fall sensitivity along with the lowest value of the false positive rate was achieved when the three parameters were fused and used with a triaxial accelerometer. Bianchi et al. [21] developed a wearable device by utilizing an accelerometer along with a pressure sensor that mounts on the waist. Different variants of fall scenarios occurring indoors as well as outdoors were tested to minimize and avoid false alarms. The results revealed that false positives occurring under general circumstances are reduced considerably with the usage of the barometric sensor. As with other usual research, the authors simulated the testing environment, and healthy young people were used for testing the device. Ease of wearing is a prime characteristic of fall detection with wearable devices because of their continuous use for a long time. A study on the wearable devices found that, in a trial with a case that involved an enclosed waist-mounted device for fall detection performed on aging adults for three months, the device was transferred to different body locations because of discomfort and bruising [22]. Thus, along with small size, comfort is also a main factor that should be focused upon. The devices should not cause discomfort even if they are used for a long time and attached to the same location. Howcroft et al. [23] analyzed the performance of using two wearable sensors together in predicting fall risks. Two sensors, i.e., pressure-sensing insoles and accelerometers, four locations of accelerometer, i.e., head, left, pelvis, and right shank, and choices of three models, i.e., support vector machine (SVM), naïve Bayesian, and neural network. The observations reported that the best input can be provided for predicting falls when gait assessment is performed using multiple sensors, such as with a hybrid of the posterior pelvis, neural network, and head and left shank accelerometers. Some researchers [24] have invented a novel approach to avert the fall of a user by governing a passive intelligent walker as per the walking attribute of the user. These sensors are connected with an aid device for walking to identify gesture movements and the sensor's distance from a person. These types of sensors usually have a short range and a high rate of false alarms, with an individual stepping away from the walker being misunderstood as a fall. Another researcher [25] worked on the prevention of bedside falls and introduced a "Bed-exit" alarm. The proposed system utilizes pressure sensors. The pressure sensors are embedded on the side rails of the user's bed to sense the movement of an individual if they move out of the bed. A threshold value is to be set for the pressure sensor which, if exceeded, leads to an alarm going off to prevent the fall. For interactions with fall prevention exercise games, the available ambient sensors are often utilized. Researchers, Pisan et al. [26] and Kayama et al. [27], proposed systems that utilize Microsoft Kinect sensors with a game invented for older adults. The proposed game helps to identify the functional and cognitive changes in the patients by carrying out different physical and cognitive tasks. Multi-tasking has been embedded because it is proven to be a reliable predictive factor for future falls. Tong et al. [28] presented an HMM (hidden Markov model) method utilizing a triaxial accelerometer for fall prediction. Additionally, the proposed work again has not been tested and analyzed on real-life scenarios and elderly people who can be an example of people who are fall prone.

The solution to wrist-worn fall detection, and its development and assessment, has been presented in this paper [29]. Several different types of signals and direction components were collaboratively utilized along with machine learning methods to find out the best approach for fall detection. The sensors included a gyroscope, magnetometer, and accelerometer, the directions utilized were vertical and non-vertical, and the signals included velocity, displacement, and acceleration. Data for the work were collected from 22 volunteers for both fall and non-fall movements. With machine learning methods, an accuracy of 99.0% was achieved along with 100% sensitivity and 97.9% specificity. Additionally, the work has been tested with threshold methods, and a 91.1% accuracy was achieved along with a 95.8% sensitivity and 86.5% specificity. In the view of practical applications, the benefits of machine learning methods have been elaborated upon by the prolonged tests of a volunteer wearing a fall detector. Work has been proposed in [16] to detect falls in aged people in indoor environments. This was an IoT-based system that takes advantage of low-power wireless sensor networks, cloud computing, and big data. For its implementation, a 6LoWPAN device wearable was used in which a 3D-axis accelerometer had been embedded, which can collect data from aged people's movements. The reading collected by the sensor was analyzed utilizing a decision tree-based model. An alert is activated if a fall is detected, and the system reacts automatically by providing notifications. Lastly, the services will be provided built on the cloud. The system provides a service that leverages these data for building up machine learning models every time a fall is detected. The work showed very effective success at achieving results within the parameters of precision and accuracy. The work presented in the survey [30] utilized a depth sensor. A unique process to identify levels of fall risk has been implemented. This procedure of level identification is an enhancement of fall detection. The proposed algorithm showed effective performance results. The different and many suggestions along with solutions are present in the form of several tools, resources, and assessments for intervention, but falling is one of the major health problems which can occur to an individual. In today's time, it is considered highly desirable to go for health care if a severe fall happens.

The proposed model [31] is a working sub-model for the real-time monitoring of heart attacks and falls of a patient. To develop this system, an Arduino UNO and Arduino NANO-based process has been included as the architecture, with pulse and accelerometer sensors. The key concept is to gather the data related to health from time to time, and the data collected are to be made available utilizing a real-time interface called Thingspeak. Within this process, the person can be invigilated from time to time without any disturbance. The proposed model is also utilized to deliver notifications at the time of emergency with GSM (global system for mobile communication) technology, which is combined with the Arduino architecture. This model will be greatly helpful for elderly people, Frankenstein syndrome patients, or patients with a history of heart attacks because of genetic disorders. Other work [32] shows a health monitoring solution that identifies the occurrence of accidental falls in the elderly. The technique of fall detection implements sound- and accelerometer-based detections for valid fall occurrence. Fall detection based on an accelerometer is instrumental for the valid detection of fall occurrence. However, it has been shown that an accelerometer individually is not enough for fall detection because an accelerometer is affected by misinterpretations of routing motion activities, categorizing them as falls. To detect the pressure of sound from a resultant fall, the utilization of sound sensors has been integrated, but the pressure of sound is not enough to be utilized as a trustworthy fall indicator. Therefore, a method for the detection of falls based on fuzzy logic has been presented to activate the sound sensor and accelerometer's output signals, and the utilization of a sound pressure detector to verify the signal provided by an accelerometer can lower the incorrect fall detection rate of every day falls from 1.37 to 0.06. Choosing a particular paradigm, given the many approaches for detecting falls and ADL, needs some parameter to ease the selection. Power consumption is one such parameter, especially when dealing with embedded systems with limited constraints. Most of the wearable as well as non-wearable devices involve classification as one of its essential steps. Generally, machine learning algorithms or threshold-based approaches are exploited for classification purposes. The low computation needs combined with the moderate classification performance of threshold-based approaches creates a trade-off with the machine learning algorithms that normally demand high computation and offer better classification performance. A solution was presented for this problem in [33] that matches the power constraints of embedded systems. The method exploited advanced signal processing to find the maximum correlation of the unknown event within the available set of fall and ADL signatures. The power requirements were reduced by adopting a modified alignment strategy along with a normalization procedure specifically targeting the computational requirements. The method was able to satisfactorily classify an unknown event belonging to a specific class of events. Paper [34] discusses UWB (ultra-wide band) sensors, which are both environmentally and practically based on radar and are non-wearable, as a solution. Specifically, we are concerned about the impact of unsupervised changes in detection techniques on UWB sensor information to detect falls. Furthermore, accelerometer sensor information is also used for assessing the oversimplification of our unsupervised method for fall detection. Planned techniques are assessed using UWB sensor information sets obtained from an Australian E-Heath research center (i.e., Living Lab) and publicly accessible accelerometer sensor information sets. Results produced capable outcomes. Work [35] shows a stance recognition-based fall discovery framework for wellbeing observations, predicated based on keen sensors worn from the body function using personal networks. If it can be determined that this has the best range limit, when incidental falls occur, it could be successfully utilized in combination with an android gadget. By aggregating the full-time information and learning of an accelerometer, cardio tachometer, and other intelligent sensors, a fall might be calculated and separated from our ordinary lifestyle. The technique concerning the planned framework has been clarified in a much more feature in the paper. The planned framework accomplishes a 99% exactness rating by utilizing exclusive sensors similar to a temperature sensor, a circulatory strain level-checking sensor, and a cardio tachometer.

The work completed in paper [36] shows how one of the projected solutions in the literature has been modified for use with a smartwatch on a wrist, solving some problems, and updating part of the procedure. The testing includes a publicly accessible dataset. The results point to numerous enhancements that can be adapted for the target population. Other work [37] is focused on designing and developing a live system capable of detecting falls in humans. When a fall occurs, it would be able to alarm the concerned person so that the after-fall damages can be minimized. This can be used to reduce the damages at construction sites and in industry as well. The setup was assembled as a low-cost gadget using a MEMS (microelectromechanical systems) motion sensor (MPU-6050) and a GSM or RF (radio frequency) to send data. The mounting location of the gadget is chosen in such a way that a minor change in the center of gravity of the subject can be noticed. The information is then processed and analyzed to detect the occurrence of falls. In this paper [38], an approach is presented that detects the fall of an elderly person while moving inside the house or indoor premise and provides their exact location. A sensor-based fall detection method is used to detect the occurrence of falls and the location is provided using an artificial neural network. The work conducted in [39] was based on the Internet of things (IoT), and focused on the development of an energy-efficient wearable sensor node. A lightweight, energy-efficient, small-size and flexible device was designed for detecting falls. The design was a consequence of an exhaustive study on the parameters that affect energy consumption in IoT devices (wearable devices). The scope of research on ambient assisted living using smartphones motivated the researchers to work in this area. It was concluded from various approaches that wearable devices perform better at identifying falls from ADLs. These systems are tested in a controlled environment and optimization is performed for a given set of sensor types, sensor positions, and subjects. A self-adaptive pervasive fall detection method is proposed in this work. The work proposed is robust to the heterogeneity of practical situations in life [40]. The authors in [39] proposed an RNN (recurrent neural network)-based human fall detection method. The ability of the network to work with acceleration measurements from sensors means that it has the appropriate tools for the task. Study [41] presented an IoT fall system for the fall detection of elderly people that uses the benefits of IoT. The proposed system shows a 3D-axis accelerometer added into a 6LoWPAN wearable device with the capacity of measuring the movements of elderly volunteers as data. Table 1 shows the specificity (SP) and sensitivity (SE) achieved by various researchers. The research work considered in this table has exploited the accelerometer sensor for detecting falls. It can be observed from the table that various researchers have succeeded at achieving 100% specificity and sensitivity by using an accelerometer to detect falls [42].

Table 1. Performance of accelerometer-based fall detection devices [4–13,15–17,19–52].

Title	Author Details	Year	Specificity	Sensitivity
Evaluation of accelerometer-based fall detection algorithms on real-world falls	F. Bagalà et al.	2012	83.3	57
Evaluation of a threshold-based tri-axial accelerometer fall detection algorithm	A.K. Bourke et al.	2007	91.6	93
Comparison of low-complexity fall detection algorithms for body attached accelerometers	M. Kangas et al.	2008	100	98
Accurate, fast fall detection using gyroscopes and accelerometer-derived posture information	Q. Li et al.	2009	92	91
Barometric pressure and triaxial accelerometry-based falls event detection	F. Bianchi et al.	2010	96.5	97.5
Assessment of waist-worn tri-axial accelerometer-based fall-detection algorithms using continuous unsupervised activities	A. Bourke et al.	2010	100	94.6
A wearable pre-impact fall detector using feature selection and support vector machine	S. Shan et al.	2010	100	100
Unsupervised machine-learning method for improving the performance of ambulatory fall-detection systems	M. Yuwono et al.	2012	99.6	98.6
Evaluation of fall detection classification approaches	H. Kerdegari et al.	2012	92	90.15
Patient Fall Detection using Support Vector Machines	C. Doukas et al.	2007	96.7	98.2
A framework for daily activity monitoring and fall detection based on surface electromyography and accelerometer signals	J. Cheng et al.	2013	97.66	95.33

3.4. Camera-Based Approaches

In fall detection and prediction systems, there is a high usage of camera-based sensors [53,54]. For monitoring the routing activities of any individual, distinct cameras are used in such systems. Along with the pros, these systems also have some cons, such as budget and privacy, and they are unable to track beyond the camera range. Another fine example of ambient sensors is proximity sensors, which are utilized for fall detection. Bian et al. [55] utilized a single-depth camera to introduce a novel approach for fall detection in which key joints of the person's body are to be analyzed. This newly developed approach utilized an infrared-based depth camera which can work in dark environments. However, the invented approach is not able to identify the falls that end with the person lying on the furniture. Paper [54] planned an integrative replica of fall motion recognition and fall severity level assessment. The detection of fall motion and the presentation of data in a continuous stream, with the time-sequential frames fifteen body joint positions, have been obtained from Kinect's 3D camera. Some features are extracted and fed into a designated machine learning model replica. Compared to existing models, which rely on inputs of the image depth, the planned method resolves the background uncertainty of the human body.

The experimental outcome confirmed that the planned method of fall detection achieved 99.97% accuracy with zero false negatives and was robust compared to the state-of-the-art approach because it utilized image depth.

The work completed in [56] suggested a method for detecting falls using the 3D skeleton data received from a Microsoft Kinect. The technique utilized the accelerated velocity of the center of mass (COM) of different body components and the skeleton data as main biomechanical features and applied long short-term memory networks (LSTM) for detecting a fall. Unlike other similar methods, it does not require the mounting of a sensor on any body part of the elderly, people preserving their privacy. The method was tested and validated on the existing dataset and was found to be effective in fall detection. Since no special mounting of sensors is required, the device can be used for detecting falls in elderly people at home. This paper [57] discusses an intelligent fall detection system based on video. The first step is to extract the silhouette of a person using the background subtraction method; a collection of features is then evaluated to estimate a fall. The head position is estimated using a new technique and its virtual velocity is computed using an FSM (finite state machine).

For the expansion of systems that are human interactive, the visual human action classification is important. The work [58] enquires about a human stage classification that is image based, with a walking support system to increase safety. The paper [59] presented a real-time system that is very fast and more accurate and able to identify falls in videos taken by cameras. A new spatial and temporal variant-based aspect is presented which comprises the geometric orientation, the location of a person, and their discriminatory motion. The datasets used for the study are different cameras that fall with two and three classes. An accuracy level in the range of 99.0 to 99.2 has been achieved. A comparison of nine methods has been conducted and the effectiveness and improvement of the presented approach with the dataset have been given in the work.

3.5. Survey/Questionnaire

The authors in their work [2] have reviewed the existing fall prediction methods and strategies for old people and patients. Based on the approaches using sensors, the techniques for detecting falls are categorized into three domains namely, "Wearable Devices", "Ambience Devices", and "Camera-Based". Each class is subdivided further based on their fundamental principle of working. The advantages and disadvantages of each category have been listed along with the remarks for further improvements. Similarly, in [8], the authors have conducted a systematic survey of existing systems for predicting falls in the elderly. The shortcomings and the challenges listed by the authors help to design effective implementation techniques for fall prevention and prediction. One of the recent surveys highlighted a crucial point regarding wearable devices, namely that 32% of the users usually stop wearing them after 6 months and almost 50% stopped their usage completely after a year [60]. Therefore, a requirement of research must be to scrutinize the functionalities of wearable devices, such as modishness, budget, reliability, and flexibility, to increase its demand among customers. Questionnaires and assessments are often a part of clinical fall risk analysis that can analyze posture, cognition, and other important fall risk factors [61]. Questionnaire and assessment analysis provides a sample and snapshot for analyzed fall risks. They are usually subjective and utilize threshold assessment scores to categorize an individual as fallers and non-fallers [62,63]. However, fall risk flow should be modeled based on a continuum, and include categories of risk, such as low, moderate, or high fall risk. Modest sensors and distinct health tools can be utilized to perform the longitudinal monitoring of aging adults who can provide an effectively accurate assessment of fall risk. Shany et al. [64] introduced the utilization of wearable devices, such as sensors, for fall risk, especially under supervised and unsupervised environments. However, discussions about the testing, validation, and maintenance of different methodologies and real-life fall implementations are not being discussed in this work.

Another work in [65] shows a methodic review according to PRISMA (preferred reporting items for systematic reviews and meta-analysis statement) principles. Twenty-two studies out of eight hundred and fifty-five were studied for this work. The features which were extracted from the study were the outcome variables, fall prediction models, sensing techniques, and assessment activities. Four major sensing technologies, i.e., cameras, pressure sensing, laser sensing, and inertial sensors, were found to be useful for predicting fall risk accurately in elderly adults. The work presented accuracy levels in the range of 47.9% to 100% because of modeling techniques and kinematic parameter variations. Several sensor technologies have been used in fall risk analysis in elderly adults. It can be said that the devices are very valuable for providing an easy-to-handle and accurate analysis. In the future, it is necessary to find out ways to diagnose fall risk by using sensor technology. One of the major concerns of healthcare in several communities, specifically with elderly people, is unintentional falls. Related surveys have found that sensors, cameras, and sensor-based approaches are used to develop systems that can classify fall detection with human beings. The work presented in [66] elaborates upon three parameters, i.e., prevention, assessment, and intervention, which are shown as a three-tier model. This work has been conducted to bring together innovative tools, proactive programs, and technology that have been constructed for fall prevention. The realization of the resources will intensify the clinician's capability to precisely assess gait and balance, with the help of which the risk of falls can decrease. Research work [67] concentrates on falls in the elderly and how elderly people can be helped with fall prevention. As per the survey, 20% of all the elderly who have fallen remained on the ground for more than an hour. Moreover, 50% of the elderly people who suffered from falls die within 6 months of it, even if there are no physical injuries. The psychological effects can also lead to death. More than 50% of elderly people suffer a fall far from home where installed fall detection systems cannot reach. One of the top reasons for fatal as well as non-fatal injuries in elderly people is due to falls.

Fall frequency within one year calculated using time-to-time monitoring has defined the status of falls for 7/153 fallers or non-fallers. Based on [68] and their analysis of 718,582 turns, prospective fallers turned less frequently, took a longer time to turn, and were not very reliable in terms of their turn angle ($p = 0.007, 0.025$, and 0.038, respectively). Prospective fallers walk slower, use up less time walking and turning, and have extra time occupied in sedentary behavior ($p = 0.043, 0.012$, and 0.015, respectively). Those who have less control over their gait and turning abilities might attempt to decrease the risk of falling by restraining exposure and implementing advisory progress strategies while turning. As there were hardly any differences in general active rates among fallers and non-fallers, turning ability and gait may lead to an elevated risk of fall. Falls of patients and other injuries related to falls remain a concern of safety. The JHFRAT (Johns Hopkins fall risk assessment) device [69] has been utilized to perform untimely risk detection, which is meant to anticipate physiological cascades in adult patients. Psychometric properties in keen care settings have not been so far completely recognized; this revision sought to fill that space. The presented results showed that JHFRAT is reliable, with negative predictive validity and high sensitivity. Positive predictive validity and specificity were lower compared to the expectation.

An assessment for the identification of fall risk [70] is usually performed in hospitals and environments, such as the laboratory. Instead of these assessment testing methods, a passive monitoring solution in the home would be a cheaper and less time-consuming option. As sensors become more readily accessible, a machine learning replica can be utilized for the huge amount of information they create. This is useful for the finding, prediction, and risk determination of falls. In this review, the increased complexity level of sensor information required analysis, and the machine learning methods used to decide the risk of falling were analyzed. The latest research on utilizing passive monitoring in house has been discussed, whereas the viability of active monitoring by utilizing wearable and vision-based sensors has been measured. The comparison of methods, such as prediction, detection of falls, and mitigation of risk, has been conducted. This study [71] proposes a technique to analyze the ways in which elderly adults at high falling risk interact with the smart rollator, i-Walker, to navigate indoor, flat environments. The smart rollator is a sensor and actuator prepared and able to collect data for several hours. In [72], a multi-parametric score based on consistent fall risk assessment tests, along with medication, the history of a patient, their motor skills, quality of sleep, and environmental factors was planned. The resulting entire fall risk score reflects entity changes in vitality and behavior, which are triggers for fall prevention interventions. The deployment and evaluation of the system has been conducted in a pilot learning program for 30 elderly patients over 4 weeks. Another paper, Ref. [73], depicts a person in motion as a scatterer using time-variant (TV) speed, TV vertical motion angles, and TV horizontal motion angles of scatterers in motion. In addition, we obtained TV angular parameters of every moving scatterer, such as the departure angle of elevation, the azimuth departure angle, the arrival angle of elevation, and the azimuth arrival angle. Moreover, TV unit vectors of the departure of transmitted wave planes and unit vectors of the arrival of the received wave planes are obtained. Additionally, showing the Doppler power spectrum uniqueness of such channels provides a closed-form explanation of the spectrogram of complex channel growth. The precision of the analysis is determined using simulations. The paper contributes an initiative for implementing to device-free monitoring of indoor activity and systems of fall detection.

Study [74] collects and analyzes technological solutions that exist for the assessment of fall risk with several sensor-based technologies. This work also presents an easy solution for fall risk assessment and provides a design based on the concept for the integration of solutions based on the sensor for the Finnish National Kanta Personal Health Record. Paper [75] shows that older adult falls result in substantial medical costs. The calculation of medical costs attributable to falls provides important data about the problem's magnitude and the potential financial outcomes of effective prevention strategies. The objective of the study [76] was to expand a fall risk mobile health (mHealth) app and to decide the applicability of a fall risk app in healthy and older adults. A fall risk app was created which carries a health history questionnaire and five progressively challenging mobility responsibilities to determine individual fall risk. An iterative design–evaluation process for semi-structured interviews was created for resolving the usability of the app on a smartphone and tablet. Participants also completed a systematic usability scale (SUS) assessment. Standing-level falls [77] are the most common reason for injury-related demise in older grown-ups and a typical cause of attendance at accident and emergency departments. In any case, these patients once in a while underwent rule-coordinated screening and mediations during or following a scene of care. Diminishing damaging falls in a maturing society starts with pre-hospital assessments and proceeds through hazard evaluations and mediations that happen after crisis division care. Even though means for preventing people from needing to access emergency services have been implemented, proof-based systems to decrease the number of falls in elderly adults rely on fall prevention, and advancements incorporate the approval of screening instruments and the consolidation of contemporary innovations, such as PDAs (personal digital assistants), to improve fall location identification rates. This work [78] included measures that speak to various elements (clinical versatility and parity, quality, physiological, postural influence, and the mean and fluctuation of distinction scores among double- and single-task walk conditions) to decide the blend of measures that were the most sensitive for distinguishing fallers from non-fallers. This study aimed to analyze a smartphone fall prevention app to identify product features [79]. Along with that, the scope of revenue generation was also explored using willingness to pay (WTP).

3.6. Threshold- and Machine Learning-Based Approach

To develop a reliable and accurate fall detector, it is desirable to have a system that is capable of effectively distinguishing ADL from falls. The authors in [80] developed a paradigm that utilizes the sensors of a smartphone. Advanced signal processing procedures were used to obtain the moving average of scalar values of the three accelerometer components. The adoption of the cross-correlation event polarized approach helped the system to behave robustly. For better classification, two different types of classification algorithms were used, one based on threshold mechanism and the other on principal component analysis (PCA). The performance of the paradigm can be analyzed on two aspects, namely, the classification of a fall and distinguishing a fall from ADL. As compared to the threshold-based approach, the method outperformed on both aspects. However, the performance was moderate for the classification of falls and satisfactory for distinguishing falls from ADL. To improve the performance of the classification of falls, a modified classifier was presented in [80]. In the modified classification approach, the posture information of the user was also gathered after the ADL detection. Using this information, it was easy to discriminate between the multiple classifications of the same event, which was made feasible when using a large dataset for assessment.

In [81], a low-cost and very accurate fall detection algorithm based on machine learning has been proposed. A new method for online feature extraction which employs the fall's time characteristics efficiently has been proposed. Along with the same, a new design of a system based on machine learning has been proposed which can achieve the numerical/accuracy complexity tradeoff. The lower computing cost of the algorithm helps to combine it with a wearable sensor as well as make the requirement of energy much lower, which increases the wearable device autonomy. The experimental results on a big open dataset show that the accuracy of the proposed algorithm is 99.9% with a computing cost of less than 500 floating-point operations per second. The fall detection systems that utilize the built-in accelerometer sensors of smartphones have been developed to overcome several limitations. One of the major drawbacks of these systems is the enhanced false alarm rate that inhibits their use as a preferred approach. In this work [82], a new technique has been proposed using data mining for monitoring falls. The accelerometer data is mined to discover sequence patterns. These patterns are utilized to formulate a robust system for monitoring falls based on the mobile platform. The proposed solution was tested on a real dataset as well as the MobiFall dataset. The results were compared with existing fall detection algorithms that are smartphone based, and it was found that the method achieved an acceptable false alarm rate. Fall detection was improved using consecutive-frame voting in this work [83]. The process starts with human detection using background subtraction. The subtraction was conducted using a combined approach that involved a mixture of the Gaussian model with an average filter model. The feature extraction section has the task of calculating orientation, aspect ratio, and area ratio from the PCA (principal component analysis) of a human silhouette. In the human centroid section, the moving objects were grouped using human centroid distance. In event classification, event postures are classified. In the end, the voting of majority results is counted from consecutive runs. The results with improved accuracy indicate that the proposed method is better than the prior work that was tested on the Le2i dataset. Most of the techniques are based on a TBA (threshold-based algorithm). However, some researchers have used machine learning-based approaches to predict falls. The hybrid approach of TBA and ML are available in some cases, but each method has its strengths and shortcomings. The work completed in [84] analyzes the TBA- and/or ML-based techniques. The work performed in [85] is capable of identifying the pattern of falls along with the task of detection. This information regarding patterns is further utilized for assistance using machine learning. The proposed method was successful at efficiently differentiating falls from non-falls, thereby increasing accuracy. An automated method for inspection is proposed in this paper [86] to check PPE (personal protective equipment) usage by steeplejacks mounted beside exterior walls for aerial work. The inclusion of the aerial operation scenario-understanding method makes the inspection a tool that can be used to take preventive measures for control. The occlusion mitigation method based on deep learning is used for PPE checking. The method was tested under various conditions. The demonstrations and experimental results proved the reliability and effectiveness of the method for fall prevention and help in adopting safe supervision. The important offering of work [87] is a non-linear model along with threshold-based classification for recognizing abnormal gait patterns with more accuracy.

Within the same paper, a dataset with some real parameters was developed to calculate fall prediction. The smartphone sensors of the gyroscope and accelerometer have been used for dataset creation. The presented approach has been implemented and an accuracy of 93.5% has been achieved, which is good compared to other approaches.

3.7. Other Approaches

Sannino et al. [88,89] proposed an approach where a tag is placed on the subject's chest for providing data. The concept of windowing was used to classify windows in fall and non-fall action categories. Consequently, a final window composition was used to determine the global action as a fall or non-fall. The technique was tested and verified on real data comprising fall and non-fall events. The testing results were convincing and justified the effectiveness of their approach. The work presented in [90] elaborates upon the multi-player fall prevention game platform and fall sensing games that were inspired by the exercise program of Otago. The results of the work showed that the game integrates well with senior care centers. Another work, Ref. [91] presented an improvement of Kalman filter-based slip estimation for characterizing slipping distance. The very impressive thing about the algorithm is the detection of accurate slip onset in a fast manner along with the cost-effective and non-intrusive features of the sensor. For the validation and demonstration of the implemented work of a slip detection and estimation model, several experiments have been conducted. The work given in [92] presented a wireless channel data-based fall-sensing system that is real time and transparent. A dynamic template matching (DTM) algorithm has been utilized to build up FallSense. The model has been tested on Wi-Fi devices and an evaluation of the same has been conducted in real environments. The results presented in the work show the outperformance of FallSense compared to other approaches in terms of parameters, such as false alarm rate, complexity, and precision. One of the top reasons for injuries among elderly people is falling. Present solutions suggest wearing fall-alert sensors, but they have been shown to be ineffective in medical research because most of the time elderly people do not wear them. These things became the reason why the new passive sensors that interpret falls using radio frequency (RF) have come into existence. This does not have any implications for elderly people, and it does not encourage them to wear any kind of device. The existing approaches cannot deal with real-world complexities, although major advances have been made in passive monitoring. These approaches perform training and testing on the same people in the same environment, and they cannot extend it to a new environment. Additionally, these approaches cannot differentiate motions from different people, which makes it easy to miss out on a fall in the presence of different motions. To handle these problems, Aryokee, a fall detection system that is RF based [93] and which utilizes a state machine-governed convolutional neural network was proposed. The fall detection system, Aryokee, works with new environments and people who are not seen in the training set. It also separates dissimilar sources of motion to improve robustness. The dataset used was of 140 people performing activities of 40 types in different environments (57 different environments). The results achieved show 92% precision and 94% recall in fall detection. The methods of fall detection based on wearable inertial devices have been explored from 2013 to 2018 [94]. First and foremost, fall definition, fall's conventional phases, the categories of falls, and the classification of falls have been introduced completely. The research work has been explained in the context of modules, such as the collection of data, pre-processing, feature extraction, and the construction of a model for wearable fall detection system frameworks. The evaluation of the fall detection method's performance has been performed by inducing the most-used technical criteria. Finally, nine datasets of fall detection have been elaborated upon, and also the predictive performance based on the datasets has been assessed.

The FLIP (flooring for injury prevention) study [95] was a superiority trial conducted over a random 4 years in 150 single rooms at a Canadian LTC (long-term care) site. Residents' rooms were randomly blocked (1:1) with compliant flooring installation (2.54 cm smart cells) or rigid control flooring (2.54 cm plywood) covered with hospital-grade vinyl in April 2013. The foremost result was a fall injury of a serious manner lasting more than 4 years which needed a visit of the emergency department and a process of treatment or a hospital diagnostic evaluation. The secondary results included minor injuries, or any injuries related to falling, fracture, and falls. Results were confirmed by blinded assessors between 1 September 2013, and 31 August 2017, and examined with treatment as the objective. The problem of fall detection has been studied elaborately for a long time. However, designing accurate embedded algorithms with affordable computing costs is still a challenge because of limited wearable hardware resources.

This work [96] presents a model that is non-stationary, and which is important for such system development. A 3D stochastic trajectory model has been designed to find the mobility patterns of the user. The designed model has a forward fall mechanism. Radio waves will be transmitted to the complete indoor propagation environment, and the fingerprints of the object scattered on the emitted waves will be collected by the receiver. The radio channel has been modeled correspondingly through a process that captures the Doppler effect based on time spent by the occupant at home. The non-stationary channel's time-frequency behavior has been studied by calculating the power spectral density of the Doppler effect and with spectrogram analysis. The derivation and simulation of instant mean Doppler shift and spread have been performed and the proposed model showed results at 5.9 GHz. The presented results are very effective at developing fall detection models which are reliable, and the model is helpful for studying the effect of several walking/falling patterns. The results are intuitive for emergent reliable fall detection techniques, though the model is functional for studying the impact of diverse patterns on the whole fall detection system performance.

This research [97] outlines a detailed technique based on CNNs (convolution neural networks) for identifying falls using non-invasive thermal vision sensors. It consists of an agile information compilation for labeling images to produce a dataset that describes numerous cases of both multiple and single occupancies. The cases mentioned comprised situations with a fallen inhabitant and standing inhabitants. They also provide information augmentation methods for optimizing the capability of classification learning and the reduction of configuration duration. Third, they define three types of CNN for analyzing the effect of the number of layers and the size of the kernel on the technique's performance. The obtained results show, in the context of single occupancy, an accuracy of 0.92, and a reduction of 0.10 in accuracy in multiple occupancies. The learning abilities of CNNs have been highlighted as outstanding for use with composite images gained from the inexpensive tools. Do the thus-produced images have more noise along with uncertain and blurred areas? The result shows that a CNN based on three layers executes stable performance, along with fast learning. The planned technique in [98] offered extracts of motion data using a best-fit approximated ellipse and a bounding box around the human body, finding a histogram projection and identifying head position over time, which is useful for producing ten features for fall identification. The above features are fed into a multilayer perceptron neural network to calculate fall categorization. The investigational outputs explain the reliability of the planned method for a high fall detection rate of 99.60% and a low false alarm rate of 2.62% when used with the UR fall detection dataset. Comparisons to state-of-the-art fall detection methods revealed the robustness of the planned method.

The study conducted in [99] focuses on the validation and improvement of existing algorithms for fall detection. The study was conducted in two phases. In the first phase, twenty subjects were recruited of ages 86.25 ± 6.66 years who had experienced high-risk falls. The data concerning their movements were recorded for 59 days in real time using the AIDE-MOI sensor. The existing algorithms were optimized using these data. Then, the evaluation of the optimized algorithm was performed for 66 days. In total, 31 real falls were recorded through the data gathered in both phases. These data were then segmented into one-minute chunks for categorization as "fall" or "non-fall". A significant improvement was observed in the sensitivity (27.3% to 80.0%) and specificity (99.9957% to 99.9978%)

of a threshold-based algorithm. A new method is described in [100] that overcomes several deficiencies of the traditional fall detection methods. The system developed is completely passive and the user is not required to wear any of the devices. The system is developed utilizing the channel state information (CSI) of Wi-Fi along with an accelerometer mounted on the ground to detect floor vibration. The proposed method also overcomes the limitations of existing methods based on the Wi-Fi CSI approach that mandates the presence of only one user in the room. The experimental results show an efficient result of 95% accuracy. A fuzzy logic-based adjustable autonomy (FLAA) model is proposed in [101,102] to handle the autonomy of multi-agent systems that are active in tough surroundings. This model focuses on the management of the autonomy of agents and enables them to make competent autonomous decisions. The autonomy is quantitatively measured and distributed among several agents using fuzzy logic based on their performance.

Figure 6 details the variation in the number of publications every two years since 1991. The results for the same are obtained through Google Scholar for the keywords "Fall Prediction" OR "Fall Detection" OR "Fall Prevention". Similarly, Figure 7 shows the publication details for certain top-level publishers every two years. From the graphs, it is evident that the task of reducing or minimizing the fall risk and its after effects has been motivating more researchers every year. Certain challenges need the focus of active researchers and show the pathways for future research.

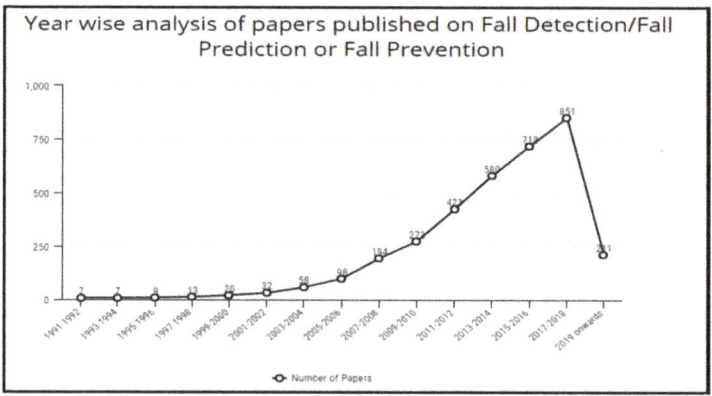

Figure 6. Variation of the number of publications (per publisher).

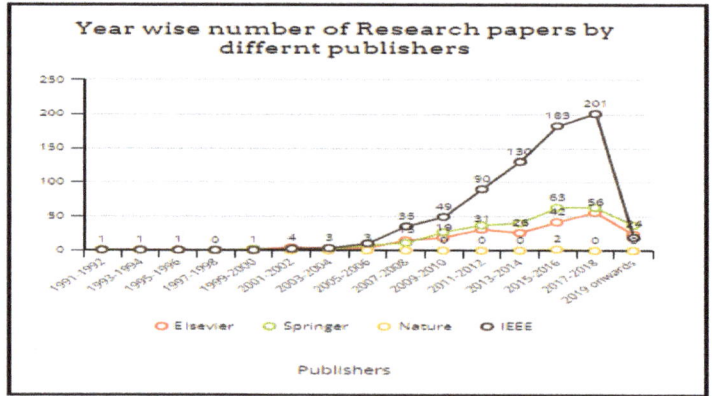

Figure 7. Variation of the number of publications (publisher-wise).

Figure 8 represents [103–105] the evaluation of the different approaches developed to detect or prevent falls. The evaluation has been conducted based on the attainment percentage of three parameters: sensitivity, specificity, and accuracy. It can be observed that in some cases, the respective authors succeeded in achieving more than a 98% value for the respective parameters [14,18,106–112].

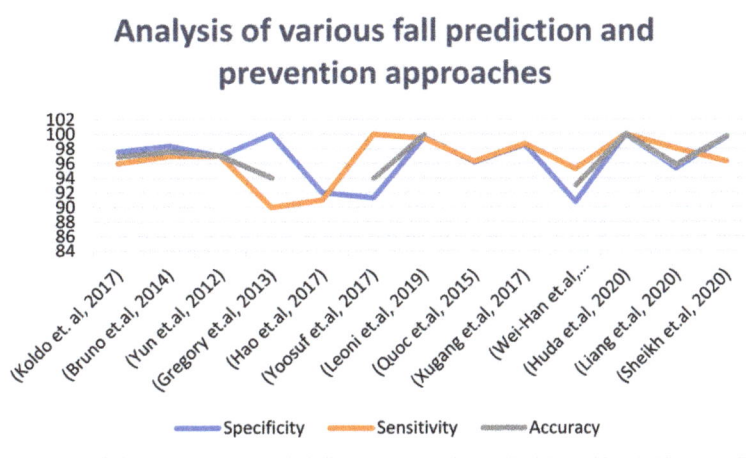

Figure 8. Qualitative analysis of various fall prediction and prevention techniques.

4. Patents

Researchers have been continuously working for the last three decades to reduce the risk and impact of falls in older people or patients. However, a comparatively fewer number of patents have been filed in this domain. The same is evident in Figure 9. The work conducted in [26] shows the number of patents filed every two years since 1991 to date. Most of the patents are filed in the USA. However, [10] describes the details of 0some of the patents granted in the USA and India. Table 2 gives an insight into some of the patents that have been granted in this domain.

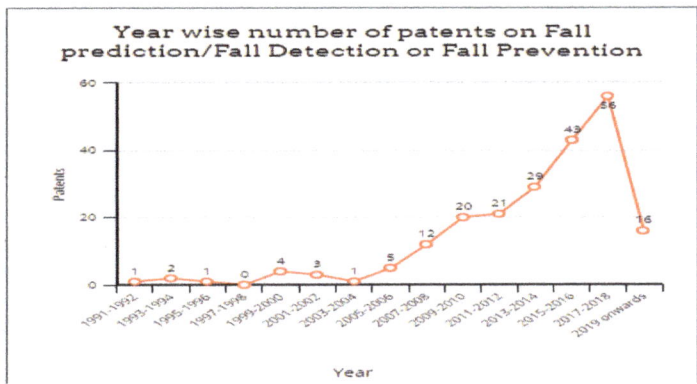

Figure 9. Patents granted on fall prediction or detection.

Table 2. Details of patents granted [113].

S. No.	Patent ID	Patent Title	Year of Approval	Inventor Name	Country
1	US10037669B2	Fall detection technology and reporting	2018	Mark Andrew Hanson, Jean-Paul Martin, Adam T. Barth, Christopher Silverman	USA
2	US8990041B2	Fall detection	2010	Mark D. Grabiner, Kenton R. Kaufman, Barry K. Gilbert	USA
3	US20160100776A1	Fall detection and fall risk detection systems and methods	2015	Bijan BolooriNajafi, Ashkan Vaziri, Ali-Reza	USA
4	US20180263534	Fall detection device and method for controlling thereof	2018	Han-sung Lee, Jae-geol Cho, Moo-rim Kim, Chang-hyun Kim	USA
5	US20180146737	Shoe system for the detection and monitoring of health, vitals, and fall detection	2018	Joseph Goodrich	USA
6	US20180007257	Automatic detection by a wearable camera	2018	Senem Velipasalar, Mauricio Casares, Akhan Almagambetov	USA
7	2316/CHE/2013	System And Method For Personal Crash/Fall Detection And Notification	2013	Abhishek H Latthe	INDIA

5. Projects and Surveys

According to the National Council of Aging, an older adult dies because of a fall every 19 minutes, and every 11 minutes, an older adult is treated in an emergency department for a fall-related injury [101]. Approximately USD 50 billion is spent on treating fall-related injuries in older adults in America. Table 3 describes some projects sanctioned in this domain along with the funding details. Having a birds' eye view of medical expenditure on falls worldwide is enough to understand the need for projects and research to be carried out in this domain. The OU College of Nursing earns a grant of USD 1 million to continue its fall prevention program. Congress was requested to allocate a budget of USD 10 million for fall prevention programs in just one financial year [112,114–123].

Table 3. Details of funded projects for fall detection or prevention.

Project Title	Investigators	Year of Sanction	Organization	Funding Details	Project Description
"Randomized Trial of a Multifactorial Fall Injury Prevention Strategy: A Joint Initiative of PCORI and the National Institute on Aging of the National Institutes of Health" [61]	Shalender Bhasin, Thomas Gill, David B. Reuben	2014	Harvard Medical School; Yale Medical School; UCLA Medical School	Budget: $33,365,602 Source: Patient-Centered Outcomes Research Institute	Behavioral Interventions, Care Coordination, Other Clinical Interventions, Other Health Services Interventions, Technology Interventions, Training and Education Interventions
"Home Safety Adaptations for the Elderly (Home SAFE)" [62]	Unspecified	2010	Fall Prevention Center of Excellence, headquartered at the University of Southern California Leonard Davis School of Gerontology	Budget: Unspecified Source: The Eisner Foundation	Home safety for older people from Fall, fire, etc. and develop and implement related strategies
"Design and Development of fall prediction and protection system for pelvis & femur fractures: Preliminary study" [63]	Dr. Dinesh Kalyanasundaram	2015	Centre for Biomedical Engineering, Indian Institute of Technology (IIT)-Delhi, Hauz Khas, New Delhi- 110 016.	Budget: Rs.26,78,162/- Source: DST INDIA	Unspecified
"WIISEL (Wireless Insole for Independent and Safe Elderly Living)" [124]	Fanny Breuil, Meritxell Garcia Milà	2007	WIISEL, 7th Framework Programme	Budget: $2.9 M Source: European Commission	To prevent falls in older people
"Development of a wireless sensor network based gait assessment system for fall prediction in elderly patients" [125]	Prof. Subrat Kar	2008	Bharti School of Telecommunication Technology and Management, Indian Institute of Technology Delhi, Hauz Khas, New Delhi-16	Budget: Rs.36,73,200/- Source: DST INDIA	Unspecified

6. Observations and Findings

The systematic study of relevant literature in the field of fall detection and prediction yields a few observations. These findings are the challenges that researchers willing to work in this domain might focus upon.

(i) The majority of the systems developed for detecting or predicting falls in elderly or ambulatory persons are not tested in the real environment. The testing of these systems is primarily performed on the volunteers, who are healthy and young, and usually in the laboratory. The lack of validation against actual users puts doubt on their performance in real life.

(ii) The final acceptance of any system by the actual users is more likely if their opinions are incorporated at the initial stage of development. Unfortunately, the requirements are not gathered by actively involving the elderly peoples initially.

(iii) Most of the projects, patents, and models developed validate their product by measuring certain parameters. There are hardly any cases where user acceptance or satisfaction is taken as the criteria for the effectiveness of the research work conducted.

(iv) A hybrid approach of wearable, as well as ambient devices under reasonable cost would be beneficial to deal with obtrusive factors.

(v) Most of the people who are under consideration are reluctant to press the panic button after a fall. It happens either because of difficulty in activating it or because they do not want to disturb their caregivers.

(vi) Nearly no studies have so far involved the inputs of actual subjects and their relatives and family members. It may be the case that not every time a person falls requires the emergency services. Similar issues can be handled if they are actively involved in the requirement gathering step.

(vii) Usually, the products are designed from a technological perspective, considering things such as power consumption, battery backup, response time, sensors mounting, etc. Medical grounds are surpassed generally by these technical debates.

(viii) In the devices with a push-button, the older people take more time to realize that they are falling rather than younger ones (who are used for testing the device). Consequently, they might not press the button in a timely manner. This is challenge for older people that needs to be addressed.

(ix) The existing systems are hardly in line with the patient confidentiality standards and regulations of the HIPPA.

7. Conclusions and Future Scope

Despite continued research over many decades into preventing and predicting falls in elderly people, some factors are still unattended to. The concerns of various governments and the reputed organizations, such as the WHO (World Health Organization), regarding the increasing incidents of falls and their impact are enough to attract researchers to this field. However, some recent research has claimed to achieve the required accuracy in predicting falls, but still they are questionable because of their testing environment. Most of the researchers have not taken into account the perceptions of the actual users regarding what they expect from the product. National governments prefer to give funding for promoting research in this field so that the budget that is spent on after-fall services can be reduced. In the future, the researchers may focus on exploiting some of the principal observations stated in this paper. A hybrid approach of proper education, IoT techniques, and clinical support is expected to achieve real goals.

Author Contributions: Conceptualization, R.T. and M.Z.; methodology, R.T. and N.N.; writing—original draft preparation, R.T. and N.N.; writing—review and editing, M.Z. and A.A.M.; visualization, R.T. and A.A.M. All authors have read and agreed to the published version of the manuscript.

Funding: This research received no external funding.

Institutional Review Board Statement: Not applicable.

Informed Consent Statement: Not applicable.

Data Availability Statement: The data presented in this study are available on request from the corresponding author.

Conflicts of Interest: The authors have no conflicts of interest. No funding was received from any source.

References

1. Igual, R.; Medrano, C.; Plaza, I. Challenges, issues and trends in fall detection systems. *Biomed. Eng. Online* **2013**, *12*, 1–24. [CrossRef]
2. Yu, X. Approaches and principles of fall detection for elderly and patient. In Proceedings of the HealthCom 2008—10th International Conference on e-Health Networking, Applications and Services, Singapore, 7–9 July 2008; pp. 42–47. [CrossRef]
3. Jiang, S.; Zhang, B.; Wei, D. The Elderly Fall Risk Assessment and Prediction Based on Gait Analysis. In Proceedings of the 2011 IEEE 11th International Conference on Computer and Information Technology, Paphos, Cyprus, 31 August–2 September 2011; pp. 176–180.
4. Jagnoor, J.; Suraweera, W.; Keay, L.; Ivers, R.; Thakur, J.S.; Gururaj, G.; Jha, P. Mortalité des enfants et des adultes résultant de chutes involontaires en Inde. *Bull. World Health Organ.* **2011**, *89*, 733–740. [CrossRef]
5. Joshi, A.; Rajabali, F.; Turcotte, K.; Beaton, M.D.; Pike, I. Fall-related deaths among older adults in British Columbia: Cause and effect of policy change. *Inj. Prev.* **2019**, *26*, 412–416. [CrossRef] [PubMed]
6. Loria, G.; Bhargava, A. Prevention of patient falls—A case study. *Apollo Med.* **2013**, *10*, 175–180. [CrossRef]
7. Rajagopalan, R.; Litvan, I.; Jung, T.-P.; Rajagopalan, R.; Litvan, I.; Jung, T.-P. Fall Prediction and Prevention Systems: Recent Trends, Challenges, and Future Research Directions. *Sensors* **2017**, *17*, 2509. [CrossRef] [PubMed]
8. CHG Hospital Beds: Patient Falls from Hospital Beds, (n.d.). Available online: http://chgbeds.blogspot.com/2012/07/patient-falls-from-hospital-beds.html (accessed on 7 August 2019).
9. White, M.L. Your Comprehensive Guide to Nursing Home Fall Injuries and Recoveries, (n.d.). Available online: https://www.grayandwhitelaw.com/library/nursing-home-fall-injury-causes-and-recoveries.cfm (accessed on 7 August 2019).
10. Critical Need to Prevent Falls as Emergency Admissions Rise | News | Nursing Times, (n.d.). Available online: https://www.nursingtimes.net/news/reviews-and-reports/critical-need-to-prevent-falls-as-emergency-admissions-rise/7021519.article (accessed on 7 August 2019).
11. Lach, H.; Reed, A.T.; Arfken, C.L.; Miller, J.P.; Paige, G.D.; Birge, S.J.; Peck, W.A. Falls in the Elderly: Reliability of a Classification System. *J. Am. Geriatr. Soc.* **1991**, *39*, 197–202. [CrossRef] [PubMed]
12. Xu, T.; Zhou, Y.; Zhu, J. New Advances and Challenges of Fall Detection Systems: A Survey. *Appl. Sci.* **2018**, *8*, 418. [CrossRef]
13. Hemmatpour, M.; Ferrero, R.; Montrucchio, B.; Rebaudengo, M. A Review on Fall Prediction and Prevention System for Personal Devices: Evaluation and Experimental Results. *Adv. Human-Comput. Interact.* **2019**, *2019*, 9610567. [CrossRef]
14. Apple Watch Series 4 with Fall Detection | s This the Right Option for You? (n.d.). Available online: https://www.medicalalertadvice.com/articles/apple-watch-fall-detection/ (accessed on 26 July 2019).
15. Steps for Preventing Falls in the Elderly | NCOA, (n.d.). Available online: https://www.ncoa.org/healthy-aging/falls-prevention/preventing-falls-tips-for-older-adults-and-caregivers/6-steps-to-protect-your-older-loved-one-from-a-fall/ (accessed on 19 July 2019).
16. Yacchirema, D.; De Puga, J.S.; Palau, C.; Esteve, M. Fall detection system for elderly people using IoT and Big Data. *Procedia Comput. Sci.* **2018**, *130*, 603–610. [CrossRef]
17. Doheny, E.P.; Walsh, C.; Foran, T.; Greene, B.R.; Fan, C.W.; Cunningham, C.; Kenny, R.A. Falls classification using tri-axial accelerometers during the five-times-sit-to-stand test. *Gait Posture* **2013**, *38*, 1021–1025. [CrossRef]
18. Hardy, E. Apple Watch Fall Detection might Get You Arrested | Cult of Mac. 2018. Available online: https://www.cultofmac.com/579077/how-apple-watch-fall-detection-might-get-you-arrested/ (accessed on 26 July 2019).
19. Wang, K.; Redmond, S.; Lovell, N. Monitoring for Elderly Care: The Role of Wearable Sensors in Fall Detection and Fall Prediction Research. In *Telemedicine and Electronic Medicine*; CRC Press: Boca Raton, FL, USA, 2015; pp. 619–652. [CrossRef]
20. Bourke, A.; Van de Ven, P.; Gamble, M.; O'Connor, R.; Murphy, K.; Bogan, E.; McQuade, E.; Finucane, P.; Olaighin, G.; Nelson, J. Evaluation of waist-mounted tri-axial accelerometer based fall-detection algorithms during scripted and continuous unscripted activities. *J. Biomech.* **2010**, *43*, 3051–3057. [CrossRef] [PubMed]
21. Bianchi, F.; Redmond, S.J.; Narayanan, M.R.; Cerutti, S.; Lovell, N.H. Barometric Pressure and Triaxial Accelerometry-Based Falls Event Detection. *IEEE Trans. Neural Syst. Rehabil. Eng.* **2010**, *18*, 619–627. [CrossRef] [PubMed]
22. Mathie, M.J.; Coster, A.; Lovell, N.H.; Celler, B.G.; Lord, S.R.; Tiedemann, A. A pilot study of long-term monitoring of human movements in the home using accelerometry. *J. Telemed. Telecare* **2004**, *10*, 144–151. [CrossRef] [PubMed]
23. Howcroft, J.; Kofman, J.; Lemaire, E. Prospective Fall-Risk Prediction Models for Older Adults Based on Wearable Sensors. *IEEE Trans. Neural Syst. Rehabil. Eng.* **2017**, *25*, 1812–1820. [CrossRef]
24. Hirata, Y.; Komatsuda, S.; Kosuge, K. Fall prevention control of passive intelligent walker based on human model. In Proceedings of the 2008 IEEE/RSJ International Conference on Intelligent Robots and Systems, Nice, France, 22–26 September 2008; pp. 1222–1228. [CrossRef]

25. Hilbe, J.; Schulc, E.; Linder, B.; Them, C. Development and alarm threshold evaluation of a side rail integrated sensor technology for the prevention of falls. *Int. J. Med. Inform.* **2010**, *79*, 173–180. [CrossRef]
26. Pisan, Y.; Marin, J.G.; Navarro, K.F. Improving lives: Using Microsoft Kinect to predict the loss of balance for elderly users under cognitive load. In Proceedings of the 9th Australasian Conference on Interactive Entertainment: Matters of Life and Death, Melbourne, Australia, 30 September–1 October 2013; pp. 1–4. [CrossRef]
27. Kayama, H.; Okamoto, K.; Nishiguchi, S.; Yamada, M.; Kuroda, T.; Aoyama, T. Effect of a Kinect-Based Exercise Game on Improving Executive Cognitive Performance in Community-Dwelling Elderly: Case Control Study. *J. Med. Internet Res.* **2014**, *16*, e61. [CrossRef] [PubMed]
28. Tong, L.; Song, Q.; Ge, Y.; Liu, M. HMM-Based Human Fall Detection and Prediction Method Using Tri-Axial Accelerometer. *IEEE Sens. J.* **2013**, *13*, 1849–1856. [CrossRef]
29. de Quadros, T.; Lazzaretti, A.E.; Schneider, F.K. A Movement Decomposition and Machine Learning-Based Fall Detection System Using Wrist Wearable Device. *IEEE Sens. J.* **2018**, *18*, 5082–5089. [CrossRef]
30. Nizam, Y.; Mohd, M.N.H.; Jamil, M.M.A. Development of a User-Adaptable Human Fall Detection Based on Fall Risk Levels Using Depth Sensor. *Sensors* **2018**, *18*, 2260. [CrossRef] [PubMed]
31. Shanmugam, M.; Singh, M. Singh, Attribution (CC-BY) 3.0 license. *J. Comput. Sci.* **2018**, *14*, 574–584. [CrossRef]
32. Er, P.V.; Tan, K.K. Non-intrusive fall detection monitoring for the elderly based on fuzzy logic. *Measurement* **2018**, *124*, 91–102. [CrossRef]
33. Andó, B.; Baglio, S.; Crispino, R.; Marletta, V. A smart inertial system for fall detection. *J. Ambient. Intell. Humaniz. Comput.* **2019**, *12*, 4503–4511. [CrossRef]
34. Mokhtari, G.; Aminikhanghahi, S.; Zhang, Q.; Cook, D.J. Fall detection in smart home environments using UWB sensors and unsupervised change detection. *J. Reliab. Intell. Environ.* **2018**, *4*, 131–139. [CrossRef]
35. Arunachalam, A.; Michael, G. An Efficient System for Posture-Recognition Based Fall Detection System and Health Monitoring, n.d. Available online: http://www.ijpam.eu (accessed on 29 November 2019).
36. Khojasteh, S.B.; Villar, J.R.; de la Cal, E.; González, V.M.; Sedano, J.; Yazgän, H.R. An Evaluation of a wrist-based wearable fall detection method. In *Hybrid Artificial Intelligent Systems, Proceedings of the International Conference on Hybrid Artificial Intelligence Systems, Oviedo, Spain, 20–22 June 2018*; Springer: Berlin/Heidelberg, Germany, 2018; pp. 377–386. [CrossRef]
37. Hayat, A.; Shan, M. Fall Detection System for Labour Safety. In Proceedings of the 2018 International Conference on Engineering, Applied Sciences, and Technology (ICEAST), Phuket, Thailand, 4–7 July 2018; pp. 1–4. [CrossRef]
38. Gharghan, S.K.; Mohammed, S.L.; Al-Naji, A.; Abu-AlShaeer, M.J.; Jawad, H.M.; Jawad, A.M.; Chahl, J. Accurate Fall Detection and Localization for Elderly People Based on Neural Network and Energy-Efficient Wireless Sensor Network. *Energies* **2018**, *11*, 2866. [CrossRef]
39. Gia, T.N.; Sarker, V.; Tcarenko, I.; Rahmani, A.M.; Westerlund, T.; Liljeberg, P.; Tenhunen, H. Energy efficient wearable sensor node for IoT-based fall detection systems. *Microprocess. Microsyst.* **2018**, *56*, 34–46. [CrossRef]
40. Krupitzer, C.; Sztyler, T.; Edinger, J.; Breitbach, M.; Stuckenschmidt, H.; Becker, C. Hips Do Lie! A Position-Aware Mobile Fall Detection System. In Proceedings of the 2018 IEEE International Conference on Pervasive Computing and Communications (PerCom), Athens, Greece, 19–23 March 2018; pp. 1–10. [CrossRef]
41. Yacchirema, D.; De Puga, J.S.; Palau, C.; Esteve, M. Fall detection system for elderly people using IoT and ensemble machine learning algorithm. *Pers. Ubiquitous Comput.* **2019**, *23*, 801–817. [CrossRef]
42. Bourke, A.K.; Van de Ven, P.; Gamble, M.; O'Connor, R.; Murphy, K.; Bogan, E.; McQuade, E.; Finucane, P.; Olaighin, G.; Nelson, J. Assessment of waist-worn tri-axial accelerometer based fall-detection algorithms using continuous unsupervised activities. In Proceedings of the 2010 Annual International Conference of the IEEE Engineering in Medicine and Biology, Buenos Aires, Argentina, 31 August–4 September 2010; pp. 2782–2785. [CrossRef]
43. Theodoridis, T.; Solachidis, V.; Vretos, N.; Daras, P. Human Fall Detection from Acceleration Measurements Using a Recurrent Neural Network. In *Precision Medicine Powered by pHealth and Connected Health, Proceedings of the International Conference on Biomedical and Health Informatics, Thessaloniki, Greece, 18–21 November 2017*; Springer: Berlin/Heidelberg, Germany, 2017; pp. 145–149. [CrossRef]
44. Bagalà, F.; Becker, C.; Cappello, A.; Chiari, L.; Aminian, K.; Hausdorff, J.M.; Zijlstra, W.; Klenk, J. Evaluation of Accelerometer-Based Fall Detection Algorithms on Real-World Falls. *PLoS ONE* **2012**, *7*, e37062. [CrossRef] [PubMed]
45. Bourke, A.; O'Brien, J.; Lyons, G. Evaluation of a threshold-based tri-axial accelerometer fall detection algorithm. *Gait Posture* **2007**, *26*, 194–199. [CrossRef]
46. Kangas, M.; Konttila, A.; Lindgren, P.; Winblad, I.; Jämsä, T. Comparison of low-complexity fall detection algorithms for body attached accelerometers. *Gait Posture* **2008**, *28*, 285–291. [CrossRef]
47. Li, Q.; Stankovic, J.A.; Hanson, M.A.; Barth, A.T.; Lach, J.; Zhou, G. Accurate, Fast Fall Detection Using Gyroscopes and Accelerometer-Derived Posture Information. In Proceedings of the 2009 Sixth International Workshop on Wearable and Implantable Body Sensor Networks, Berkeley, CA, USA, 3–5 June 2009; pp. 138–143. [CrossRef]
48. Shan, S.; Yuan, T. A wearable pre-impact fall detector using feature selection and Support Vector Machine. In Proceedings of the IEEE 10th International Conference On Signal Processing Proceedings, Beijing, China, 24–28 October 2010; pp. 1686–1689. [CrossRef]

49. Yuwono, M.; Moulton, B.D.; Su, S.W.; Celler, B.G.; Nguyen, H.T. Unsupervised machine-learning method for improving the performance of ambulatory fall-detection systems. *Biomed. Eng. Online* **2012**, *11*, 9. [CrossRef]
50. Kerdegari, H.; Samsudin, K.; Ramli, A.R.; Mokaram, S. Evaluation of fall detection classification approaches. In Proceedings of the 2012 4th International Conference on Intelligent and Advanced Systems (ICIAS2012), Kuala Lumpur, Malaysia, 12–14 June 2012; pp. 131–136. [CrossRef]
51. Doukas, C.; Maglogiannis, I.; Tragas, P.; Liapis, D.; Yovanof, G. Patient Fall Detection using Support Vector Machines. In Proceedings of the IFIP International Conference on Artificial Intelligence Applications and Innovations, Athens, Greece, 19–21 September 2007; pp. 147–156. [CrossRef]
52. Cheng, J.; Chen, X.; Shen, M. A Framework for Daily Activity Monitoring and Fall Detection Based on Surface Electromyography and Accelerometer Signals. *IEEE J. Biomed. Health Inform.* **2013**, *17*, 38–45. [CrossRef] [PubMed]
53. Vallabh, P.; Malekian, R. Fall detection monitoring systems: A comprehensive review. *J. Ambient. Intell. Humaniz. Comput.* **2017**, *9*, 1809–1833. [CrossRef]
54. Patsadu, O.; Watanapa, B.; Dajpratham, P.; Nukoolkit, C. Nukoolkit, Fall Motion Detection with Fall Severity Level Estimation by Mining Kinect 3D Data Stream. *Int. Arab J. Inf. Technol.* **2018**, *15*, 378–388.
55. Bian, Z.-P.; Hou, J.; Chau, L.-P.; Magnenat-Thalmann, N. Fall Detection Based on Body Part Tracking Using a Depth Camera. *IEEE J. Biomed. Health Inform.* **2015**, *19*, 430–439. [CrossRef] [PubMed]
56. Xu, T.; Zhou, Y. Elders' fall detection based on biomechanical features using depth camera. *Int. J. Wavelets Multiresolut. Inf. Process.* **2018**, *16*, 1840005. [CrossRef]
57. Sehairi, K.; Chouireb, F.; Meunier, J. Elderly fall detection system based on multiple shape features and motion analysis. In Proceedings of the 2018 IEEE International Conference on Intelligent Systems and Computer Vision (ISCV), Fez, Morocco, 2–4 April 2018; pp. 1–8. [CrossRef]
58. Taghvaei, S.; Kosuge, K. Image-based fall detection and classification of a user with a walking support system. *Front. Mech. Eng.* **2017**, *13*, 427–441. [CrossRef]
59. Ali, S.F.; Khan, R.; Mahmood, A.; Hassan, M.T.; Jeon, A.M. Using Temporal Covariance of Motion and Geometric Features via Boosting for Human Fall Detection. *Sensors* **2018**, *18*, 1918. [CrossRef]
60. Melillo, P.; Castaldo, R.; Sannino, G.; Orrico, A.; de Pietro, G.; Pecchia, L. Wearable technology and ECG processing for fall risk assessment, prevention and detection. In Proceedings of the 2015 37th Annual International Conference of the IEEE Engineering in Medicine and Biology Society (EMBC), Milan, Italy, 25–29 August 2015; pp. 7740–7743. [CrossRef]
61. Preventing Serious Falls Among Older Adults: A Project Supported by PCORI and the National Institute on Aging of the National Institutes of Health—The STRIDE Study. 2019. Available online: https://www.pcori.org/research-results/2014/preventing-serious-falls-among-older-adults-project-supported-pcori-and (accessed on 27 July 2019).
62. HomeSAFE | Fall Prevention Center of Excellence, (n.d.). Available online: http://stopfalls.org/resources/homesafe/ (accessed on 27 July 2019).
63. Projects Sanctioned during 2015–2016, n.d. Available online: http://dst.gov.in/sites/default/files/2015-16.pdf (accessed on 27 July 2019).
64. Shany, T.; Redmond, S.; Narayanan, M.R.; Lovell, N. Sensors-Based Wearable Systems for Monitoring of Human Movement and Falls. *IEEE Sens. J.* **2011**, *12*, 658–670. [CrossRef]
65. Sun, R.; Sosnoff, J.J. Novel sensing technology in fall risk assessment in older adults: A systematic review. *BMC Geriatr.* **2018**, *18*, 1–10. [CrossRef] [PubMed]
66. Khanuja, K.; Joki, J.; Bachmann, G.; Cuccurullo, S. Gait and balance in the aging population: Fall prevention using innovation and technology. *Maturitas* **2018**, *110*, 51–56. [CrossRef] [PubMed]
67. Krooneman, J.M. Designing a Fall Detection System for Elderly. Bachelor's Thesis, University of Twente, Enschede, The Netherlands, 2018.
68. Leach, J.M.; Mellone, S.; Palumbo, P.; Bandinelli, S.; Chiari, L. Natural turn measures predict recurrent falls in community-dwelling older adults: A longitudinal cohort study. *Sci. Rep.* **2018**, *8*, 4316. [CrossRef] [PubMed]
69. Poe, S.S.; Dawson, P.B.; Cvach, M.; Burnett, M.; Kumble, S.; Lewis, M.; Thompson, C.B.; Hill, E.E. The Johns Hopkins Fall Risk Assessment Tool: A Study of Reliability and Validity. *J. Nurs. Care Qual.* **2018**, *33*, 10–19. [CrossRef] [PubMed]
70. Forbes, G.; Massie, S.; Craw, S. Fall prediction using behavioural modelling from sensor data in smart homes. *Artif. Intell. Rev.* **2019**, *53*, 1071–1091. [CrossRef]
71. Cortés-Martínez, A. Human-Smart Rollator Interaction for Gait Analysis and Fall Prevention Using Learning Methods and the i-Walker. Ph.D. Thesis, Polytechnic University of Catalonia, Barcelona, Spain, 2018.
72. Haescher, M.; Matthies, D.J.; Srinivasan, K.; Bieber, G. Mobile Assisted Living: Smartwatch-based fall risk assessment for elderly people. In Proceedings of the 5th International Workshop on Sensor-Based Activity Recognition and Interaction, Berlin, Germany, 20–21 September 2018. [CrossRef]
73. Abdelgawwad, A.; Paetzold, M. A Framework for Activity Monitoring and Fall Detection Based on the Characteristics of Indoor Channels. In Proceedings of the 2018 IEEE 87th Vehicular Technology Conference (VTC Spring), Porto, Portugal, 3–6 June 2018; pp. 1–7. [CrossRef]
74. Immonen, M.S.; Similä, H.; Lindholm, M.; Korpelainen, R.; Jämsä, T. Technologies for fall risk assessment and conceptual design in personal health record system. *Finn. J. eHealth eWelfare* **2019**, *11*, 53–67. [CrossRef]

75. Florence, C.S.; Bergen, G.; Atherly, A.; Burns, E.; Stevens, J.; Drake, C. Medical Costs of Fatal and Nonfatal Falls in Older Adults. *J. Am. Geriatr. Soc.* **2018**, *66*, 693–698. [CrossRef]
76. Hsieh, K.L.; Fanning, J.T.; A Rogers, W.; A Wood, T.; Sosnoff, J.J. A Fall Risk mHealth App for Older Adults: Development and Usability Study. *JMIR Aging* **2018**, *1*, e11569. [CrossRef]
77. Carpenter, C.R.; Cameron, A.; Ganz, D.A.; Liu, S. Older Adult Falls in Emergency Medicine—A Sentinel Event. *Clin. Geriatr. Med.* **2018**, *34*, 355–367. [CrossRef]
78. Commandeur, D.; Klimstra, M.; MacDonald, S.; Inouye, K.; Cox, M.; Chan, D.; Hundza, S. Difference scores between single-task and dual-task gait measures are better than clinical measures for detection of fall-risk in community-dwelling older adults. *Gait Posture* **2018**, *66*, 155–159. [CrossRef]
79. Rasche, P.; Mertens, A.; Brandl, C.; Liu, S.; Buecking, B.; Bliemel, C.; Horst, K.; Weber, C.D.; Lichte, P.; Knobe, M. Satisfying Product Features of a Fall Prevention Smartphone App and Potential Users' Willingness to Pay: Web-Based Survey Among Older Adults. *JMIR mHealth uHealth* **2018**, *6*, e75. [CrossRef] [PubMed]
80. Ando, B.; Baglio, S.; Lombardo, C.O.; Marletta, V.; Pergolizzi, E.A.; Pistorio, A. An event polarized paradigm for ADL detection in AAL context. *IEEE Trans. Instrum. Meas.* **2014**, *64*, 1079–1082. [CrossRef]
81. Saleh, M.; Jeannes, R.L.B. Elderly Fall Detection Using Wearable Sensors: A Low Cost Highly Accurate Algorithm. *IEEE Sens. J.* **2019**, *19*, 3156–3164. [CrossRef]
82. Pipanmaekaporn, L.; Wichinawakul, P.; Kamolsantiroj, S. Mining Acceleration Data for Smartphone-based Fall Detection. In Proceedings of the 2018 10th International Conference on Knowledge and Smart Technology (KST), Chiang Mai, Thailand, 31 January–3 February 2018; pp. 74–79. [CrossRef]
83. Poonsri, A.; Chiracharit, W. Improvement of fall detection using consecutive-frame voting. In Proceedings of the 2018 International Workshop on Advanced Image Technology (IWAIT), Chiang Mai, Thailand, 7–10 January 2018; pp. 1–4. [CrossRef]
84. Khel, M.A.B.; Ali, M. Technical Analysis of Fall Detection Techniques. In Proceedings of the 2019 2nd International Conference on Advancements in Computational Sciences (ICACS), Lahore, Pakistan, 18–20 February 2019. [CrossRef]
85. Hussain, F.; Ehatisham-Ul-Haq, M.; Azam, M.A.; Khalid, A. Elderly Assistance Using Wearable Sensors by Detecting Fall and Recognizing Fall Patterns. In Proceedings of the 2018 ACM International Joint Conference and 2018 International Symposium on Pervasive and Ubiquitous Computing and Wearable Computers, Singapore, 8–12 October 2018; pp. 770–777. [CrossRef]
86. Fang, Q.; Li, H.; Luo, X.; Ding, L.; Luo, H.; Li, C. Computer vision aided inspection on falling prevention measures for steeplejacks in an aerial environment. *Autom. Constr.* **2018**, *93*, 148–164. [CrossRef]
87. Hemmatpour, M.; Ferrero, R.; Gandino, F.; Montrucchio, B.; Rebaudengo, M. Nonlinear Predictive Threshold Model for Real-Time Abnormal Gait Detection. *J. Health Eng.* **2018**, *2018*, 1–9. [CrossRef] [PubMed]
88. Fortino, G.; Gravina, R. Fall-MobileGuard: A Smart Real-Time Fall Detection System. In Proceedings of the 10th EAI International Conference on Body Area Networks, Sydney, Australia, 28–30 September 2015. [CrossRef]
89. Sannino, G.; De Falco, I.; De Pietro, G. Detection of falling events through windowing and automatic extraction of sets of rules: Preliminary results. In Proceedings of the 2017 IEEE 14th International Conference on Networking, Sensing and Control (ICNSC), Falerna, Italy, 16–18 May 2017; pp. 661–666. [CrossRef]
90. Silva, J.; Oliveira, E.; Moreira, D.; Nunes, F.; Caic, M.; Madureira, J.; Pereira, E. Design and Evaluation of a Fall Prevention Multiplayer Game for Senior Care Centres. In Proceedings of the International Conference on Entertainment Computing, Poznan, Poland, 17–20 September 2018; pp. 103–114. [CrossRef]
91. Trkov, M.; Chen, K.; Yi, J.; Liu, T. Inertial Sensor-Based Slip Detection in Human Walking. *IEEE Trans. Autom. Sci. Eng.* **2019**, *16*, 1399–1411. [CrossRef]
92. Gu, Y.; Zhang, Y.; Huang, M.; Ren, F. Your WiFi Knows You Fall: A Channel Data-driven Device-free Fall Sensing System. In Proceedings of the 2018 5th IEEE International Conference on Cloud Computing and Intelligence Systems (CCIS), Nanjing, China, 23–25 November 2018; pp. 943–947. [CrossRef]
93. Tian, Y.; Lee, G.-H.; He, H.; Hsu, C.-Y.; Katabi, D. RF-Based Fall Monitoring Using Convolutional Neural Networks. *Proc. ACM Interact. Mob. Wearable Ubiquitous Technol.* **2018**, *2*, 1–24. [CrossRef]
94. Hu, L.S.; Wang, S.Z.; Chen, Y.Q.; Gao, C.L.; Hu, C.Y.; Jiang, X.L.; Chen, Z.Y.; Gao, X.Y. Fall detection algorithms based on wearable device: A review. *Zhejiang Daxue Xuebao J. Zhejiang Univ. Eng. Sci.* **2018**, *52*, 1717–1728. [CrossRef]
95. Mackey, D.C.; Lachance, C.C.; Wang, P.T.; Feldman, F.; Laing, A.C.; Leung, P.M.; Hu, X.J.; Robinovitch, S.N. The Flooring for Injury Prevention (FLIP) Study of compliant flooring for the prevention of fall-related injuries in long-term care: A randomized trial. *PLoS Med.* **2019**, *16*, e1002843. [CrossRef] [PubMed]
96. Borhani, A.; Patzold, M. A Non-Stationary Channel Model for the Development of Non-Wearable Radio Fall Detection Systems. *IEEE Trans. Wirel. Commun.* **2018**, *17*, 7718–7730. [CrossRef]
97. Quero, J.M.; Burns, M.; Razzaq, M.A.; Nugent, C.; Espinilla, M. Detection of Falls from Non-Invasive Thermal Vision Sensors Using Convolutional Neural Networks. *Proceedings* **2018**, *2*, 1236. [CrossRef]
98. Lotfi, A.; Albawendi, S.; Powell, H.; Appiah, K.; Langensiepen, C. Supporting Independent Living for Older Adults; Employing a Visual Based Fall Detection Through Analysing the Motion and Shape of the Human Body. *IEEE Access* **2018**, *6*, 70272–70282. [CrossRef]
99. Scheurer, S.; Koch, J.; Kucera, M.; Bryn, H.; Bärtschi, M.; Meerstetter, T.; Nef, T.; Urwyler, P. Optimization and Technical Validation of the AIDE-MOI Fall Detection Algorithm in a Real-Life Setting with Older Adults. *Sensors* **2019**, *19*, 1357. [CrossRef]

100. Ramezani, R.; Xiao, Y.; Naeim, A. Sensing-Fi: Wi-Fi CSI and accelerometer fusion system for fall detection. In Proceedings of the 2018 IEEE EMBS International Conference on Biomedical & Health Informatics (BHI), Las Vegas, NV, USA, 4–7 March 2018; pp. 402–405. [CrossRef]
101. Mostafa, S.A.; Mustapha, A.; Mohammed, M.A.; Ahmad, M.S.; Mahmoud, M.A. A fuzzy logic control in adjustable autonomy of a multi-agent system for an automated elderly movement monitoring application. *Int. J. Med Inform.* **2018**, *112*, 173–184. [CrossRef] [PubMed]
102. Intellectual Property India, (n.d.). Available online: https://ipindiaservices.gov.in/PublicSearch/PublicationSearch/Search (accessed on 23 July 2019).
103. Casilari, E.; Luque, R.; Morón, M.-J. Analysis of Android Device-Based Solutions for Fall Detection. *Sensors* **2015**, *15*, 17827–17894. [CrossRef] [PubMed]
104. Fall Detection System Market Will Reflect Significant Growth Prospects during 2019–2029—Zebvo, (n.d.). Available online: https://www.zebvo.com/2019/09/25/fall-detection-system-market-will-reflect-significant-growth-prospects-during-2019-2029/ (accessed on 23 December 2019).
105. Apple Watch, (n.d.). Available online: https://en.wikipedia.org/wiki/Apple_Watch (accessed on 26 July 2019).
106. Use Fall Detection with Apple Watch Series 4—Apple Support, (n.d.). Available online: https://support.apple.com/en-in/HT208944 (accessed on 26 July 2019).
107. Aziz, O.; Klenk, J.; Schwickert, L.; Chiari, L.; Becker, C.; Park, E.J.; Mori, G.; Robinovitch, S.N. Validation of accuracy of SVM-based fall detection system using real-world fall and non-fall datasets. *PLoS ONE* **2017**, *12*, e0180318. [CrossRef]
108. Sucerquia, A.; López, J.D.; Vargas-Bonilla, J.F. Real-life/real-time elderly fall detection with a triaxial accelerometer. *Sensors* **2018**, *18*, 1101. [CrossRef]
109. Habib, M.A.; Mohktar, M.S.; Kamaruzzaman, S.B.; Lim, K.S.; Pin, T.M.; Ibrahim, F. Smartphone-Based Solutions for Fall Detection and Prevention: Challenges and Open Issues. *Sensors* **2014**, *14*, 7181–7208. [CrossRef]
110. De Miguel, K.; Brunete, A.; Hernando, M.; Gambao, E. Home Camera-Based Fall Detection System for the Elderly. *Sensors* **2017**, *17*, 2864. [CrossRef]
111. Aguiar, B.; Rocha, T.; Silva, J.; Sousa, I. Accelerometer-based fall detection for smartphones. In Proceedings of the 2014 IEEE International Symposium on Medical Measurements and Applications (MeMeA), Lisbon, Portugal, 11–12 June 2014; pp. 1–6.
112. Li, Y.; Ho, K.C.; Popescu, M. A Microphone Array System for Automatic Fall Detection. *IEEE Trans. Biomed. Eng.* **2012**, *59*, 1291–1301. [CrossRef] [PubMed]
113. Google Scholar, (n.d.). Available online: https://scholar.google.co.in/scholar?hl=en&as_sdt=0,5&as_vis=1&q=%22Fall+prediction%22+OR+%22Fall+Detection%22+OR+%22Fall+prevention%22 (accessed on 23 July 2019).
114. Koshmak, G.A.; Linden, M.; Loutfi, A. Evaluation of the android-based fall detection system with physiological data monitoring. In Proceedings of the 2013 35th Annual International Conference of the IEEE Engineering in Medicine and Biology Society (EMBC), Osaka, Japan, 3–7 July 2013; pp. 1164–1168.
115. Wang, H.; Zhang, D.; Wang, Y.; Ma, J.; Wang, Y.; Li, S. RT-Fall: A Real-Time and Contactless Fall Detection System with Commodity WiFi Devices. *IEEE Trans. Mob. Comput.* **2016**, *16*, 511–526. [CrossRef]
116. Nizam, Y.; Mohd, M.N.H.; Jamil, M.M.A. Human Fall Detection from Depth Images using Position and Velocity of Subject. *Procedia Comput. Sci.* **2017**, *105*, 131–137. [CrossRef]
117. Santos, G.L.; Endo, P.T.; De Monteiro, K.H.C.; Da Rocha, E.S.; Silva, I.; Lynn, T. Accelerometer-Based Human Fall Detection Using Convolutional Neural Networks. *Sensors* **2019**, *19*, 1644. [CrossRef] [PubMed]
118. Huynh, Q.T.; Nguyen, U.D.; Irazabal, L.B.; Ghassemian, N.; Tran, B.Q. Optimization of an Accelerometer and Gyroscope-Based Fall Detection Algorithm. *J. Sens.* **2015**, *2015*, 452078. [CrossRef]
119. Xi, X.; Tang, M.; Miran, S.M.; Luo, Z. Evaluation of Feature Extraction and Recognition for Activity Monitoring and Fall Detection Based on Wearable sEMG Sensors. *Sensors* **2017**, *17*, 1229. [CrossRef]
120. Chen, W.-H.; Ma, H.-P. A fall detection system based on infrared array sensors with tracking capability for the elderly at home. In Proceedings of the 2015 17th International Conference on E-health Networking, Application & Services (HealthCom), Boston, MA, USA, 14–17 October 2015; pp. 428–434. [CrossRef]
121. Hashim, H.A.; Mohammed, S.L.; Gharghan, S.K. Accurate fall detection for patients with Parkinson's disease based on a data event algorithm and wireless sensor nodes. *Measurement* **2020**, *156*, 107573. [CrossRef]
122. Ma, L.; Liu, M.; Wang, N.; Wang, L.; Yang, Y.; Wang, H. Room-Level Fall Detection Based on Ultra-Wideband (UWB) Monostatic Radar and Convolutional Long Short-Term Memory (LSTM). *Sensors* **2020**, *20*, 1105. [CrossRef] [PubMed]
123. Nooruddin, S.; Islam, M.; Sharna, F.A. An IoT based device-type invariant fall detection system. *Internet Things* **2019**, *9*, 100130. [CrossRef]
124. WIISEL, (n.d.). Available online: http://www.wiisel.eu/ (accessed on 27 July 2019).
125. No, C.S. Chandrasekhar Rao, List of Projects Sanctioned during 2007–2008 under STAWS Scheme Including New Initiatives, n.d. Available online: http://dst.gov.in/sites/default/files/staws-07-08.pdf (accessed on 27 July 2019).

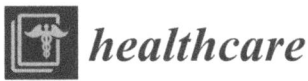

Commentary

Digital Contact Tracing and COVID-19: Design, Deployment, and Current Use in Italy

Noemi Scrivano [1], Rosario Alfio Gulino [1] and Daniele Giansanti [2,*]

[1] Facoltà di Ingegneria, Università di Tor Vergata, 00133 Roma, Italy; noemi-scrivano@hotmail.com (N.S.); rosario.gulino.uni.tv@hotmail.com (R.A.G.)
[2] Centro Tisp, Istituto Superiore di Sanità, 00161 Roma, Italy
* Correspondence: daniele.giansanti@iss.it; Tel.: +39-06-49902701

Abstract: The technological innovation of digital contact tracing (DCT) has certainly characterized the COVID-19 pandemic, as compared to the previous ones. Based on the first studies, considerable support was expected from smartphone applications ("apps") for DCT. This commentary focuses on digital contact tracing. Its contributions are threefold: (a) Recall the initial expectations of these technologies and the state of diffusion. (b) Deal with the introduction of the app "Immuni" in Italy, while also highlighting the initiatives undertaken at the government level. (c) Report the state of diffusion and use of this App. The commentary ends by proposing some reflections on the continuation of this investigation in Italy.

Keywords: eHealth; medical devices; digital health; mHealth; cyber-risk; contact tracing; digital health; app; pandemic; COVID-19

Citation: Scrivano, N.; Gulino, R.A.; Giansanti, D. Digital Contact Tracing and COVID-19: Design, Deployment, and Current Use in Italy. *Healthcare* 2022, 10, 67. https://doi.org/10.3390/healthcare10010067

Academic Editor: Norbert Hosten

Received: 21 October 2021
Accepted: 28 December 2021
Published: 30 December 2021

Publisher's Note: MDPI stays neutral with regard to jurisdictional claims in published maps and institutional affiliations.

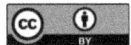

Copyright: © 2021 by the authors. Licensee MDPI, Basel, Switzerland. This article is an open access article distributed under the terms and conditions of the Creative Commons Attribution (CC BY) license (https://creativecommons.org/licenses/by/4.0/).

1. Introduction

In the *health domain*, contact tracing (CT) is defined by the World Health Organization [1] to be composed of three activities:

(a) Contact identification,
(b) Contact listing, and
(c) Contact follow-up.

In this pandemic, unlike the previous ones, we have been able to rely on strong technological innovation in mobile technology as we know it today, which is based on smartphones (available in their current configuration starting from 2007 [2]). Immediately at the beginning of the pandemic, the potential of mobile technology as a strategic support tool for controlling the spread of the pandemic, emerged through modeling studies. Ferretti et al. [3] demonstrated that the use of digital contact tracing (DCT) [3] could control the diffusion of the COVID-19 (transforming the three components of the CT into the three components of the DCT). Indeed, in some cases, DCT seems irreplaceable. Just think of super diffusion events, or when it is impossible for a person to remember all the recent contacts.

Subsequently, DCT has been considered as a powerful and strategic tool capable of transforming the traditional CT with a practical, effective, speedy, and reliable digital approach. Solutions with a different technological approach have been developed quickly in the first few months of the pandemic. Apps were deployed using GPS or Bluetooth (with different technological variants) for DCT, with different approaches to privacy [4]. DCT also used other solutions, such as in China [5]. A national app was not developed here. WeChat and Alipay were used in China to convey a security code (*Healthcode*) for DCT. In the following months, the use of DCT has spread, and, to date, there is consolidated scientific literature on this experience of using technology in the *health domain*.

The purpose of the commentary is: (*a*) to recall the state of diffusion of DCT to date. (*b*) To highlight the initiatives undertaken at the government level for the *running in* of the Italian DCT based on the App, "Immuni". (*c*) To report the state of diffusion and use. The remainder of this commentary is arranged in three sections, followed by concluding perspectives.

Section 2 (The digital contact tracing: the state of diffusion of the technology) takes stock of the diffusion of technology in the health domain. Section 3 (The Italian national app, "Immuni", for digital contact tracing: the running-in and the initiatives supporting the diffusion) deals with the introduction of the App, "Immuni", and the government initiatives undertaken in Italy. Section 4 (State of diffusion and use of the app, "Immuni") reports and discusses the state of diffusion and use of DCT in Italy.

2. The Digital Contact Tracing: Design, Deployment, and Current Use

A search on Pubmed (as of 5 October 2021) with the key *((Contact tracing [Title/Abstract]) AND (App))* returned 176 results, of which 172 (97.73%) were published between 2020–2021. Before the pandemic DCT had been used in the field of tuberculosis [6] and hepatitis [7]. Among these articles, 21 are reviews or overviews, as they were found by the search terms *((Contact tracing [Title/Abstract]) AND (App)) AND (review)*, 20 of which were released from the last two years. A total of 13 reviews and overviews are very recent, as they appeared in 2021. They deal with heterogeneous aspects of DCT development. They concern *census, privacy, functionality, integrations with other systems, integration acceptance, quality, effectiveness, and other issues.*

To date, more than 78 countries have developed COVID-19 DCT apps to limit the spread of the coronavirus [8]. An analysis of the literature shows that Bluetooth is one of the major technologies used in DCT [9]. Europe, for example, proposed at least two digital contact tracing application models, one described based on privacy-preserving proximity tracing [10] with calculations on the mobile phone, and the other based on pan-European privacy-preserving proximity tracing [11], with calculations on a central server. The approach relating to the collection of information (to be entered into the system) was different between the different apps. For example, The Norwegian, Singaporean, Georgian, and New Zealand apps were among those that collected the most personal information from users, whereas some apps, such as the Swiss app and the Italian ("Immuni") app, did not collect any user information [9].

The study proposed in [12] reviewed the functionalities and effectiveness of the free mobile health applications available in the Google Play and App stores in some nations during the COVID-19 outbreak [12]. The analysis revealed that various applications have been developed for different functions, such as contact tracing, awareness building, appointment booking, online consultation, etc. However, the study highlighted that only a few applications have integrated various functions and features (e.g., self-assessment, consultation, support, and access to information). No apps were identified that had built-in social media features. Very few apps were dedicated to raising awareness and sharing information about the COVID-19 pandemic. The study [12] suggested developing integrated mobile health applications with most of the features, including DCT. The study reported in [13] considered the quality of the apps for DCT. It used the mobile app rating scale to assess the app quality. It highlighted that European national health authorities have generally released high quality COVID-19 contact tracing apps, about functionality, aesthetics, and information quality. However, the study reported that the engagement-oriented design generally was of lower quality. A lot of both *technological and medical knowledge* has been collected. There are now studies, such as [14], which derive and summarize best practices for the design of the ideal digital contact tracing apps.

3. The Italian National App, "Immuni", for Digital Contact Tracing: The *Running-In* and the Initiatives Supporting the Diffusion

Italy released its own national app called *"Immuni"*. The use (download and data entry) is on a voluntary basis [15].

Italian politicians have opted for a centralized and non-regionalized approach for the use of an app for DCT. A government app was therefore developed after an appropriate public selection of various proposals [16]. Updated information and project data, with a high-level description, are available in [15,17]. In brief, this app uses Bluetooth low energy technology to distinguish proximity events between citizens using a smartphone with the app installed.

The introduction of the app, "Immuni", was accompanied by dissemination initiatives for all the actors involved: *health domain workers, contact tracing operators*, and the *population*.

Public dissemination documents have been provided at the national level for *health domain workers* (including stakeholders).

The Istituto Superiore di Sanità, the Italian National Institute of Health, has proposed (and continues to propose) guidelines during the pandemic, on various issues related to the epidemic. These guidelines are called *Istituto Superiore di Sanità Covid Report* and they are all available in the Italian language [18]. Many of these reports are also available in the English language [19].

During the *start-up* period of the *Italian Digital Contact Tracing*, three reports [20–22], dedicated or strongly correlated to DCT were proposed. The last had two versions: the first one was in May 2020, and the last one in October 2020. These three reports [20–22] dealt with three aspects of the *health domain* that are closely related to DCT: the traditional CT [20], DCT [22], and the impact of ethics in DCT [21]. This is to inform, update, and raise awareness among workers in the *health domain*.

The *first report* [20] highlighted how contact tracing is a key component of COVID-19 prevention and control strategies. Furthermore, the report explained the aim of contact tracing to rapidly identify secondary cases and prevent further transmission of infection, and described the key phases of contact tracing in Italy.

The *second report* [21] highlighted that DCT raises multiple relevant ethical issues involving various areas: organization of health services, public health, clinical medicine, social medicine, epidemiology, technology, law, and many other areas. Furthermore, it reported some crucial elements from an ethical point of view, which included the evaluation of effectiveness, the separation of personal data from public health data, transparency, information, and the solidarity dimension (for example, helping the less capable with technologies) that must characterize any public health action.

The *third report* [22] had three perspectives. The first one introduced contact tracing, starting from the definition of the World Health Organization and independently from the digital techniques. The second point of view highlighted the innovations of mobile technology, based on smartphones connected to DCT. The third point of view dealt with the diffusion and evolution of these apps through an analysis of state-of-the-art technology.

The Istituto Superiore di Sanità coordinated online courses at a national level and proposed them to the contact-tracing operators [23]. Specific training was also provided on the app, "Immuni". The remote training methods allowed both the enlargement of the prospective number of the trained subjects and maintained social distancing. *The general population also* received information on the app, "Immuni" through the mass media (the internet, radio, newspapers, and public posters).

4. Deployment and Current Use of the App, "Immuni"

The section analyzes the deployment and use of the app, also taking into consideration parameters relating to the digital divide, the estimates of truly positive subjects based on seroprevalence, and economic indicators. Table 1 reports the description of the topic considered, the source referring to it, and the relative indexed scientific references (web, report, and study) accessed at the date of writing the piece (5 October 2021). The acronyms used are also shown in the list of acronyms before the references. References are available in [24–26] (Table 1) and provide the numerical data related to: (a) the daily numerical downloads; (b) the daily number of *diagnosed positives* to the virus, who accepted data storage; and (c) the number of notifications. Based on this data, we observe that *16,167,210* downloads were carried out; *25,720* positive users registered voluntarily; and *111,791* notifications were sent. The manufacturer says that the detection is partial, as all notifications for iOS devices are detected and only a third of those sent by Android have the necessary technology available to safely detect them.

Table 1. Summary table with the description of the data considered, the direct or indirect source, and the references (* accessed at the date of writing, 5 October 2021).

Description	Sources (Direct or Indirect)	Reference and Year
Statistics on people owning smartphones in Italy.	CENSIS (Italian national body designated for social research) reports	N. 31 (2019), N. 32 (2021)
Statistics on the use of the app "Immuni" (downloading, uploading of diagnosed positive subjects, etc.)	GitHub and app "Immuni" Webs	N. 15–17, N. 24–26, N. 33–34 (*)
Statistics on *gross domestic product* per capita (GDP)	Eurostat (European body designed for European statistics) reports	N. 35–36 (Updated 3 march 2021)
Statistics on Italian population	ISTAT (Italian national body designated for social research) reports	N. 27 (*)
Serological investigation on COVID-19 In Italy	ISTAT (Italian national body designated for social research) reports	N. 28–29 (2021)
Statistics on COVID-19 in Italy	Data from Italian Ministry of health	N. 28 (*)

It is interesting to compare these data with the national population. The Italian population amounts to *59,257,566* [27] (Table 1); therefore, a fraction of *16,167,210/59,257,566 = 0.2728* of the Italian population downloaded the app (*27.28%*). The number of *diagnosed positive subjects* (*DPS*) since the start of the pandemic is *4,683,646* [28] (Table 1). The number of DPS is much lower [29,30] than the number of *really positive subjects* (RPS). The ability to diagnose positive subjects depends on many factors, ranging from medical knowledge and up to citizen participation and diagnostic power. It changes from nation to nation. In Italy, a national survey was conducted [30] to estimate the RPS. From 25 May to 15 July 2020, the seroprevalence investigation on SARS-CoV-2 was carried out in accordance with the provisions of the law decree 10 May 2020 n. 30 "Urgent measures in the field of epidemiological and statistical studies on SARS-CoV-2", converted into law on 2 July 2020.

The latest updated data from the national survey conducted by the Italian Ministry of Health [29,30] (Table 1) estimated that the number of *RPS* is up to six times greater that *DPS*:

$$RPS = 6 \times DPS \tag{1}$$

Given that new and updated epidemiological investigations could lead to corrections of this value, we can parametrize this relationship.

$$RPS = K \times DPS \tag{2}$$

Considering that the study was conducted at the beginning of the pandemic, when diagnostic capabilities and resources were still limited, we can consider the value of *K* = 6 as the maximum value. We need also to consider the impact of the *Digital Divide* on the percentage of population, reported above 27.28%, who downloaded the app. We must count the individuals who do not own a smartphone and consider them. In Italy, according to the data of the national census, conducted shortly before the pandemic, 73.8% [31] (Table 1) of the population had a smartphone. In this case, the ratio between the app downloads and the population that own smartphones is 0.37. According to the data of the latest national census (available on 6 October 2021), this value had increased to 83.3% [32] (Table 1). In this second case, the ratio between the app downloads and the population that own smartphones is 0.33.

Figure 1 shows the ratio between the *diagnosed positive subjects uploaded* (DPSU) in the DCT system and the RPS for different values of K in three cases: (a) without considering the impact of the digital divide (not considered, R1). (b) Considering the two different estimates of the digital divide at 73.8% (R2) and 83.3% (R3). The best estimate considering the digital divide indicates a value never higher than 7.5 ‰, while the best estimate without considering the digital divide indicates a value never higher than 5.0 ‰.

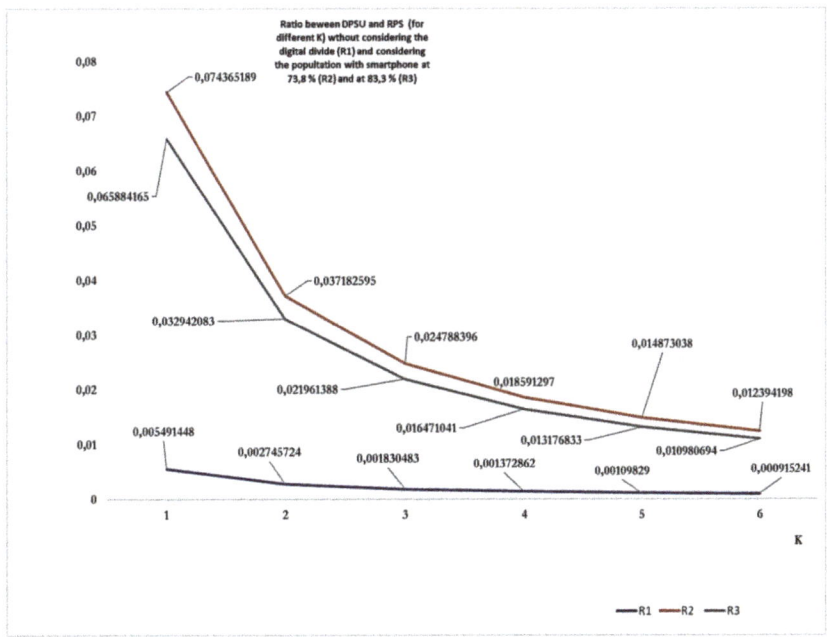

Figure 1. Ratio between the DPSU in the DCT system and the RPS (for different values of K): without the different impact of the digital divide (not considered, R1); considering the two different estimates of the digital divide at 73.8% (R2) and 83.3% (R3).

We can also identify the percent of downloads (%D) for each region [33,34] (Table 1). Table 2 shows these values for people with an age over 14 years. The region with the highest %D was Emilia Romagna, with 22.3%. The region with the lowest %D was Calabria, with 12.2%. An interesting result emerges if we consider the data relating to %D at a regional level compared to the *gross domestic product per capita (GDP)* [35,36] (Figure 2). Table 2 shows that: (a) the Italian regions with the largest GDP ($\geq$80) all have a %D > 15%. (b) Regions with a lower GDP (<65) performed a %D <15%. (c) The regions with an intermediate GDP (65 $\leq$ GDP < 80 demonstrated a different behavior (Molise demonstrated %D <15%, Sardegna and Basilicata demonstrated %D > 15%).

Table 2. Tabular representation of percent of downloads for each region and GDP.

Region	Percent of Downloads for Each Region	GDP
Abruzzo	21.5	GDP ≥ 80
Basilicata	16.9	65 ≤ GDP < 80
Calabria	12.2	GDP < 65
Campania	13.3	GDP < 65
Emilia-Romagna	22.3	GDP ≥ 80
Friuli Venezia Giulia	15.8	GDP ≥ 80
Lazio	21.7	GDP ≥ 80
Liguria	18.3	GDP ≥ 80
Lombardia	20.1	GDP ≥ 80
Marche	19.2	GDP ≥ 80
Molise	14.9	65 ≤ GDP < 80
Piemonte	17.5	GDP ≥ 80
Puglia	14.6	GDP < 65
Sardegna	19.8	6 ≤ GDP < 80
Sicilia	12.5	GDP < 65
Toscana	21.8	GDP ≥ 80
Provincia autonoma di Trento	19.4	GDP ≥ 80
Provincia autonoma di Bolzano	16.7	GDP ≥ 80
Umbria	20.7	GDP ≥ 80
Valle d'Aosta	20.0	GDP ≥ 80
Veneto	16.4	GDP ≥ 80

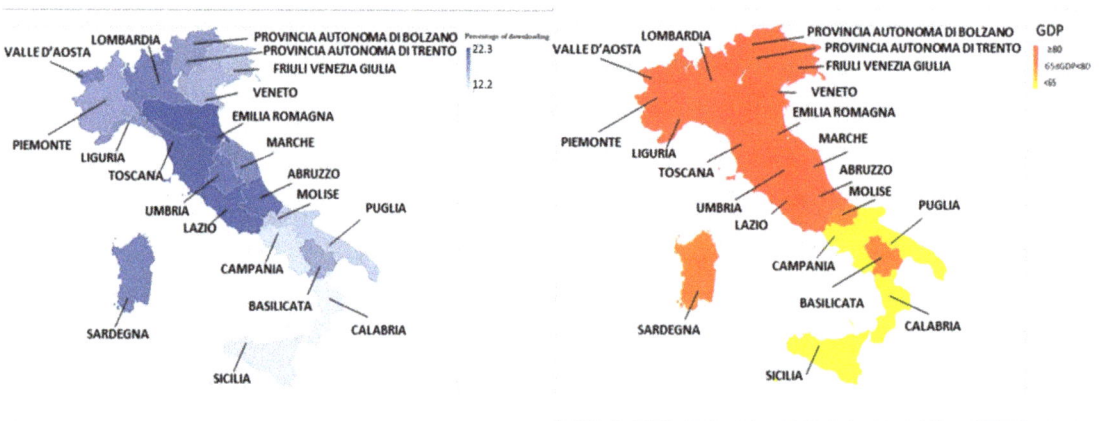

Figure 2. Graphic representation of percent of downloads for each region and GDP.

5. Discussion and Conclusions

5.1. Our Contributions

The technological innovation of DCT has certainly characterized this pandemic compared to the previous ones. Considerable support was expected from the apps for DCT, based on the first studies [3]. Now, many months after the start of the use of this technology, scholars are wondering [37] what has been the real contribution of these apps to contact tracing and the fight against the pandemic. In our contribution, we first recalled the evolution of the technology, the development and diffusion that these apps have had worldwide, accompanied by a conspicuous and noteworthy increase in scientific output. Then we focused on the Italian DCT and retraced the introduction of the "Immuni" app. We highlighted that the introduction of this app was accompanied by awareness-raising initiatives for *health domain workers* and *contact-tracing operators* [20–23]. We have finally taken stock of the current deployment and uptake in Italy, noting underlying factors.

5.2. The Limits in the Deployment and the Current Use of DCT in Italy

Despite the initiatives undertaken, the deployment and the current use in Italy have shown limits. Only about a quarter of the population downloaded the app. A very low number of DPS (a fraction of the RPS, which was estimated to be even six times higher) uploaded their data. This number is around 7.5 ‰, if we consider the digital divide, and around 5.0 ‰ if we do not consider the digital divide. Among the factors that contributed to a higher/lower downloading, although not by much, we identified the digital divide and, at the regional level, the GDP, which accounts for several sub-factors (e.g., social factors, infrastructure, technology, education, and health).

5.3. The Impact of the Digital Divide

A notable part of the population certainly could not take advantage of these technologies due to the digital divide. The digital divide is a very key aspect and depends on two very important parameters: *literacy* [38] and access to *infrastructures* [39]. This value, with reference to the access to mobile technology in the period immediately preceding the pandemic, was equal to 26.2% [31] and then decreased to 16.7% [32]. We do not have information regarding the intention of this lost population group to join DCT. However, assuming a uniformity of behavior within the population, the contribution of this group would not have changed the conclusions.

Information on the social demographic influence on the digital divide is not directly available due to privacy. However, previous studies based on questionnaires reveal that some categories (e.g., elderly) were not familiar with the Italian DCT [40]. In Italy, important initiatives to minimize the digital divide were undertaken in this period, both in terms of *literacy* and *infrastructure*. National cashback programs on reimbursement with debit and credit cards, managed by an app, motivated the approach and familiarization with mobile technology [41]. The possibility of providing shopping vouchers [42] to individuals from low socio-economic groups, dedicated to the purchase of mobile devices and the internet, is an initiative that has improved access to *infrastructures*.

All of these initiatives have contributed to bridging the digital divide, thereby increasing the number of citizens with smartphones from 73.8% to 83.3%. However, as we have seen, this has not consistently improved the use of DCT.

5.4. Factors Influencing Adoption of the App Based on the Literature

The evidence that we report in the analysis is consistent with what is emerging in the recent reviews available from scientific literature. Our study has begun to highlight some factors that have influenced the distribution of the app. The scientific literature has highlighted how, in general, there are more *design factors*, connected to the technological choice, and more *transversal factors* concerning acceptability and desirability (Table 3 provides a summary). Of course, these factors are also interconnected (e.g., desirability is linked to design factors). As far as the *design factors* are concerned, we highlight how the

"Immuni" app is an app based on *proximity tracing* with *a high level of privacy*, dedicated almost exclusively to DCT.

Table 3. Articles on DCT recalled with a brief description of their focus.

Ref	Cited Article	Brief Description of the Focus
[8]	Garousi V, Cutting D, Felderer M. Mining user reviews of COVID contact-tracing apps: An exploratory analysis of nine European apps. J Syst Softw. 2021	Authors went to the field to review the referees relating to these apps to understand what the users were not satisfied with.
[9]	Elkhodr M, Mubin O, Iftikhar Z, Masood M, Alsinglawi B, Shahid S, Alnajjar F. Technology, Privacy, and User Opin-ions of COVID-19 Mobile Apps for Contact Tracing: Systematic Search and Content Analysis. J Med Internet Res. 2021 Feb 9;23(2):e23467. doi: 10.2196/23467. PMID: 33493125; PMCID: PMC7879719 Nov 4:111136. doi: 10.1016/j.jss.2021.111136. Epub ahead of print. PMID:34751198; PMCID: PMC8566091	Reviewed different apps for DCT, highlighted that *the app, "Immuni", is one of the apps with the greatest respect for privacy, with a very low amount of data collected*.
[12]	Alanzi T. A Review of Mobile Applications Available in the App and Google Play Stores Used During the COVID-19 Outbreak. J Multidiscip Healthc. 2021 Jan 12;14:45–57. doi: 10.2147/JMDH.S285014. PMID: 33469298; PMCID: PMC7812813	Highlighted that a large integration of functionalities are lacking in the apps developed for the COVID-19.
[13]	Kahnbach L, Lehr D, Brandenburger J, Mallwitz T, Jent S, Hannibal S, Funk B, Janneck M. Quality and Adoption of COVID-19 Tracing Apps and Recommendations for Development: Systematic Interdisciplinary Review of European Apps. J Med Internet Res. 2021 Jun 2;23(6):e27989. doi: 10.2196/27989. PMID: 33890867; PMCID: PMC8174558	The study faced the quality in the apps for DCT. It used the mobile app rating scale to assess the app quality.
[14]	O'Connell J, Abbas M, Beecham S, Buckley J, Chochlov M, Fitzgerald B, Glynn L, Johnson K, Laffey J, McNicholas B, Nuseibeh B, O'Callaghan M, O'Keeffe I, Razzaq A, Rekanar K, Richardson I, Simpkin A, Storni C, Tsvyatkova D, Walsh J, Welsh T, O'Keeffe D. Best Practice Guidance for Digital Contact Tracing Apps: A Cross-disciplinary Review of the Literature. JMIR Mhealth Uhealth. 2021 Jun 7;9(6):e27753. doi: 10.2196/27753. PMID: 34003764; PMCID: PMC8189288	Authors reviewed the desiderable requirements that a DCT app must have to be successful and have made them explicit.
[37]	Maccari L, Cagno V. Do we need a contact tracing app? Comput Commun. 2021 Jan 15;166:9–18. doi: 10.1016/j.comcom.2020.11.007. Epub 2020 Nov 19. PMID:33235399; PMCID: PMC7676320	It has been underlined that the proximity detection using BLTE gave a low contribute to the detection of cases.
[43]	.Kolasa K, Mazzi F, Leszczuk-Czubkowska E, Zrubka Z, Péntek M. State of the Art in Adoption of Contact Tracing Apps and Recommendations Regarding Privacy Protection and Public Health: Systematic Review. JMIR Mhealth Uhealth. 2021 Jun 10;9(6):e23250. doi: 10.2196/23250. PMID: 34033581; PMCID: PMC8195202	Showed that apps with high levels of compliance with standards of data privacy (and "Immuni" is one of them) tend to fulfill public health interests to a limited extent and DCT with a lower level of data privacy protection allow for the collection of more data.
[44]	Oyibo K, Sahu KS, Oetomo A, Morita PP. Factors Influencing the Adoption of Contact Tracing Applications: Protocol for a Systematic Review. JMIR Res Protoc. 2021 Jun 1;10(6):e28961. doi: 10.2196/28961. PMID: 33974551; PMCID: PMC8171387	The study proposed protocols for the correct identification of the factors influencing DCT.
[45]	Anglemyer A, Moore TH, Parker L, Chambers T, Grady A, Chiu K, Parry M, Wilczynska M, Flemyng E, Bero L. Digital contact tracing technologies in epidemics: a rapid review. Cochrane Database Syst Rev. 2020 Aug 18;8(8):CD013699. doi: 10.1002/14651858.CD013699. PMID: 33502000; PMCID:PMC8241885	The study on the Cochrane database system review traced both the reflections and the future directions and efforts in DCT. The outcome from randomized controlled trials (RCTs), cluster-RCTs, quasi-RCTs, cohort studies, cross-sectional studies, and modeling studies in general populations was considered.

The scientific literature on these specific points connected to the *design factors* has produced clear evidence of:

- *The limits of the proximity tracing*

    In general, we note [37] the limit of *proximity technologies*, using Bluetooth, in discovering cases of COVID-19. It has been underlined in [37] that the proximity detection using low energy Bluetooth was a small contribution to the detection of cases of COVID-19.

- *High levels of compliance with standards of data privacy are limiting*

    Some studies have shown that the app, "Immuni", is one of the apps with the greatest respect for privacy, with a very low amount of data collected [9]. Some studies confirm that apps with high levels of compliance with standards of data privacy (and "Immuni" is one of them) tend to fulfill public health interests to a limited extent and DCT with a lower level of data privacy protection allow for the collection of more data [43].

- *High level of integration of functions could improve the use*

We have seen how the integrations of greater functionality with DCT (including connection functions with social media) have been lacking in the apps developed for COVID-19 [12]. An expansion of the offer of functions could probably improve the use of the "Immuni" app. It should be noted that the app, "Immuni", is already moving in this direction, allowing, for example, one to download the vaccination certificate.

There are many transversal factors that still need to be explored. It is important to focus on protocols for the clear identification of these factors. Furthermore, it is also important both to investigate the desirable requirements that an app for DCT must have and design bottom-up mechanisms to understand the failure factors. We have rephrased. In addition, on these aspects, the scientific literature is supporting us and could be extended to the Italian DCT experience:

- Some works are moving towards the definition of protocols for the correct identification of the factors [44].
- Some authors have focused on the desirable requirements that a DCT app must have to be successful and have made them explicit [14].
- Other authors went to the field to review the reports on the app stores relating to these apps [8] to understand what the users were not satisfied with.

5.5. Final Reflections and Further Work

A recent study available on the Cochrane database [45] traced both the reflections and the future directions and efforts in DCT. We strongly share this position based on the outcome from randomized controlled trials, cluster-randomized controlled trials, quasi-randomized controlled trials, cohort studies, cross-sectional studies, and modeling studies in general populations (all very important sources for evidence-based medicine).

The key takeaways from this review are as follows:

- There is very low-certainty evidence that DCT may produce more reliable counts of contacts and reduce time to complete contact tracing.
- Stronger primary research on the effectiveness of contact tracing technologies is needed.
- Future studies should better consider the access, acceptability, and equity.
- Studies should focus on the relationships between acceptability of DCT and the impact of the privacy that can hamper the diffusion of this technology.

We believe that a field survey could help us a lot to face the above-listed key takeaways and to focus on all the emerging issues to understand which factors have influence, what are the design suggestions of the population, and what is lacking in acceptability. Certainly, electronic questionnaires, designed for the population, could be useful [40], as they have already been used in the USA for many issues related to the pandemic [46]. Our idea is, because they have already been used, to continue this path by proposing a dedicated national questionnaire, also based on a *community engaged approach*, involving all the actors (*health domain workers, contact tracing operators*, and the general population) that for the apps, such as "Immuni", could give useful feedbacks for the improvement of their use [47].

Author Contributions: Conceptualization, D.G.; methodology, D.G.; software, all; validation, D.G. and R.A.G.; formal analysis, N.S. and R.A.G.; investigation, all; resources, D.G.; data curation, D.G.; writing—original draft preparation, D.G.; writing—review and editing, N.S. and R.A.G.; supervision, D.G.; project administration, D.G. All authors have read and agreed to the published version of the manuscript.

Funding: This research received no external funding.

Institutional Review Board Statement: Not applicable.

Informed Consent Statement: Not applicable.

Data Availability Statement: Data sharing not applicable.

Conflicts of Interest: The authors declare no conflict of interest.

Abbreviations

CT	Contact tracing
DCT	Digital contact tracing
RPS	Really positive subjects
DPS	Diagnosed positive subjects
DPSU	Diagnosed positive subjects uploaded
%D	Percent of downloads
GDP	Gross domestic product per capita

References

1. WHO. Contact Tracing during an Outbreak of Ebola Virus Disease. Available online: https://www.who.int/csr/resources/publications/ebola/contact-tracing-during-outbreak-of-ebola.pdf (accessed on 30 December 2021).
2. The Brief History of Smartphones. Available online: https://www.thoughtco.com/history-of-smartphones-4096585 (accessed on 15 December 2021).
3. Ferretti, L.; Wymant, C.; Kendall, M.; Zhao, L.; Nurtay, A.; Abeler-Dörner, L.; Parker, M.; Bonsall, D.G.; Fraser, C. Quantifying SARS-CoV-2 transmission suggests epidemic control with digital contact tracing. *Science* **2020**, *368*, eabb6936. [CrossRef] [PubMed]
4. Liang, F. COVID-19 and Health Code: How Digital Platforms Tackle the Pandemic in China. *Soc. Media + Soc.* **2020**, *6*, 2056305120947657. [CrossRef] [PubMed]
5. Kleinman, R.A.; Merkel, C. Digital contact tracing for COVID-19. *CMAJ* **2020**, *192*, E653–E656. [CrossRef] [PubMed]
6. Iribarren, S.J.; Schnall, R.; Stone, P.W.; Carballo-Diéguez, A. Smartphone Applications to Support Tuberculosis Prevention and Treatment: Review and Evaluation. *JMIR Mhealth Uhealth* **2016**, *4*, e25. [CrossRef] [PubMed]
7. Ruscher, C.; Werber, D.; Thoulass, J.; Zimmermann, R.; Eckardt, M.; Winter, C.; Sagebiel, D. Dating apps and websites as tools to reach anonymous sexual contacts during an outbreak of hepatitis A among men who have sex with men, Berlin, 2017. *Eurosurveillance* **2019**, *24*, 1800460. [CrossRef] [PubMed]
8. Garousi, V.; Cutting, D.; Felderer, M. Mining user reviews of COVID contact-tracing apps: An exploratory analysis of nine European apps. *J. Syst. Softw.* **2021**, *184*, 111136. [CrossRef] [PubMed]
9. Elkhodr, M.; Mubin, O.; Iftikhar, Z.; Masood, M.; Alsinglawi, B.; Shahid, S.; Alnajjar, F. Technology, Privacy, and User Opinions of COVID-19 Mobile Apps for Contact Tracing: Systematic Search and Content Analysis. *J. Med. Internet Res.* **2021**, *23*, e23467. [CrossRef] [PubMed]
10. Dp-3/Documents. Available online: https://github.com/DP-3T/documents (accessed on 15 December 2021).
11. Pan European Privacy-Preserving Proximity Tracing. Available online: https://github.com/pepp-pt (accessed on 15 December 2021).
12. Alanzi, T. A Review of Mobile Applications Available in the App and Google Play Stores Used During the COVID-19 Outbreak. *J. Multidiscip. Healthc.* **2021**, *14*, 45–57. [CrossRef] [PubMed]
13. Kahnbach, L.; Lehr, D.; Brandenburger, J.; Mallwitz, T.; Jent, S.; Hannibal, S.; Funk, B.; Janneck, M. Quality and Adoption of COVID-19 Tracing Apps and Recommendations for Development: Systematic Interdisciplinary Review of European Apps. *J. Med. Internet Res.* **2021**, *23*, e27989. [CrossRef] [PubMed]
14. O'Connell, J.; Abbas, M.; Beecham, S.; Buckley, J.; Chochlov, M.; Fitzgerald, B.; Glynn, L.; Johnson, K.; Laffey, J.; McNicholas, B.; et al. Best Practice Guidance for Digital Contact Tracing Apps: A Cross-disciplinary Review of the Literature. *JMIR Mhealth Uhealth* **2021**, *9*, e27753. [CrossRef] [PubMed]
15. Immuni. Available online: https://www.immuni.italia.it/ (accessed on 15 December 2021).
16. MID—Sottogruppo di Lavoro 6. *Report Sulle Attività Svolte dal Sottogruppo di Lavoro Impegnato Nell'individuazione di "Tecnologie per il Governo Dell'emergenza" (in Particolare Contact-Tracing) Mediante Valutazione di 319 Soluzioni Tecnologiche Pervenute con Call for Contribution dal 24 al 26 Marzo*; Ministero della Innovazione Tecnologica e della Digitalizzazione: Rome, Italy, 2020. Available online: https://innovazione.gov.it/assets/docs/SGdL6%20-%20Relazione.pdf (accessed on 30 December 2021).
17. Immuni Documentation. Available online: https://github.com/immuni-app/immuni-documentation (accessed on 15 December 2021).
18. Rapporti Covid in italiano. Available online: https://www.iss.it/rapporti-covid-19 (accessed on 15 December 2021).
19. Rapporti Covid in inglese. Available online: https://www.iss.it/rapporti-iss-covid-19-in-english (accessed on 15 December 2021).
20. Filia, A.; Urdiales, A.M.; Rota, M.C. Guida per la ricerca e gestione dei contatti (contact tracing) dei casi di COVID-19. In *Versione del 25 Giugno 2020*; Rapporto ISS COVID-19, n. 53/2020; Istituto Superiore di Sanità: Rome, Italy, 2020.
21. ISS Bioethics COVID-19 Working Group. *Digital Support for Contact Tracing during the Pandemic: Ethical and Governance Considerations*; Version of September 17, 2020, Rapporto ISS COVID-19 n. 59/2020—English version; Istituto Superiore di Sanità: Rome, Italy, 2020.

22. Giansanti, D.; D'Avenio, G.; Rossi, M.; Spurio, A.; Bertinato, L.; Grigioni, M. *Technologies Supporting Proximity Detection: Reflections for Citizens, Professionals and Stakeholders in the COVID-19 Era*; Version of October 29, 2020, Rapporto ISS COVID-19 n. 54/2020 Rev.—English version; Istituto Superiore di Sanità: Rome, Italy, 2020.
23. Emergenza Epidemiologica COVID-19: Elementi per il Contact Tracing. Available online: https://www.eduiss.it/pluginfile.php/544990/course/summary/165F20_Programma%20senza%20firme%20%28psicologi%29.pdf (accessed on 15 December 2021).
24. Web Immuni. Immuni-Dashboard-Data/Dati/Andamento-Download.csv. Available online: https://github.com/immuni-app/immuni-dashboard-data/blob/master/dati/andamento-download.csv (accessed on 15 December 2021).
25. WeB GITHUB. Immuni-Dashboard-Data/Dati/Andamento-Dati-Nazionali.csv. Available online: https://github.com/immuni-app/immuni-dashboard-data/blob/master/dati/andamento-dati-nazionali.csv (accessed on 15 December 2021).
26. Web Immuni. The Numbers of Immune. Available online: https://www.immuni.italia.it/dashboard.html (accessed on 15 December 2021).
27. Web Tuttitalia.it. Popolazione per età, sesso e stato civile 2021. Available online: https://www.tuttitalia.it/statistiche/popolazione-eta-sesso-stato-civile-2021/ (accessed on 15 December 2021).
28. Web Lab. Coronavirus, la situazione in Italia. Available online: https://lab.gedidigital.it/gedi-visual/2020/coronavirus-i-contagi-in-italia/ (accessed on 15 December 2021).
29. Web Istat. Indagine sierologica su Covid-19 condotta da Ministero della Salute e Istat. Available online: https://www.istat.it/it/archivio/242676 (accessed on 15 December 2021).
30. Web Itatt. PRIMI RISULTATI DELL'INDAGINE DI SIEROPREVALENZA SUL SARS-CoV-2. Available online: https://www.istat.it/it/files/2020/08/ReportPrimiRisultatiIndagineSiero.pdf (accessed on 15 December 2021).
31. Web Censis. I Media Digitali e la fine Dello Star System. Available online: https://www.censis.it/comunicazione/i-media-digitali-e-la-fine-dello-star-system (accessed on 15 December 2021).
32. Web Censis. I Media dopo la Pandemia. Available online: https://www.censis.it/comunicazione/i-media-dopo-la-pandemia-1 (accessed on 15 December 2021).
33. Web GitHub. Available online: https://user-images.githubusercontent.com/7631137/97900742-65047900-1d3b-11eb-9d0f-67f20ce73398.png (accessed on 15 December 2021).
34. Web GitHub. Download per Regione #4. Available online: https://github.com/immuni-app/immuni-dashboard-data/issues/4 (accessed on 15 December 2021).
35. Web Ansa. Pil Bolzano sopra la media Ue, Calabria la peggiore d'Italia. Available online: https://www.ansa.it/europa/notizie/la_tua_europa/notizie/2021/03/03/pil-bolzano-sopra-la-media-ue-calabria-la-peggiore-ditalia_57a18efa-5918-4fb4-80fe-9763b36783b9.html (accessed on 15 December 2021).
36. Web Eurostat. Regional GDP per Capita Ranged from 32% to 260% of the EU Average in 2019. Available online: https://ec.europa.eu/eurostat/web/products-eurostat-news/-/ddn-20210303-1 (accessed on 15 December 2021).
37. Maccari, L.; Cagno, V. Do we need a contact tracing app? *Comput. Commun.* **2021**, *166*, 9–18. [CrossRef] [PubMed]
38. Neter, E.; Brainin, E.; Baron-Epel, O. Group differences in health literacy are ameliorated in ehealth literacy. *Health Psychol. Behav. Med.* **2021**, *9*, 480–497. [CrossRef] [PubMed]
39. van Deursen, A.J.; van Dijk, J.A. The first-level digital divide shifts from inequalities in physical access to inequalities in material access. *New Media Soc.* **2019**, *21*, 354–375. [CrossRef] [PubMed]
40. Giansanti, D.; Veltro, G. The Digital Divide in the Era of COVID-19: An Investigation into an Important Obstacle to the Access to the mHealth by the Citizen. *Healthcare* **2021**, *9*, 371. [CrossRef] [PubMed]
41. Partecipa al Cashback con L'app, IO. Available online: https://io.italia.it/cashback/ (accessed on 18 August 2021).
42. Ansa IT Economia. Available online: https://www.ansa.it/bannernews/notizie/breaking_news_eco/2020/12/18/-manovraun-cellulare-per-1-anno-con-isee-sotto-20mila-euro-_14e1c456-f1f4-4630-9cc5-ff8ab26d596c.html (accessed on 18 August 2021).
43. Kolasa, K.; Mazzi, F.; Leszczuk-Czubkowska, E.; Zrubka, Z.; Péntek, M. State of the Art in Adoption of Contact Tracing Apps and Recommendations Regarding Privacy Protection and Public Health: Systematic Review. *JMIR Mhealth Uhealth* **2021**, *9*, e23250. [CrossRef] [PubMed]
44. Oyibo, K.; Sahu, K.S.; Oetomo, A.; Morita, P.P. Factors Influencing the Adoption of Contact Tracing Applications: Protocol for a Systematic Review. *JMIR Res. Protoc.* **2021**, *10*, e28961. [CrossRef] [PubMed]
45. Anglemyer, A.; Moore, T.H.; Parker, L.; Chambers, T.; Grady, A.; Chiu, K.; Parry, M.; Wilczynska, M.; Flemyng, E.; Bero, L. Digital contact tracing technologies in epidemics: A rapid review. *Cochrane Database Syst. Rev.* **2020**, *8*, CD013699. [CrossRef] [PubMed]
46. Salomon, J.A.; Reinhart, A.; Bilinski, A.; Chua, E.J.; La Motte-Kerr, W.; Rönn, M.; Reitsma, M.; Morris, K.A.; LaRocca, S.; Farag, T.; et al. The U.S. COVID-19 Trends and Impact Survey, 2020–2021: Continuous real-time measurement of COVID-19 symptoms, risks, protective behaviors, testing and vaccination. *MedRxiv* **2021**. [CrossRef]
47. Smith, S.A.; Whitehead, M.S.; Sheats, J.; Mastromonico, J.; Yoo, W.; Coughlin, S.S. A Community-engaged approach to developing a mobile cancer prevention App: The mCPA Study Protocol. *JMIR Res. Protoc.* **2016**, *5*, e34. [CrossRef] [PubMed]

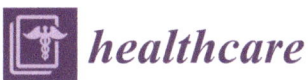

Article

Fuzzy Cognitive Scenario Mapping for Causes of Cybersecurity in Telehealth Services

Thiago Poleto [1], Victor Diogho Heuer de Carvalho [2], Ayara Letícia Bentes da Silva [1], Thárcylla Rebecca Negreiros Clemente [3], Maísa Mendonça Silva [4], Ana Paula Henriques de Gusmão [5], Ana Paula Cabral Seixas Costa [4] and Thyago Celso Cavalcante Nepomuceno [3],*

1 Departamento de Administração, Universidade Federal do Pará, Belém 66075-110, Brazil; thiagopoleto@ufpa.br (T.P.); ayara.ufpa@gmail.com (A.L.B.d.S.)
2 Campus do Sertão, Universidade Federal de Alagoas, Delmiro Gouveia 57480-000, Brazil; victor.carvalho@delmiro.ufal.br
3 Centro Acadêmico do Agreste, Universidade Federal de Pernambuco, Caruaru 55014-900, Brazil; tharcylla.clemente@ufpe.br
4 Departamento de Engenharia de Produção, Universidade Federal de Pernambuco, Recife 52171-900, Brazil; maisa@cdsid.org.br (M.M.S.); apcabral@cdsid.org.br (A.P.C.S.C.)
5 Departamento de Engenharia de Produção, Universidade Federal de Sergipe, Aracaju 49100-000, Brazil; anapaulagusmao@cdsid.org.br
* Correspondence: thyago.nepomuceno@ufpe.br; Tel.: +55-81-98705-2702

Abstract: Hospital organizations have adopted telehealth systems to expand their services to a portion of the Brazilian population with limited access to healthcare, mainly due to the geographical distance between their communities and hospitals. The importance and usage of those services have recently increased due to the COVID-19 state-level mobility interventions. These services work with sensitive and confidential data that contain medical records, medication prescriptions, and results of diagnostic processes. Understanding how cybersecurity impacts the development of telehealth strategies is crucial for creating secure systems for daily operations. In the application reported in this article, the Fuzzy Cognitive Maps (FCMs) translated the complexity of cybersecurity in telehealth services into intelligible and objective results in an expert-based cognitive map. The tool also allowed the construction of scenarios simulating the possible implications caused by common factors that affect telehealth systems. FCMs provide a better understanding of cybersecurity strategies using expert knowledge and scenario analysis, enabling the maturation of cybersecurity in telehealth services.

Keywords: cybersecurity; fuzzy cognitive maps; telehealth; scenario analysis; planning

Citation: Poleto, T.; Carvalho, V.D.H.d.; Silva, A.L.B.d.; Clemente, T.R.N.; Silva, M.M.; Gusmão, A.P.H.d.; Costa, A.P.C.S.; Nepomuceno, T.C.C. Fuzzy Cognitive Scenario Mapping for Causes of Cybersecurity in Telehealth Services. *Healthcare* **2021**, *9*, 1504. https://doi.org/10.3390/healthcare9111504

Academic Editors: Tin-Chih Toly Chen and Daniele Giansanti

Received: 16 September 2021
Accepted: 2 November 2021
Published: 5 November 2021

Publisher's Note: MDPI stays neutral with regard to jurisdictional claims in published maps and institutional affiliations.

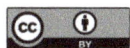

Copyright: © 2021 by the authors. Licensee MDPI, Basel, Switzerland. This article is an open access article distributed under the terms and conditions of the Creative Commons Attribution (CC BY) license (https://creativecommons.org/licenses/by/4.0/).

1. Introduction

The Brazilian Ministry of Health created the national telehealth system in 2007 with the initial objective of promoting family health remotely by using Information and Communication Technologies (ICT). One factor that justifies implementing this system is delivering healthcare to people living in remote communities where the nearest hospital care is distant. Bernardes et al. [1] stated that based on data from the Brazilian Institute of Geography and Statistics, only 24% of the country's population live in large cities, which adds to telehealth's importance as a public policy.

During the first semester of 2020, telehealth, also called telemedicine strategies, became essential in Brazil and many other countries due to the COVID-19 pandemic pressure on the limited hospital resources and the related response from public authorities imposing quarantine campaigns and mobility interventions worldwide. According to Nepomuceno et al. [2], when many potentially infected patients require regular or intensive care at the same time, hospitals with limited resources end up overloaded, the probability of propagation increases, and, as a result, the health systems collapse due to the lack of technical resources, fatigue, and overloading health teams. COVID-19 lockdown and social distance strategies in many have presented an opportunity for both doctors and patients to use telemedicine as a new manner of engagement and treatment in many regions [3,4].

The Telehealth Guidelines established by the Ministry of Health through Decree-Law No. 9795, of 17 May 2019, are mainly intended to improve user satisfaction and the quality of services provided to citizens through the Unified Health System [5]. The related systems have confidential data such as patient health histories, drug prescriptions, and medical diagnoses. Such data can be the target of cyberattacks, highlighting the importance of well-defined strategies for their protection. According to Kruse et al. [6], there was a 22% increase in cyberattacks in 2015, compromising about 112 million medical information records.

It is emphasized that cybersecurity should not be analyzed only as a compliance practice given the occurrence of specific events causing additional costs [7,8], but should be designed in a structured and contingent way to consider all systems from the conception of telemedicine systems and services to be offered [9,10]. Deficiencies in the ICT infrastructure of these services contribute significantly to the increase of harmful attacks on health organizations that also adopt the strategy of promoting their services remotely [11]. Thus, the ICT infrastructure is a crucial factor in developing cybersecurity analysis to implement telehealth systems [12–15]. The importance of considering vulnerabilities is often associated with the risk of losses, corruptions, inappropriate changes, and theft of data, with information and documents that affect the integrity of medical diagnoses delivered to the patient, which can cause serious damage to the health of the individual [16]. In general, these situations allow threats to be exploited and are often caused by cyberattacks from malicious systems or people [17]. Zain et al. [18] identified four main situations verified in cyberattacks which can occur in telehealth services, such as (i) when the data is destroyed or becomes unavailable, (ii) when an unauthorized system or person accesses the database, (iii) when an unauthorized system or person obtains access to the service and makes improper changes, and (iv) when an unauthorized system or person inserts counterfeit objects into the database. These situations are possible failures or threats in the data transmission process, which can be accidental or purposeful.

In telehealth services, the main challenge of the physicians is protecting the privacy of data. However, most of these professionals do not receive adequate training, and they are subject to situations that may compromise the performance of healthcare. This context requires preventive actions and security tools due to the sensitive data in healthcare systems such as digital signatures, professional credentials, financial data, patient diagnostic images, among others [19]. It is worth mentioning that this concern becomes even more complex when considering cyberattacks, especially due to the different interactions that occur on the Internet [20]. Furthermore, failure to comply with legal regulations may result in financial or criminal penalties [21,22]. For this, the IT professionals must make strategic decisions to define security policies and ensuring authenticity, integrity, and confidentiality of the database, besides ensuring business sustainability.

Little research has been carried out in the context of cybersecurity in telehealth and on attacks on related systems to analyze the damaging effects of information stored on patients' clinical health. Poleto et al. proposed a framework for cybersecurity risk management in telemedicine [23]. New studies focus can be oriented towards cybersecurity aspects, determining causal relationships either to prevent attacks or to solve problems that have already occurred, ensuring the security of services and, consequently, the activities and associated practices. The use of tools to support the identification of these security factors in telehealth services is beneficial for this purpose; however, the analytical process can be complex, and it requires high cognitive effort from the professionals involved, whether analysts or decision-makers, towards the planning of different assessment scenarios, helping to choose the best security measures.

Most of these strategic decisions are involved in business sustainability process [24], which can define action plans to ensure the telehealth services operation. The ICT management process assists in directing how medical centers can use IT to manage technologic art of ensuring the existence and continuity of a nation's information society, guaranteeing and protecting in cyberspace all of its information assets and critical infrastructure.

The interaction with the ICT manager was essential for analyzing concepts that influence cyberattacks in telehealth systems, especially in the testimony of their possible consequences associated with the system's vulnerabilities. The data relevance reinforces the importance of guaranteeing the network's health since, in the case of loss of confidentiality, it can cause moral damage to all involved, especially to patients [31,32]. Despite many studies identifying threats regarding cybersecurity in distributed systems, there is still a gap in the literature related to the causes that trigger ecosystem cybersecurity occurrences in telehealth systems.

In addition to the discussion with the information security expert, a total of fifteen variables (concepts) influencing the cyberattacks occurrences in telehealth services were identified, which had support in the literature [33]. These concepts can be considered the weaknesses that affect the operational performance in telehealth systems. Table 1 presents a description of these concepts that the ICT manager has validated, three meetings were held and the time was 1 h.

Table 1. Description of variables involved in the study in telehealth services.

Main Concepts	Description	Fuzzy Interpretation	References
C1: Insecure network protocols	Due to insecure network protocols, (HTTP), attackers can enter the organization's network	−1: Low incompatibility network protocol 0: Average incompatibility network protocol 1: High incompatibility network protocol	[34]
C2: Sensitive data encryption	Involve custom code development that brings encryption into the individual application data fields	−1: Low Information Security maintenance 0: Average Information Security maintenance 1: High Information Security maintenance	[35]
C3: Mobile health apps failure	Operational failures occur in telehealth due to users not being prepared to adopt information security protocols.	−1: Low Operational failures occur in telehealth 0: Average Operational failures occur in telehealth 1: High Operational failures occur in telehealth	[36]
C4: Cybersecurity certification	Provides a rationale for why the auditable events are deemed to be adequate to support the after-fact investigations of security incidents into operational telehealth server	−1: Absolute abandonment of auditable events. 0: Average attention to auditable events. 1: Priority attention to auditable events	[37]
C5: Outsourcing of IT cloud services	Provides help desks, tech support, and provider to protect the confidentiality of the outsourced information.	−1: No supporting communication security. 0: A few supporting communication security. 1: Priority attention to communication security	[38]
C6: IT governance	Provides security strategies aligned with and supporting the business objectives	−1: Absolute abandonment of IT Governance. 0: Average attention to IT Governance. 1: Priority attention to IT Governance	[39]
C7: Controls for wireless communication	Establishment of policies and procedures for the effective implementation of selected security and control enhancements into telehealth.	−1: Absolute abandonment of policy access. 0: Average attention to policy access. 1: Priority attention to policy access	[40]
C8: Mobile connected medical devices	Lack of updates or lack of patching, a common threat that can have a significant impact on the healthcare organization	−1: Low Information Security maintenance 0: Average Information Security maintenance 1: High Information Security maintenance	[5]
C9: Supplier eligibility criteria	Establish security baseline requirements and translate them into eligibility criteria when selecting suppliers	−1: No supporting supplier eligibility 0: A few supporting Supplier eligibility 1: Plenty of supporting supplier eligibility	[41]
C10: Medical system configuration error	Medical platforms are software that needs to be installed on a practice or health system's local server	−1: No supporting medical systems. 0: A few supportive medical systems. 1: Priority attention of medical systems.	[42]
C11: Big data privacy in healthcare	Big data has considerable potential to improve patient outcomes and predict outbreaks of epidemics	−1: Low Information Security maintenance 0: Average Information Security maintenance 1: High Information Security maintenance	[43]
C12: Augmented reality	Provide remote clinicians, such as surgeons, to guide physicians, paramedics, and other staff to perform emergency procedures in telehealth	−1: No supporting augmented reality 0: A few supporting augmented reality 1: Plenty of supporting augmented reality	[44]
C13: IT Investment	Provides IT investments during the pandemic, accelerating the use of telemedicine services	−1: No supporting IT Investment 0: A few supporting IT Investment 1: Plenty of supporting IT Investment	[35]
C14: Patient's errors	Providers should educate patients about cybersecurity and the steps they should take to improve the overall safety of their interactions online	−1: No supporting education. 0: A few supporting education. 1: Plenty of supporting education	[45]
C15: Incident response plan	Systems and devices eventually fail due to inaccurate coding, improper handling, or just tear and wear	−1: No supporting incident plan. 0: A few supporting incident plan. 1: Plenty of supporting incident plans	[6]

The concepts allow complex and critical ecosystem threats to be exploited in a telehealth system. However, the lack or inefficiency of information security planning makes it challenging to identify cybersecurity. This inefficiency also requires tools and methodologies to minimize cybersecurity consequences, which can cause large-scale damage to business sustainability [20].

An FCM diagram was built using the ICT manager's knowledge with the cybersecurity expert's support through an interview. A cognitive structure with subjective information was generated using the central concepts previously discussed, enabling performance analysis of the telehealth system. This information is associated with the concepts of critical infrastructures—which refers to facilities, services, goods, and systems that will have a severe social and economic impact if their performance is degraded or if they are suspended or destroyed. The visual representation of the expert-based FCM created based on the concepts is shown in Figure 1.

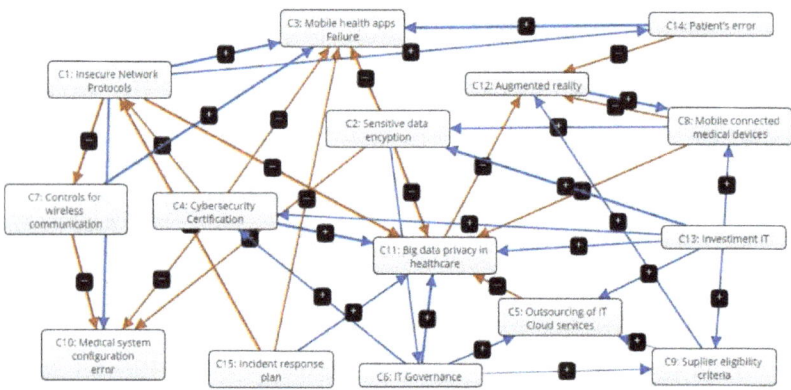

Figure 1. Model FCM cybersecurity in the telehealth university hospital.

The FCM diagram's construction aims at verifying the computed values of intensity in the concepts related to cybersecurity in telehealth. The causal relationship between concepts is indicated by an arrow and the positive symbol (+).

The framework of Figure 1 is meant to map the cybersecurity relationships (networks) within the scope of telehealth management by using a Fuzzy Cognitive Map. This process consisted of three phases: 1. Nodes: The key concepts from an Expert Panel; 2. Map: Cause-and-effect relationship in each of the arcs and a graphical representation of the network; and 3. Model: Numerical values and computational simulation. Once the cybersecurity in the telehealth management model is formulated, the subsequent simulation tasks (what-if scenarios) is carried out, with assumptions that modify the input variables (Value Repositories and Constraints), to finally check what impact these changes have on the performance of cybersecurity in the telehealth.

Outputs of Scenario Analysis

The interpretations of the FCM diagram's relationships are important for the strategic planning process of the hospital's ICT department. With these implications, ICT managers can define preference concept actions and develop information security plans capable of minimizing the consequences caused by the vulnerabilities. Each analysis compares the steady-state promoted by the FCM with the scenarios defined by the ICT manager based on the main concepts. Therefore, it is possible to highlight the best and worst scenarios of cyberattacks in the hospital's telehealth system, considering the concepts of the present study. Table 2 shows the levels of centrality and preferred state for the concepts of cybersecurity in telehealth.

solutions. For this, it is opportune to present methodologies to support organizational diagnoses to identify these possible causes of threats in telehealth systems. One of these methodologies is Fuzzy Cognitive Maps (FCMs) [25], which represents scientific knowledge and strategic decision making in systems using elements of a mental map, based on fuzzy logic computation.

This context into account, this article proposes an analytical approach based on Fuzzy Cognitive Maps (FCM) aimed at the mental representation of experts on causal relationships within a set of concepts related to cybersecurity that impact telehealth systems, providing support for strategic planning and decision-making. FCM can represent all relationships intelligibly, enabling creating scenarios and reducing cognitive effort by allowing their analysis through objective graphic elements, and representing interesting support to improve information asset protection concerning patient information management. This article aims to demonstrate the results of applying FCMs in favor of cybersecurity in a telehealth system, seeking to identify variables that can be used for cybersecurity planning, in addition to simulating involved scenarios. The remaining of this paper is organized as follows: Section 2 presents the Materials and Methods, explaining the mechanism of the proposed approach. Section 3 undertakes an application that validates the proposed approach. Section 4 is the discussion of the main findings; conceptual and practical implications are in Section 5. Finally, Section 6 draws some conclusions, indicates some study limitations, and suggests future research lines.

2. Materials and Methods

According to Tsadiras [26], FCM analysis allows identifying strategies cybersecurity in a system having a more significant impact on other factors and provides possible scenarios by varying the degree of intensity of these variables in a complex problem. Moreover, incorporating the subjectivity and knowledge of an expert leads to a constructivist methodology and provides a complement to information security planning in hospitals.

Protecting patients' private data in telehealth services can be severely damaged by malicious interventions, such as altering or stealing data and information. Other factors, such as data privacy and credibility, can affect the image of the medical center. In Brazil, telehealth services have been valued in recent years and this has encouraged governmental decisions regarding (i) the prioritization of telemedicine infrastructure; (ii) the systematization of the teleassistance process, with the development of clinical data cybersecurity protocols; and (iii) the structuring of security planning to provide the quality and confidentiality of the data and services offered by telehealth in hospitals.

The present research's motivation is based on the following question: what are the main cybersecurity factors affecting telehealth? In response to this question, the following issues will be discussed: (i) the role of stakeholders in the cybersecurity decision process at a hospital; (ii) the use of FCM as an integrated methodology to analyze cybersecurity, to develop planning policies, and to assess the impacts of such decisions in hospital.

First, we identified the main security concepts that occur in telehealth services. For this, an informative and analytical list of concepts that may influence cybersecurity planning in telehealth at a hospital was created. Considering that the planning decisions are strategic, a manager in the ICT area of a hospital assumed the expert's role in eliciting the concepts in the cybersecurity context. Two technical meetings were held with the hospital's ICT manager, each having an average duration of two hours, coordinated by a facilitator who is an expert in information security and responsible for analyzing the results. During the interview, the study's objectives and the research procedure were presented, allowing for a better understanding of the study by the ICT manager. As a result, the list of the main concepts and the description of the leading information about security strategies adopted to treat and prevent problems caused by cyberattacks in telehealth services were obtained, considering the ICT manager's perception [27].

This list consisted of grouping the concepts that affect cybersecurity and analyzing the cause and effect relationship between them. For this, the Mental Modeler software was used to obtain the expert's cognitive map [28]. The ICT manager identified causal connections between the nodes, which required defining the type of relationship (positive or negative), between w_i and w_j, and the intensity of each one over the other. The dynamic analysis of the FCM focuses on evaluating the system's behavior when the cause and effect relationships between the selected concepts are changed, enabling the evaluation of different scenarios [29].

The information was collected to support developing a strategic plan dedicated to cybersecurity in telehealth at hospital. Moreover, to analyze the changes that may impact cybersecurity, the construction of scenarios involves using the identified relationships among the concepts. Consequently, the scenarios can be considered roadmaps for developing and improving the model that describes the problem in a learning process. This study's cognitive structure allowed for greater transparency in cybersecurity planning of telehealth services and theoretical contributions, directed to strategic decisions, and promoting organizational learning [30].

FCM Procedure

A FCM can be described as a fuzzy graph containing the concepts to be casually assigned in the nodes and the relationships in the edge arrows [25]. The procedure for creating the FCM can be defined in three main steps [27]:

First Step: clarify the FCM purpose and if it is not well defined the search for causal relationships will make the formation of the FCM unfeasible.

Second Step: identify the relevant concepts that influence the decision to be taken.

Third Step: find the causal relationships between the concepts defined in the previous step, so that these relationships need to be abstracted from the decision maker's definitions, through instruments such as questionnaires and interviews.

Thus, from a mathematical point of view, an FCM can be described as a set of nodes (concepts) C_i with $i = 1, \ldots, n$, being the number of concepts in the problem and all these concepts together represent a vector of state $A = [A_1, \ldots, A_n]$. The value of each concept is influenced by the values of the concepts that are related to it along with the corresponding causal weight and for the concept system to evolve, the vector A needs to be passed repeatedly over the connection matrix W [31].

The associated mathematical formula is given in Equation (1) [32]:

$$A_I^{(K+1)} = f\left(A_i^k + \sum_{\substack{j \neq i \\ j = 1}}^{N} A_j^k W_{ji} \right) \quad (1)$$

where:

$A_I^{(K+1)}$ is the value of concept C_i at step $k + 1$;

A_j^k is the value of the concept C_j in step k;

W_{ji} is the weight of the relationship between C_j and C_i; and

$f(x)$ is a sigmoid threshold function defined by Equation (2):

$$f = \frac{1}{1 + e^{-\lambda x}} \quad (2)$$

where λ is a positive constant in a determined interval and $f(x)$ lies between [0, 1].

3. Results

The proposed FCM model considers a holistic view to analyze cybersecurity concepts within telehealth in a hospital in the Amazon region. In the model, minimal changes were necessary to expand the notion and technical specifications for adequate cybersecurity planning. First, the concept of cybersecurity was explained to the ICT manager—it refers to the

Table 2. Degree of the centrality of IT manager preference concepts.

Main Concepts Cybersecurity in Telehealth	Indegree	Outdegree	Centrality	Preferred State
C1: Insecure network protocols	1.01	2.69	3.71	Decrease
C2: Sensitive data encryption	0.95	1.88	2.83	Increase
C3: Mobile health apps failure	3.26	0.00	3.25	Decrease
C4: Cybersecurity certification	0.65	1.67	2.32	Increase
C5: Outsourcing of IT cloud services	0.88	0.33	1.22	Increase
C6: IT governance	0.27	1.34	1.61	Increase
C7: Controls for wireless communication	0.56	1.05	1.61	Increase
C8: Mobile connected medical devices	0.91	0.97	1.88	Increase
C9: Supplier eligibility criteria	0.41	0.35	0.77	Increase
C10: Medical system configuration error	1.68	0.00	1.68	Decrease
C11: Big Data privacy in healthcare	3.82	0.34	4.17	Decrease
C12: Augmented reality	1.10	0.52	1.62	Increase
C13: Investments IT	0.00	2.39	2.39	Increase
C14: Patient's error	0.32	0.89	1.13	Decrease
C15: Incident response plan	0.00	1.48	1.48	Increase

The analysis based on the FCM modeling results allows the ICT manager to build different scenarios of strategic consequences. The construction of the scenarios offers contributions in the simulation of possible implications caused by common factors that affect telehealth systems in a specific way. In addition, these scenarios can support the decision process in the strategic planning of actions to prevent or mitigate vulnerabilities that could compromise the performance of telehealth systems. Planning of mitigation actions, when done without due care can negatively influence the possibility of occurrences of attacks analyzed in Figure 2. The matrix representation of the fuzzy cognitive map (the Wij Weight matrix) obtained after expert interviews and process of modeling change its configuration depending on the experts' corrections. Based on the current literature, it was found that if a negative value is specified in the initial concept state of the estimation vector, then the modeling results influenced by the factors would be inverted, meaning that hostile factors contribute to cybersecurity.

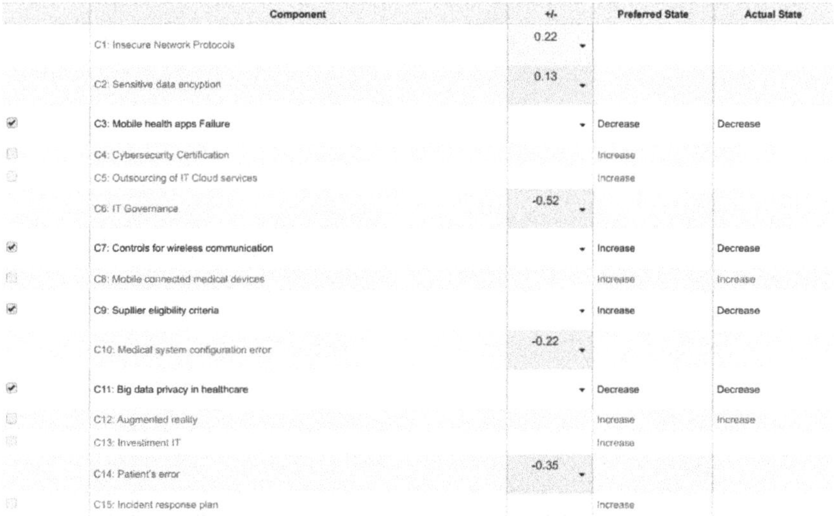

	Component	+/-	Preferred State	Actual State
	C1: Insecure Network Protocols	0.22		
	C2: Sensitive data encyption	0.13		
☑	C3: Mobile health apps Failure		Decrease	Decrease
☐	C4: Cybersecurity Certification		Increase	
☐	C5: Outsourcing of IT Cloud services		Increase	
	C6: IT Governance	-0.52		
☑	C7: Controls for wireless communication		Increase	Decrease
☐	C8: Mobile connected medical devices		Increase	Increase
☑	C9: Suplier eligibility criteria		Increase	Decrease
	C10: Medical system configuration error	-0.22		
☑	C11: Big data privacy in healthcare		Decrease	Decrease
☐	C12: Augmented reality		Increase	Increase
☐	C13: Investment IT		Increase	
	C14: Patient's error	-0.35		
☐	C15: Incident response plan		Increase	

Figure 2. Final equilibrium states by the value of nodal element C1 (insecure network protocols), C2 (Sensitive data encryption), C6 (IT Governance), C10 (Medical system configuration error), and C14 (Patient's error).

The main components in telehealth systems, according to ICT expert, judged in the range [−1] to [1], are "Mobile health apps failure" (C3) and "Controls for wireless Communication" (C7) [6]. On the other hand, regarding "Supplier eligibility criteria" (C9) and "Big Data privacy in healthcare" (C11) [46]. Figure 3 illustrates the telehealth scenario analysis.

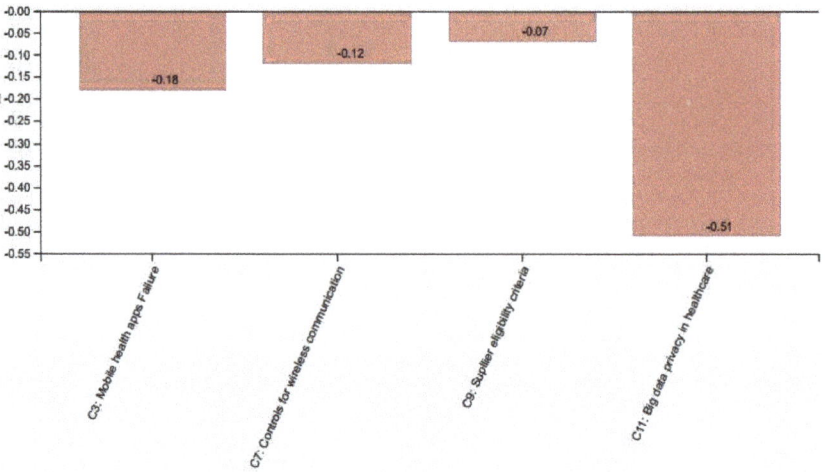

Figure 3. Scenario I: analysis cybersecurity in telehealth.

Scenario I analyzes the impact of the set of the main concept "Mobile health apps failure" (C3) scoring −0.18, "Controls for wireless Communication" (C7) scoring 0.12, "Supplier eligibility criteria" (C9) with scoring −0.07, and "Big Data privacy in healthcare" (C11) scoring −0.51 on the vulnerabilities pointed out in the telehealth system. This scenario highlights the association with the consequence of exploiting vulnerabilities when these factors are identified. These results confirm how changes and wrong configurations can be overflowing the infrastructure of telehealth servers [47–49].

Further, configurations and composition of the servers responsible for the processing and storage of data and information can increase the probability of attacks that deflect the destination of the data and manipulate the system's functionalities. Thus, it is necessary to monitor the data origin and destination points, checking what actions are being carried out, as well as to understand the collaboration policies between providers of these ICT services and systems' users (patients or physicians) so that the university hospital can minimize the damage on the services provided.

In Scenario II, the main components are "Medical System configuration error" (C10) and "IT Investments" (C13). Although each business has its budget destined for investments, procrastinating investment to adequate technology, or using poor quality devices can increase the probability of inefficiency in the answering service and reinforce problems in devices used in telehealth systems. In this context, the effect of cybersecurity is more significant because the malicious action activates defense planning. These situations are generally recorded when the telehealth system comes with records of malware and logical attacks [50]. The analysis related to this Scenario II is represented in Figures 4 and 5.

	Component	+/-	Preferred State	Actual State
☐	C1: Insecure Network Protocols		Decrease	Increase
☑	C2: Sensitive data encryption	▼ Increase		Decrease
☐	C3: Mobile health apps Failure		Decrease	Increase
☑	C4: Cybersecurity Certification	▼ Increase		Decrease
☑	C5: Outsourcing of IT Cloud services	▼ Increase		Decrease
☑	C6: IT Governance	▼ Increase		Decrease
☐	C7: Controls for wireless communication		Increase	Decrease
☐	C8: Mobile connected medical devices		Increase	Decrease
☐	C9: Supplier eligibility criteria		Increase	Decrease
	C10: Medical system configuration error	−0.22 ▼		
☐	C11: Big data privacy in healthcare		Decrease	Decrease
☐	C12: Augmented reality		Increase	Increase
	C13: Investment IT	−0.3 ▼		
☐	C14: Patient's error		Decrease	Increase
☐	C15: Incident response plan		Increase	

Figure 4. Final equilibrium states by the value of nodal element C10 (Medical system configuration error) and C13 (IT Investment).

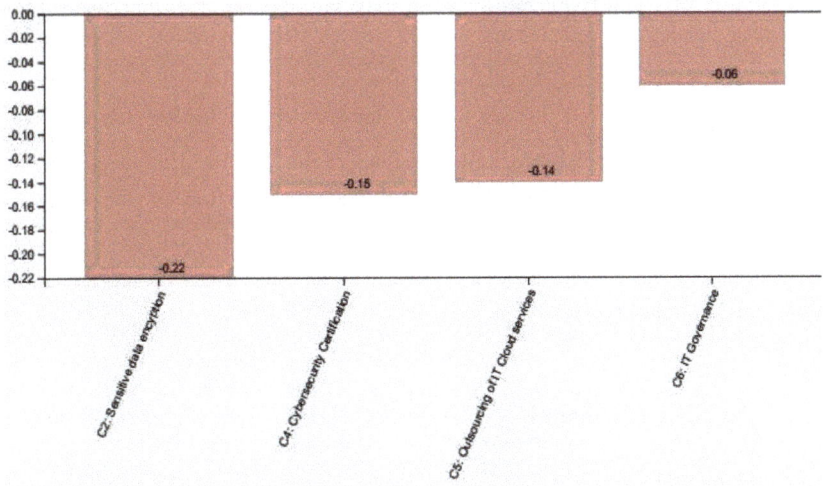

Figure 5. Scenario II: analysis cybersecurity in telehealth.

In Scenario II, as shown in Figure 5, the main concepts are "Sensitive data encryption" (C2 with −0.22) occurrence, "Cybersecurity certification" (C4 with −0.15), "Outsourcing of IT Cloud services" (C5 with −0.14), and "IT Governance" (C6 with −0.06) occurrence. This scenario highlights the concern about controlling the ICT services that are essential for the organization. In medical centers, personal data relating to the patients' health status should receive greater attention and should be considered requirements for developing specific security policies. The results show that it is possible to view different vulnerability types regarding patient care in the two scenarios. Based on the analysis, it is important to consider that in addition to the value of the information, other criteria must be incorporated in the process of defining the protection requirements of telehealth systems, such as the ability to identify and record system's threats and vulnerabilities. However, these criteria were not analyzed in the present study. Despite this limitation, it is essential to know in advance the asset's value to be protected to identify threats and vulnerabilities to return consistent results, which is why cybersecurity planning is needed.

4. Discussion

Recent studies argue that the increase in cybersecurity investments has not resulted in more adequate security levels in many areas. This discrepancy can be justified by the lack of consistent information security management [41]. According to Sivaprakash et al. [51], in a comparison made between healthcare and financial organizations, in terms of data management and protection, both types of organizations are concerned and incorporate strategic actions to control and protect data generated in their environments. However, managers do not have adequate training to deal with cyber threats in healthcare organizations [6]. In contrast, financial organizations have been investing in cybersecurity for about twenty years, aligning cybersecurity with the organization's objectives.

The need for data sharing in heterogeneous public and private healthcare organizations and the lack of continuous and standardized communication in cybersecurity show importance in the responses under the threats and vulnerabilities of the systems, involving medical actors, patients, and ICT analysts [52]. In this context, the ICT professionals have access to data about patients and their clinical status (clinical historic, vital parameters, physical examination data, among other data) that are useful for planning and the decision-making process in telehealth services. However, the provision of healthcare assistance cannot be analyzed as an isolated process but in line with organizational planning as a whole. From this perspective, this study can help the senior manager and the IT manager to understand the vulnerabilities that can affect telehealth systems' operational performance that contribute as a resource to support cybersecurity planning and ensuring the achievement and enhancement of the efficiency of the information protection in medical centers.

The value of the information is not the only criterion used to define the protection requirements. The measure of the ability to identify threats can be a more consistent indicator of this definition. When the asset's value is known, the greater the likelihood of efficiency in the process, hence the need for cybersecurity planning. Annual audits, for example, are a way of ensuring minimum compliance with cybersecurity requirements. The determination of an approved regulatory and supervisory body requires organizations to adopt information security procedures and standards to be used as maturity indicators, ensuring an effective cybersecurity policy for telehealth services. The lack of an information security policy is directly reflected in telehealth services' operational performance.

Our findings show that without imposing any restrictions on cybersecurity, it is possible to allow significant occurrences and negative impacts to reduce telehealth services' efficiency [53]. The visualization tools allow a better understanding of the causal relationships between the factors and the vulnerabilities considered. FCM is a modeling method for complex systems that use simulations based on the mental map of human reasoning to operate on systems' representation. Thus, the application of FCM shows the modeling ability to operate ambiguous and vague terms, simulating a sense of words and supporting decision-making and strategic planning of actions related to information security in the health area, a fact reinforced in a previous work of ours (see [54]), which has been expanded by the present article.

4.1. University Hospitals and Telehealth Cyber Security Strategies

Regarding the objective unit of the case study, university hospitals, it is noted a strategic decision-making application of actions in an ad hoc stage in relation to cybersecurity risks and necessary measures for prevention and mitigation. This is because, in the university hospital's perspective where the analysis was applied, planning, information security is considered an essential requirement to be fulfilled within the overall information technology planning. On the other hand, although managers understand the importance of this type of security, it is noteworthy they still do not have the most appropriate tools capable of supporting their decision-making process for related planning, seeking to identify empirically the causal relationships between the various existing elements or concepts, and prioritize them according to their impact on the continuity of telehealth services. At some instance this has been sufficient for mitigating some risks and technological treats.

Resorting to most appropriate tools, however, may offer additional opportunity for managerial continuous improvement. Tools such as FCM, despite popular in many sectors of economic activity and other areas for decision-making, seem to be unknown or underused instruments for cybersecurity managers in Brazil, taking this conclusion specifically within the context of university hospitals. The development of the case study reported here also suggests they can be used relatively easily and efficiently so that these managers can develop plans more in line with the reality they know well, as they develop daily activities on them. Above all, FCM constitute a knowledge management tool capable of externalizing the experiences contained in these managers' minds, encoding this experience in an intelligible and accessible way for use in cybersecurity and information security planning.

4.2. Comparison with Other Methods/Approaches Found in Literature

In Table 3, a synthesis of the works containing similar methods used in the literature to support the development of this article will be presented. It contains the objectives and main similarities and differences, as well as a synthesis of this work, for comparative purposes.

Table 3. Literature comparison.

Reference	Objective	Main Similarities	Main Differences
[10]	Develop and validate a telehealth privacy and security self-assessment questionnaire to be applied with providers.	It applies expert assessment that can be used to identify vulnerabilities in telehealth systems.	It does not establish causal relationships among the identified elements. The applied procedure is based in the application of questionnaires and psychometric analysis.
[12]	Present a big data risk model using Failure Mode and Effects Analysis (FMEA) and Grey Theory.	It provides a structured approach to assess risk factors, facilitating the assessment and providing a vision of risks relations.	The work uses Different methods (Failure Mode and Effects Analysis and Grey Theory).
[13]	Propose a risk model for information security that identify and evaluate the events' sequence in scenarios related to the abuses of information technology systems.	The model allows ranking the risks based on their criticality, supporting the definitions of preventive or corrective actions. Use of Fuzzy Theory elements.	It does not establish causal relationships among the identified elements. Use of Event Tree Analysis.
[14]	Propose an approach to information security risk management based on Failure Mode and Effects Analysis (FMEA) and Fuzzy Theory.	The approach applies identification of risk elements/concepts, prioritizing risk dimensions according to the risk's criticality, to support defining preventive or corrective actions. Use of Fuzzy Theory elements.	It does not establish causal relationships among the identified elements. Use of Failure Mode and Effects Analysis.
[15]	Propose a model to evaluate cybersecurity risk using Fault Tree Analysis, Decision Theory and Fuzzy Theory.	The model analyses risk scenarios also using elements from Fuzzy Theory, supporting the identification of vulnerabilities in cybersecurity linking them with potential consequences.	Use of Fault Tree Analysis, with elements from decision theory.
[23]	Propose a framework for cybersecurity risk management in telemedicine.	Identification of causes, consequences, and preventive measures for security threats, using scenario analysis.	Different methods (fault tree analysis and event tree analysis).
[29]	Propose a quantitative assessment framework to evaluate nuclear power plant risks related to cyber-attacks.	Assessment of cybersecurity risk elements, using scenarios, and providing risk information to develop preventive or corrective strategies.	Use of difficulty and consequences of cyber-attacks in the assessment, use of Bayesian belief networks and probabilistic safety assessment methods.
	Objective	Main characteristics	Main characteristics compared to other models/approaches
This work	Propose an analytical approach using Fuzzy Cognitive Maps (FCM) representing experts' opinions about causal relationships of concepts related to cybersecurity in telehealth systems, providing support for strategic planning and decision-making	Use of expert knowledge creating a graphical representation about expert reasoning about cybersecurity threats, aiding to prioritize them according to scenarios. Support to cybersecurity strategies development by understanding the causal relationships between the concepts.	The approach applied in this study do not consider the probabilistic component involved in risk analysis, in its mathematical formulation to generate de graphs from FCM. Most of the methods or approaches previously presented deal with probabilistic data about the security threats.

5. Conceptual and Practical Implications

Our results highlight cybersecurity issues in telehealth services that deserve special attention, whether from a conceptual or practical point of view since sensitive data circulates through any type of information system. In this sense, exploring the system's possible vulnerabilities is fundamental to adopting preventive or corrective measures [55].

This issue is even more delicate in telehealth services and systems since certain information may be under medical confidentiality and can compromise patients' physical and psychological integrity should they be improperly exposed [56]. The conceptual point of view about using FCM in telehealth systems is linked to how this tool can influence the planning and adoption of security measures in these systems. Here we can establish the following question: how should these systems be thought of, from their planning through their implementation, finally reaching their full functioning, to ensure that this sensitive information is protected efficiently and effectively?

Our model demonstrates that several concepts related to threats in systems and types of cyberattacks, always considering the participation of experts, whose understanding of the relationships between these concepts is represented through the graph resulting from the application of the FCM. These relationships are still supported by obtaining a measure of strength extracted from a fuzzy context that represents vagueness in the definitions made by these experts when eliciting his knowledge.

Here it can be connected with knowledge engineering, which states that eliciting or extracting expert (tacit) knowledge is a bottleneck and a critical issue in systems development [57]. In this analogy, the FCM acts as a formal means for this knowledge to be acquired and recorded, allowing the engineers and systems analysts involved with telehealth systems projects to correct existing security breaches and design plans for action contingency of possible cyberattacks.

From the perspective of telehealth systems actors, whether health professionals or patients, concepts such as confidentiality, consistency, and availability of information, together with the use of these systems only by authorized personnel and the presence of functions to reduce errors [58], deserve mention in this discussion, to add or enforce security requirements. In addition to the professionals responsible for designing, implementing, and managing information systems and ensuring information security, users also deserve to be heard since they are the final subjects to whom the system was designed [10].

Therefore, the applied methodology can be extended to obtain new security perceptions about the telehealth system, reinforcing those already elicited from experts. These two perspectives, in fact, require feedback: (i) on the knowledge of experts providing technical elements for the design and implementation of systems and information security measures; and (ii) on the opinion of the end-users, being evaluated based on these technical elements, to reinforce them or identify new requirements.

Based on our empirical results, referring to vulnerabilities, forms of cyber-attacks, and user concerns, can be analyzed through the FCM. The results obtained should be discussed by the security project team in a post-conceptualization stage. While other works have their approach focused on more technical elements related to the security guarantee in telehealth systems, the value of the methodology used in this work is at a more managerial and strategic level, ensuring the visualization of the related concepts for making decisions about themselves.

This part of the discussion aims to determine what should be implemented as a priority since the conceptual elements detected through the methodology are likely to be in large numbers. Trade-offs will emerge in this type of valuation, such as less time spent on systems valuation instead of information and more time spent assigning values to the assets involved [59].

The following question arises: what is the most appropriate way to evaluate these concepts and to choose what will be implemented as a priority? Each team must carry out the evaluations according to what is defined by the organization, and the users' opinions deserve attention, complementing the information security requirements. Nevertheless, it is essential to note that the information collected mainly from the users can provide valuable feedback to the project development team. FCMs have the advantage of showing defuzzified numerical values referring to the relationships between the evaluated elements [60,61]. These indicators can be combined with other more common elements in evaluating alternatives to be implemented, such as the cost and time involved. Moreover, FCMs make it possible for decisions to be made by analyzing varied scenarios built based on the subjective opinions of the people involved [31], ensuring the inclusion of elements described in a technical and non-technical way, the latter related to the perspectives of users.

Furthermore, practical implications at a higher level, leaving aside the view on more technical elements, the use of FCM favors the creation of information security and cybersecurity policies. Analyzing the existing relationships between guidelines, requirements, and rules—elements that constitute these policies and lead to information security compliance [55]—is a process potentially facilitated by using the explored methodology. On the other hand, the definition of these policies implies the determination of a pattern of user behavior towards security in telehealth systems, since the behavioral factor alone has a more considerable influence than technical security elements in related systems and services [62] since the focus of the analysis now becomes the users' conduct as a "breach breaker" of security in the system.

In summary, the practical implications of the use of FCMs fall on implementing the telehealth system, providing security requirements to be implemented, whether defined by the experts' perspective or considering users' opinions. Also, the conduct of users of the system must be in line with security policies, which are also definitions that can be carried out with the support of the methodology.

6. Conclusions

In general, telehealth, precisely its technological, economic, and environmental characteristics, substantially contribute to society and is expected to provide health services to thousands of people limited by geographical constraints. Given this context, telehealth can benefit from the scenario-planning approach because it plays an essential role in future development related to planning policies against cyberattacks.

This paper presented an application of FCM that analyzes information security factors related to telehealth. The FCM model allowed the causal inference of direct chaining and numerical data-based updates and cybersecurity experts' opinions. Preliminary results are encouraging concerning the FCM approach's possibilities to decision-makers/ICT managers, enabling a good insight into the impact of cyberattacks on telehealth and ensuring a more focused view of the necessary protective actions. These results show the possibility of obtaining scenario planning in cybersecurity, highlighting the most critical telehealth factors. The analytical process should be carried out annually or semiannually to analyze the impact of improvements in information security, with possible improvements addressing identified critical points.

Although our focus is on the main concepts of aligning cybersecurity in telehealth, it should be noted that the construction of FCM allowed the identification of new concepts. In particular, the problem of image privacy of medical exam results can affect patients' integrity. Moreover, new concepts were included in the FCM, as they are rarely considered in security practice, which allowed it to be formalized in a way that contributed to reducing the variables omitted in the decision on cybersecurity.

The tools proposed by previous FCM literature were suitable for the cybersecurity scenario due to the ability to capture the ICT experts' knowledge by modeling dynamic simulation systems and improving support against cyberattacks. COVID-19 has dramatically impacted telehealth functionality and required adaptation in coping with circumstances that continued to change relative to safety measures, limiting customer interactions and reducing employee availability. The COVID-19 pandemic has generated remarkable and unique societal and economic events leveraged by cyber-criminals. Our analysis of telehealth has shown the causes of cybersecurity in telehealth services.

With many new perspectives brought by the current pandemic, we believe this new paradigm for cybersecurity in telehealth also came to stay in the post-pandemic (hopefully) new future. FCMs can be adjusted according to iterative scenarios to support accurate decision-making representing subjectivity in the business model of healthcare units. In addition, it can increase the transparency of analyses, including information hidden to IT managers. The post-pandemic is an important consideration to accommodate many legal aspects generated during the pandemic, specially related to the computerization of various services or intensification of current computerized services, as it is the case with telehealth. Therefore, this kind of application is essential for helping hospital managers concerned with the maintenance of telemedicine services during the planning phases, which are not limited to the pandemic context.

It is worth noting that telemedicine has become an efficient and effective way to develop the necessary care in a critical period such as the COVID-19 pandemic, avoiding hospital overload with high demands of patients seeking care, and avoiding contamination by the disease amidst clusters of people. Our perception leads us to believe that cybersecurity measures in telehealth systems have entered as mandatory components in ICT planning for hospital institutions, ensuring the security of patient information and ensuring that services continue to run without interruptions and external interference, such as hacker attacks. The FCMs are a helpful instrument for university hospital managers concerned with the maintenance of their telemedicine services, and regardless of the pandemic context, they deserve to be applied in the associated planning phase.

Therefore, the added value of using FCMs in cybersecurity in telemedicine is none other than supporting the planning of strategies to combat security breaches, always preventing sensitive and sensitive patient information from being accessed or intercepted by inappropriate persons. In the planning practice, it is a new tool for managers to use, in the planning practice, helping in their decisions about actions to avoid or correct security problems.

Future work should aggregate other methods to assist ICT managers in deciding upon actions such as using fuzzy sets theory to translate the judgments of health units' managers into crisp values for an accurate support that can minimize cybersecurity problems in telehealth [63], and combining multicriteria methods with other operational methodologies for conflict resolution, resource management and risk assessment in telemedicine [53,55,64]. More specifically, the research leading to this article, for the time being, has implications for the construction and improvement of a framework aimed at identifying risks associated with cybersecurity in telemedicine, carrying out tests for its validation in Brazilian university hospitals.

Concerning the continuation of this research, it is possible to define the need to assess how university hospitals, in a study of multiple cases, are prepared to deal with cybersecurity threats, clarifying what the main strategies adopted are, in addition to how the planning process is developed for these strategies, gathering data with a set of these hospitals. Another indication is the development of a meta-analysis study comparing quantitative results of other works containing methods applied with the same purpose as the one applied in this study, helping mainly to determine which methods are most suitable to support the planning process in cybersecurity in telehealth.

For these two last indications of further research, as we did not aimed at evaluating a general context for cybersecurity, and evaluating the performance of many different healthcare institutions to know how well they are in preparing to face telehealth cybersecurity threats, they are beyond of the scope of our current application. Therefore, these limitations can be addressed in future extensions of the current analysis.

Author Contributions: Conceptualization, T.P., V.D.H.d.C., and A.L.B.d.S.; methodology, A.P.H.d.G. and T.R.N.C.; software, A.L.B.d.S.; validation, T.P., V.D.H.d.C., and T.C.C.N.; formal analysis, M.M.S. and T.R.N.C.; writing—review and editing, T.C.C.N. and V.D.H.d.C.; visualization, A.P.C.S.C. and T.R.N.C.; project administration, T.P., V.D.H.d.C., and A.L.B.d.S.; funding acquisition, T.P. All authors have read and agreed to the published version of the manuscript.

Funding: This research received no external funding.

Institutional Review Board Statement: Not applicable.

Informed Consent Statement: Not applicable.

Data Availability Statement: The data presented in this study are available on request from the corresponding author.

Acknowledgments: This research was partially supported by the Universidade Federal do Pará (PROPESP/UFPA), the Universidade Federal de Alagoas (UFAL), the Universidade Federal de Pernambuco (UFPE), and the Grupo de Pesquisa em Sistemas de Informação e Decisão (GPSID). The authors would like to acknowledge the Coordenação de Aperfeiçoamento de Pessoal de Nível Superior—Brazil (CAPES) and the Conselho Nacional de Desenvolvimento Científico e Tecnológico—Brazil (CNPq) for their financial support.

Conflicts of Interest: The authors declare no conflict of interest.

References

1. Bernardes, A.C.F.; Coimbra, L.C.; Serra, H.O. Utilização do Programa Telessaúde no Maranhão como ferramenta para apoiar a Educação Permanente em Saúde. *Rev. Panam. Salud Públ.* **2018**, *42*, 1–9. [CrossRef]
2. Nepomuceno, T.C.C.; Silva, W.M.N.; Nepomuceno, T.C.; Barros, I.K.F. A DEA-Based Complexity of Needs Approach for Hospital Beds Evacuation during the COVID-19 Outbreak. *J. Healthc. Eng.* **2020**, *2020*, 1–9. [CrossRef]
3. Woods, D.W.; Moore, T. Does Insurance Have a Future in Governing Cybersecurity? *IEEE Secur. Priv.* **2020**, *18*, 21–27. [CrossRef]
4. Sokol, R.; Suter, S.; Pierce, B.; Council, L.; Grossman, E.; Roland, L.; Roll, D.; Mintzer, E. A novel transition: Lessons learned during rapid implementation and evolution of telehealth group based opioid treatment (t-GBOT) during the COVID-19 pandemic. *Healthcare* **2021**, *9*, 100559. [CrossRef]
5. Maldonado, J.M.S.d.V.; Marques, A.B.; Cruz, A. Telemedicine: Challenges to dissemination in Brazil. *Cad. Saude Publ.* **2016**, *32*, 1–11. [CrossRef]
6. Kruse, C.S.; Krowski, N.; Rodriguez, B.; Tran, L.; Vela, J.; Brooks, M. Telehealth and patient satisfaction: A systematic review and narrative analysis. *BMJ Open* **2017**, *7*, e016242. [CrossRef]
7. Rubio, J.E.; Alcaraz, C.; Roman, R.; Lopez, J. Current cyber-defense trends in industrial control systems. *Comput. Secur.* **2019**, *87*, 101561. [CrossRef]
8. Sittig, D.F.; Belmont, E.; Singh, H. Improving the safety of health information technology requires shared responsibility: It is time we all step up. *Healthcare* **2018**, *6*, 7–12. [CrossRef] [PubMed]
9. Ahmed, Y.; Naqvi, S.; Josephs, M. Cybersecurity Metrics for Enhanced Protection of Healthcare IT Systems. In Proceedings of the 2019 13th International Symposium on Medical Information and Communication Technology (ISMICT), Olso, Norway, 8–10 May 2019; pp. 1–9.
10. Zhou, L.; Thieret, R.; Watzlaf, V.; DeAlmeida, D.; Parmanto, B. A Telehealth Privacy and Security Self-Assessment Questionnaire for Telehealth Providers: Development and Validation. *Int. J. Telerehabil.* **2019**, *11*, 3–14. [CrossRef]
11. Alami, H.; Gagnon, M.; Ali, M.; Ahmed, A.; Fortin, J. Digital health: Cybersecurity is a value creation lever, not only a source of expenditure. *Health Policy Technol.* **2019**, *8*, 319–321. [CrossRef]
12. Mendonça Silva, M.; Poleto, T.; Silva, L.C.E.; Henriques De Gusmao, A.P.; Cabral Seixas Costa, A.P. A grey theory based approach to big data risk management using FMEA. *Math. Probl. Eng.* **2016**, *2016*, 1–15. [CrossRef]
13. De Gusmão, A.P.H.; Silva, E.L.C.; Silva, M.M.; Poleto, T.; Costa, A.P.C.S. Information security risk analysis model using fuzzy decision theory. *Int. J. Inf. Manag.* **2016**, *36*, 25–34. [CrossRef]
14. Silva, M.M.; De Gusmão, A.P.H.; Poleto, T.; Silva, L.C.E.; Costa, A.P.C.S. A multidimensional approach to information security risk management using FMEA and fuzzy theory. *Int. J. Inf. Manag.* **2014**, *34*, 733–740. [CrossRef]
15. De Gusmão, A.P.H.; Silva, M.M.; Poleto, T.; Silva, L.C.; Costa, A.P.C.S. Cybersecurity risk analysis model using fault tree analysis and fuzzy decision theory. *Int. J. Inf. Manag.* **2018**, *43*, 248–260. [CrossRef]
16. Sun, Q.; Zhang, K.; Shi, Y. Resilient Model Predictive Control of Cyber–Physical Systems Under DoS Attacks. *IEEE Trans. Ind. Inform.* **2020**, *16*, 4920–4927. [CrossRef]
17. Nifakos, S.; Chandramouli, K.; Nikolaou, C.K.; Papachristou, P.; Koch, S.; Panaousis, E.; Bonacina, S. Influence of human factors on cyber security within healthcare organisations: A systematic review. *Sensors* **2021**, *21*, 5119. [CrossRef] [PubMed]
18. Zain, J.; Clarke, M. Security in telemedine: Issues in watermarking medical images. In Proceedings of the 3rd International Conference: Sciences of Electronic, Technologies of Information and Telecommunications, Susa, Tunisia, 27–31 March 2005.

19. Faragallah, O.S.; Afifi, A.; El-Shafai, W.; El-Sayed, H.S.; Naeem, E.A.; Alzain, M.A.; Al-Amri, J.F.; Soh, B.; El-Samie, F.E.A. Investigation of Chaotic Image Encryption in Spatial and FrFT Domains for Cybersecurity Applications. *IEEE Access* **2020**, *8*, 42491–42503. [CrossRef]
20. Lim, E.Y.S. Data Security and Protection for Medical Images. In *Biomedical Information Technology*; Elsevier: Amsterdam, The Netherlands, 2008; pp. 249–257.
21. Andriole, K.P. Security of electronic medical information and patient privacy: What you need to know. *J. Am. Coll. Radiol.* **2014**, *11*, 1212–1216. [CrossRef]
22. Nagasubramanian, G.; Sakthivel, R.K.; Patan, R.; Gandomi, A.H.; Sankayya, M.; Balusamy, B. Securing e-health records using keyless signature infrastructure blockchain technology in the cloud. *Neural Comput. Appl.* **2018**, 639–647. [CrossRef]
23. Poleto, T.; Silva, M.M.; Clemente, T.R.N.; de Gusmão, A.P.H.; Araújo, A.P.d.B.; Costa, A.P.C.S. A Risk Assessment Framework Proposal Based on Bow-Tie Analysis for Medical Image Diagnosis Sharing within Telemedicine. *Sensors* **2021**, *21*, 2426. [CrossRef]
24. Barney, J.B.; Hesterly, W.S. *Strategic Management and Competitive Advantage: Concepts and Cases*; Pearson: Essex, UK, 2015.
25. Kosko, B. Fuzzy cognitive maps. *Int. J. Man. Mach. Stud.* **1986**, *24*, 65–75. [CrossRef]
26. Tsadiras, A.K. Comparing the inference capabilities of binary, trivalent and sigmoid fuzzy cognitive maps. *Inf. Sci.* **2008**, *178*, 3880–3894. [CrossRef]
27. Kim, H.S.; Lee, K.C. Fuzzy implications of fuzzy cognitive map with emphasis on fuzzy causal relationship and fuzzy partially causal relationship. *Fuzzy Sets Syst.* **1998**, *97*, 303–313. [CrossRef]
28. Gray, S.; Zanre, E.; Gray, S. Fuzzy Cognitive Maps as Representations of Mental Models and Group Beliefs. In *Fuzzy Cognitive Maps for Applied Sciences and Engineering*; Springer: Berlin/Heidelberg, Germany, 2014; pp. 29–48.
29. Park, J.W.; Lee, S.J. A quantitative assessment framework for cyber-attack scenarios on nuclear power plants using relative difficulty and consequence. *Ann. Nucl. Energy* **2020**, *142*, 107432. [CrossRef]
30. Hanafizadeh, P.; Ghamkhari, F. Elicitation of Tacit Knowledge Using Soft Systems Methodology. *Syst. Pract. Action Res.* **2019**, *32*, 521–555. [CrossRef]
31. Papageorgiou, E.I. Learning Algorithms for Fuzzy Cognitive Maps—A Review Study. *IEEE Trans. Syst. Man Cybern. Part C Appl. Rev.* **2012**, *42*, 150–163. [CrossRef]
32. Papageorgiou, E.I.; Subramanian, J.; Karmegam, A.; Papandrianos, N. A risk management model for familial breast cancer: A new application using Fuzzy Cognitive Map method. *Comput. Methods Programs Biomed.* **2015**, *122*, 123–135. [CrossRef]
33. Pogliani, M.; Quarta, D.; Polino, M.; Vittone, M.; Maggi, F.; Zanero, S. Security of controlled manufacturing systems in the connected factory: The case of industrial robots. *J. Comput. Virol. Hacking Tech.* **2019**, *15*, 161–175. [CrossRef]
34. Komporozos-Athanasiou, A. Information Technology Outsourcing in the Service Economy: Client maturity and knowledge/power asymmetries. In *Information Technology in the Service Economy: Challenges and Possibilities for the 21st Century*; Barrett, M., Davidson, E., Middleton, C., DeGross, J.I., Eds.; IFIP—The International Federation for Information Processing; Springer US: New York, NY, USA, 2008; Volume 267, pp. 301–310. ISBN 978-0-387-09767-1.
35. Panaousis, E.; Fielder, A.; Malacaria, P.; Hankin, C.; Smeraldi, F. Cybersecurity games and investments: A decision support approach. *Lect. Notes Comput. Sci. (Subser. Lect. Notes Artif. Intell. Lect. Notes Bioinform.)* **2014**, *8840*, 266–286. [CrossRef]
36. Dondossola, G.; Garrone, F.; Szanto, J. Cyber risk assessment of power control systems—A metrics weighed by attack experiments. In Proceedings of the IEEE Power Energy Society General Meeting, Detroit, MI, USA, 24–28 July 2011; pp. 1–9. [CrossRef]
37. Alshaikh, M. Developing cybersecurity culture to influence employee behavior: A practice perspective. *Comput. Secur.* **2020**, *98*, 1–10. [CrossRef]
38. Adepu, S.; Kandasamy, N.K.; Zhou, J.; Mathur, A. Attacks on smart grid: Power supply interruption and malicious power generation. *Int. J. Inf. Secur.* **2020**, *19*, 189–211. [CrossRef]
39. Hu, G.; Xiao, D.; Xiang, T.; Bai, S.; Zhang, Y. A Compressive Sensing based privacy preserving outsourcing of image storage and identity authentication service in cloud. *Inf. Sci.* **2017**, *387*, 132–145. [CrossRef]
40. Wang, P.; Govindarasu, M. Cyber-Physical Anomaly Detection for Power Grid with Machine Learning. In *Industrial Control Systems Security and Resiliency*; Springer: Berlin/Heidelberg, Germany, 2019; pp. 31–49.
41. Lu, N.; Zhang, Y.; Shi, W.; Kumari, S.; Choo, K.-K.R. A secure and scalable data integrity auditing scheme based on hyperledger fabric. *Comput. Secur.* **2020**, *92*, 101741. [CrossRef]
42. Namavar Jahromi, A.; Hashemi, S.; Dehghantanha, A.; Choo, K.-K.R.; Karimipour, H.; Newton, D.E.; Parizi, R.M. An improved two-hidden-layer extreme learning machine for malware hunting. *Comput. Secur.* **2020**, *89*, 101655. [CrossRef]
43. Butpheng, C.; Yeh, K.-H.; Xiong, H. Security and Privacy in IoT-Cloud-Based e-Health Systems—A Comprehensive Review. *Symmetry* **2020**, *12*, 1191. [CrossRef]
44. Xiang, Y.; Wang, L.; Liu, N. Coordinated attacks on electric power systems in a cyber-physical environment. *Electr. Power Syst. Res.* **2017**, *149*, 156–168. [CrossRef]
45. Zachrison, K.S.; Boggs, K.M.; Hayden, E.M.; Espinola, J.A.; Camargo, C.A. Understanding Barriers to Telemedicine Implementation in Rural Emergency Departments. *Ann. Emerg. Med.* **2020**, *75*, 392–399. [CrossRef]
46. Sturm, L.D.; Williams, C.B.; Camelio, J.A.; White, J.; Parker, R. Cyber-physical vulnerabilities in additive manufacturing systems: A case study attack on the STL file with human subjects. *J. Manuf. Syst.* **2017**, *44*, 154–164. [CrossRef]

47. Nepomuceno, T.C.C.; Nepomuceno, K.T.C.; Costa, A.P.C.S. Contractual Misincentives in the Outsourcing of Information Technology: A Principal-Agent Approach. In *Global Encyclopedia of Public Administration, Public Policy, and Governance*; Springer International Publishing: Cham, Switzerland, 2020; pp. 1–10.
48. Nepomuceno, T.C.C.; de Moura, J.A.; Costa, A.P.C.S. Modeling sequential bargains and personalities in democratic deliberation systems. *Kybernetes* 2018, *47*, 1906–1923. [CrossRef]
49. Wang, M.; Xu, B. Observer-based guaranteed cost control of Cyber-Physical Systems under DoS jamming attacks. *Eur. J. Control.* 2019, *48*, 21–29. [CrossRef]
50. Hong, J.; Liu, C.C.; Govindarasu, M. Integrated anomaly detection for cyber security of the substations. *IEEE Trans. Smart Grid* 2014, *5*, 1643–1653. [CrossRef]
51. Sivaprakash, A.; Rajan, S.N.E.; Selvaperumal, S. Privacy Protection of Patient Medical Images using Digital Watermarking Technique for E-healthcare System. *Curr. Med. Imaging Former. Curr. Med. Imaging Rev.* 2019, *15*, 802–809. [CrossRef]
52. Jalali, M.S.; Razak, S.; Gordon, W.; Perakslis, E.; Madnick, S. Health care and cybersecurity: Bibliometric analysis of the literature. *J. Med. Internet Res.* 2019, *21*, e12644. [CrossRef] [PubMed]
53. Nepomuceno, T.C.C.; Daraio, C.; Costa, A.P.C.S. Combining multi-criteria and directional distances to decompose non-compensatory measures of sustainable banking efficiency. *Appl. Econ. Lett.* 2020, *27*, 329–334. [CrossRef]
54. Poleto, T.; de Oliveira, R.C.P.; da Silva, A.L.B.; de Carvalho, V.D.H. Using Fuzzy Cognitive Map Approach for Assessing Cybersecurity for Telehealth Scenario. In *Trends and Innovations in Information Systems and Technologies, WorldCIST 2020, Proceedings of the Advances in Intelligent Systems and Computing, Budva, Montenegro, 7–10 April 2020*; Rocha, A., Adeli, H., Reis, L., Costanzo, S., Orovic, I., Moreira, F., Eds.; Springer: Berlin/Heidelberg, Germany, 2020; Volume 1160, pp. 828–837.
55. Koohang, A.; Nowak, A.; Paliszkiewicz, J.; Nord, J.H. Information Security Policy Compliance: Leadership, Trust, Role Values, and Awareness. *J. Comput. Inf. Syst.* 2020, *60*, 1–8. [CrossRef]
56. Alami, H.; Gagnon, M.-P.; Fortin, J.-P.; Kouri, R.P. La télémédecine au Québec: État de la situation des considérations légales, juridiques et déontologiques. *Eur. Res. Telemed./La Rech. Eur. Téléméd.* 2015, *4*, 33–43. [CrossRef]
57. Gaines, B.R. Knowledge acquisition: Past, present and future. *Int. J. Hum. Comput. Stud.* 2013, *71*, 135–156. [CrossRef]
58. Handayani, P.W.; Hidayanto, A.N.; Pinem, A.A.; Hapsari, I.C.; Sandhyaduhita, P.I.; Budi, I. Acceptance model of a Hospital Information System. *Int. J. Med. Inform.* 2017, *99*, 11–28. [CrossRef] [PubMed]
59. Bergström, E.; Lundgren, M.; Ericson, Å. Revisiting information security risk management challenges: A practice perspective. *Inf. Comput. Secur.* 2019, *27*, 358–372. [CrossRef]
60. Anninou, A.P.; Groumpos, P.P.; Polychronopoulos, P. Modeling health diseases using Competitive Fuzzy Cognitive Maps. In *Proceedings of the IFIP Advances in Information and Communication Technology*; Springer: Berlin/Heidelberg, Germany, 2013; Volume 412, pp. 88–95.
61. Mirghafoori, S.H.; Morovati Sharifabadi, A.; Karimi Takalo, S. Development of causal model of sustainable hospital supply chain management using the Intuitionistic Fuzzy Cognitive Map (IFCM) method. *J. Ind. Eng. Manag.* 2018, *11*, 588. [CrossRef]
62. Pérez-González, D.; Preciado, S.T.; Solana-Gonzalez, P. Organizational practices as antecedents of the information security management performance. *Inf. Technol. People* 2019, *32*, 1262–1275. [CrossRef]
63. de Carvalho, V.D.H.; Poleto, T.; Nepomuceno, T.C.C.; Costa, A.P.P.C.S. A study on relational factors in information technology outsourcing: Analyzing judgments of small and medium-sized supplying and contracting companies' managers. *J. Bus. Ind. Mark.* 2021. ahead of publishing. [CrossRef]
64. Papageorgiou, E.I.; Hatwágner, M.F.; Buruzs, A.; Kóczy, L.T. A concept reduction approach for fuzzy cognitive map models in decision making and management. *Neurocomputing* 2017, *232*, 16–33. [CrossRef]

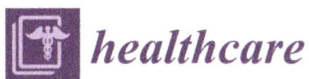

Article

Hospitals' Cybersecurity Culture during the COVID-19 Crisis

Anna Georgiadou [1,*], Ariadni Michalitsi-Psarrou [1], Fotios Gioulekas [2], Evangelos Stamatiadis [2], Athanasios Tzikas [2], Konstantinos Gounaris [2], Georgios Doukas [1], Christos Ntanos [1], Luís Landeiro Ribeiro [3] and Dimitris Askounis [1]

[1] Decision Support Systems Laboratory, National Technical University of Athens, Iroon Polytechniou 9, 15780 Athens, Greece; amichal@epu.ntua.gr (A.M.-P.); gdoukas@epu.ntua.gr (G.D.); cntanos@epu.ntua.gr (C.N.); askous@epu.ntua.gr (D.A.)
[2] 5th Regional Health Authority of Thessaly & Sterea, Mezourlo, 41110 Larissa, Greece; fogi@dypethessaly.gr (F.G.); vstam@dypethessaly.gr (E.S.); atzi@uhl.gr (A.T.); kgounaris@ghv.gr (K.G.)
[3] Projeto Desenvolvimento Manutenção Formação e Consultadoria-PDMFC, Rua Fradesso da Silveira n. 4, Piso 1 B, 1300-609 Lisbon, Portugal; luis.ribeiro@pdmfc.com
* Correspondence: ageorgiadou@epu.ntua.gr

Abstract: The coronavirus pandemic led to an unprecedented crisis affecting all aspects of the concurrent reality. Its consequences vary from political and societal to technical and economic. These side effects provided fertile ground for a noticeable cyber-crime increase targeting critical infrastructures and, more specifically, the health sector; the domain suffering the most during the pandemic. This paper aims to assess the cybersecurity culture readiness of hospitals' workforce during the COVID-19 crisis. Towards that end, a cybersecurity awareness webinar was held in December 2020 targeting Greek Healthcare Institutions. Concepts of cybersecurity policies, standards, best practices, and solutions were addressed. Its effectiveness was evaluated via a two-step procedure. Firstly, an anonymous questionnaire was distributed at the end of the webinar and voluntarily answered by attendees to assess the comprehension level of the presented cybersecurity aspects. Secondly, a post-evaluation phishing campaign was conducted approximately four months after the webinar, addressing non-medical employees. The main goal was to identify security awareness weaknesses and assist in drafting targeted assessment campaigns specifically tailored to the health domain needs. This paper analyses in detail the results of the aforementioned approaches while also outlining the lessons learned along with the future scientific routes deriving from this research.

Keywords: cybersecurity culture; COVID-19; security assessment; phishing; health domain

Citation: Georgiadou, A.; Michalitsi-Psarrou, A.; Gioulekas, F.; Stamatiadis, E.; Tzikas, A.; Gounaris, K.; Doukas, G.; Ntanos, C.; Landeiro Ribeiro, L.; Askounis, D. Hospitals' Cybersecurity Culture during the COVID-19 Crisis. *Healthcare* **2021**, *9*, 1335. https://doi.org/10.3390/healthcare9101335

Academic Editor: Daniele Giansanti

Received: 25 August 2021
Accepted: 1 October 2021
Published: 7 October 2021

Publisher's Note: MDPI stays neutral with regard to jurisdictional claims in published maps and institutional affiliations.

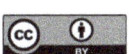

Copyright: © 2021 by the authors. Licensee MDPI, Basel, Switzerland. This article is an open access article distributed under the terms and conditions of the Creative Commons Attribution (CC BY) license (https://creativecommons.org/licenses/by/4.0/).

1. Introduction

Coronavirus disease 2019 (COVID-19) is an infectious disease caused by severe acute respiratory syndrome coronavirus 2 (SARS-CoV-2) [1]. It was originally identified in December 2019 in Wuhan [2], from where it spread worldwide, leading to a pandemic, as denoted by the World Health Organization (WHO), in March 2020 [3]. Since then, there have been 198,778,175 confirmed cases of COVID-19, including 4,235,559 casualties [4]. As of 14 June 2021, a total of 2,310,082,345 vaccine doses have been administered, attempting to armor humans against this virus.

Even though epidemiologists argue that the health crisis is close to being over, the same does not apply to its political, societal, economic, and technical side-effects. Special circumstances created by this extraordinary crisis led to what is known as the "Great Shutdown" or "Great Lockdown" [5–8], radically altering our daily reality. Digital transformation and adaptation were forced in almost all aspects of the business world. Remote working, commonly known as "tele-working" or "working from home", became a necessity even for sectors where it was considered prohibited up until now [9,10].

The accruing anxiety and generic crisis conditions provided a fertile ground for opportunistic criminals to act. A significant cyber-crime increase was denoted during the pandemic [11–13], with a noticeable preference towards the health sector [14–16]. Phishing, ransomware, and distributed denial-of-service attacks are only a sample of the reported cyber-crime incidents during the COVID-19 crisis [17–21].

Cybersecurity has been one of the emerging technological challenges of this century for the health domain [22], being among each country's critical infrastructures. Over the last years, extensive research has been conducted aiming to identify vulnerabilities and gaps in the cyber-resilience of hospitals and healthcare facilities [23–26]. Various assessment methodologies have been applied towards pinpointing mitigation techniques and cyber-defense strategies [27–32]. Yet, scientific contribution and professional evolution failed to protect the health sector during a crisis which dictated its devotion to its main purpose of curing patients and saving lives.

Most of the security agencies, organizations and experts worldwide have issued recommendations and proposed safeguard measures to assist individuals and corporations defend against cyber-crime [11,33–35]. Security officers have become aware of the great cybersecurity perils they are facing. Therefore, the vast majority of them has designed and conducted a series of security awareness training programs carefully trimmed to the needs and the busy schedule of their workforce.

This paper presents the effort made by the IT and security experts of European health representative organizations during the pandemic aiming to endorse the cybersecurity awareness of healthcare employees. Towards that end, a virtual workshop was designed and held on the 16 December 2020 in Greece [36]. The effectiveness of the security awareness training program was assessed in a two-phase evaluation: a questionnaire filled directly after the workshop voluntarily by the participants and a phishing campaign held four months later.

This paper presents our research approach on evaluating the security readiness of the healthcare personnel during the COVID-19 pandemic, based on a holistic cybersecurity culture framework. Section 2 offers background information related to both the framework and the participating health domain representatives. Section 3 unfolds our methodological approach using a sequential switching between training and assessment steps. In Section 4, we analyze our two-phase security evaluation while underlying important results. Section 5 collectively summarizes our key findings, whereas, in Section 6, we outline a number of considerations and limitations regarding the proposed methodology. Finally, Section 7 concludes our research presentation by outlining areas of further research and potential future applications.

2. Background
2.1. Cybersecurity Culture Framework

Cybersecurity Culture Framework was developed in the context of the EnergyShield [37], a European Union (EU) project targeting cybersecurity in the Electrical Power and Energy System (EPES). It was officially introduced in 2020 [38], presenting an evaluation and assessment methodology of both individuals' and organizations' security culture readiness. It is based on a combination of **organizational** and **individual** security factors structured into **dimensions** and **domains**. Its main goal is to examine organizational security policies and procedures in conjunction with employees' individual characteristics, behavior, attitude, and skills. Each security metric introduced by the framework is assessed using a variety of evaluation techniques, such as surveys, tests, simulations, and serious games.

The framework was later on correlated both with the hybrid MITRE ATT&CK Model for an OT Environment, consisted of a combination of the Enterprise and the ICS threat model [39] and with an enriched version of the Management and Education of the Risk of Insider Threat (MERIT) model [40], developed by the Secret Service and the Software Engineering Institute CERT Program at Carnegie Mellon University. Research related to both scientific directions focused on mapping the end-users' socio-cultural behavior to specific cyber-threats.

During the COVID-19 crisis, the aforementioned framework was used to design a cybersecurity culture assessment campaign targeting critical infrastructures [41]. Its revealing findings [42] provided significant feedback to the participating EU organizations. Insights and recommendations towards enforcing their cybersecurity resilience were offered, further contributing to this research domain.

This scientific effort inspired SPHINX, an EU project aiming to enhance the cyber protection of the Health and Care IT Ecosystem [43], and triggered a collaboration activity with EnergyShield. The following paragraph presents how the cybersecurity culture framework assisted SPHINX security specialists in the design of a two-phase security awareness campaign targeting health sector personnel.

2.2. Cybersecurity Assessment

Approximately two months prior to the global outbreak of the COVID-19 crisis, a cybersecurity awareness assessment was conducted among Greek, Portuguese, and Romanian healthcare employees [44] in the context of the SPHINX EU Project. The findings on the IT workforce, doctors, nurses, auxiliary staff, laboratory personnel and administrative clerks indicated the necessity of performing targeted training and campaigns to mitigate the increasing number of phishing and fraud attacks and fortify hospital assets.

More specifically, the result analysis revealed that limited investment had been made in cybersecurity appliances procurement, software upgrades and hardware. Although an individual cybersecurity unit was not fully deployed in the surveyed organizations, all IT departments had firewalls, antivirus solutions, as well as backup mechanisms. Furthermore, it was noticed that the IT departments did not regularly keep log files of cybersecurity-related events or login actions. Cybersecurity-related key performance indicators (KPIs) were not being monitored. Notwithstanding, the IT workforce reported that penetration tests or associated training on cybersecurity concepts had not been conducted to assist them in reaching a higher level of readiness.

Additionally, a significant percentage of the non-IT staff stated that they were unaware of information security policies, albeit they could comprehend when a computer was hacked or infected and knew whom to contact. Moreover, many of them reported that they did not know what an email fraud is or how to identify it. Most importantly, the vast majority considered that organizational security policies would help improve their own work while indicating the necessity to attend sufficient cybersecurity training programs and/or general data protection regulation (GDPR) [45] seminars targeted exclusively to the operations of their healthcare institution.

Within this context, the SPHINX consortium defined and organized specific training activities and awareness webinars to increase the level of cybersecurity. To this end, apart from the dissemination of information material to the healthcare organizations with important indications and cybersecurity alerts, a webinar was explicitly designed and held to improve the cybersecurity skills of the IT employees during the COVID-19 period. The webinar took place in Greece, presenting state-of-the-art security practices, methods, tools, and standards to the healthcare environments. The cybersecurity culture framework, developed in the context of the EnergyShield project, was used to evaluate the effectiveness of the aforementioned training program, as presented in detail in the following paragraphs.

3. Methodology

In September 2019, a three-month cybersecurity awareness survey was held by the SPHINX consortium. After assessing 28 and 449 responses from IT and non-IT healthcare employees in Greek Healthcare Institutions [44], respectively, it was deduced that certain actions toward introducing advanced cybersecurity methods, tools, and standards were required. Therefore, an internal awareness campaign initiated by the IT departments to the rest of the healthcare staff was executed verbally or via dissemination actions. On the 16 December 2020, an IT-dedicated webinar took place [36]. The specific webinar's effectiveness was assessed via a two-step methodology: a questionnaire filled directly after its conclusion voluntarily by the attendees and a phishing campaign held from the 26 April 2021 until the 28 May 2021. The aforementioned methodological approach is being graphically represented in Figure 1.

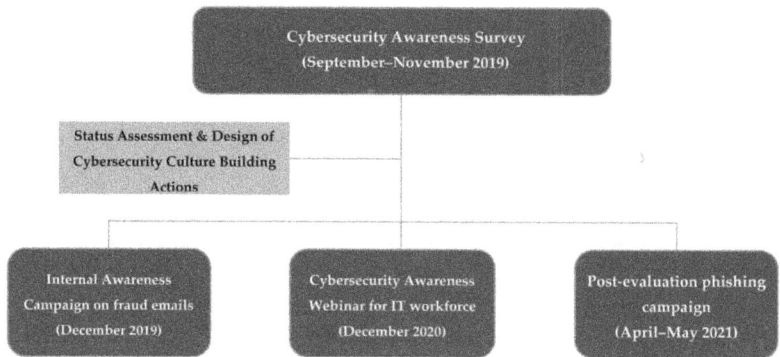

Figure 1. Cybersecurity Awareness Methodology.

3.1. Cybersecurity Awareness Campaign

As described in the previous paragraphs, an intensive awareness campaign through the IT departments of Greek Healthcare institutions was initiated, in December 2019, focusing on actions and precautions that each healthcare employee should undertake to protect the data they handle. A variety of communication means were employed, including:

1. A certified GDPR training program provided by the Greek National Centre of Public Administration and Local Government to public servants.
2. A flyer with important cybersecurity notes and indications which was distributed to all departments and clinics. In compliance with the Directive (EU) 2016/1148 of the European Parliament and of the Council of 6 July 2016 concerning measures for a high common level of network and information systems security across the Union, the flyer informed its readers that healthcare organizations have to comply with certain cybersecurity rules regarding their network and information systems. Consequently, the healthcare workforce was advised to:

- Change the access passwords frequently without disclosing them;
- Always keep backup of critical data (if possible);
- Avoid opening emails and following links from unknown senders without first checking the sender's emails;
- Never allow unauthorized third parties to use the organizations' workstations;
- Always lock their screens prior to leaving the office;
- Avoid plugging in a USB stick on the PCs without the approval of the IT department.

3.2. Cybersecurity Awareness Webinar

In December 2020, a cybersecurity awareness webinar was specifically designed trimmed to the needs of the Greek IT health domain departments. The webinar was made publicly available (upon registration) to every EU healthcare IT employee interested in participating. Instructors from the European Union Agency for Cybersecurity (ENISA), academic institutions and cybersecurity industry representatives from the SPHINX consortium were involved. The webinar presented aspects from ISO 27001 [46] as a path to the directive on security of network and information systems (NIS directive) compliance [47]. Moreover, it highlighted the key points to cybersecurity risk assessment in hospitals along with procurement guidelines for healthcare cybersecurity. Furthermore, various practical methods and techniques were presented to assist IT employees in their daily activities to control cybersecurity while topics in the state-of-the-art firewalls, antivirus configurations, backup mechanisms as part of the network topologies were covered.

After the webinar's conclusion, the participants were requested to respond to a questionnaire, voluntarily and anonymously, in order to measure the comprehension level of the concepts presented. The questionnaire included questions on demographics, information security and policies, network security and data management (Appendix A). From a total of 113 attendees from various EU countries and institutions, 62 were employed in Greek Hospitals' IT departments (approximately 30% of the total permanent IT workforce of Greek healthcare organizations in the public sector [48]), and 30 of them answered the optional questionnaire.

3.3. Phishing Awareness Campaign

Based on the 2020 HIMSS Healthcare Cybersecurity Survey, security incidents continue to plague healthcare organizations of all types and sizes, with phishing being the most common of all [49]. Phishing is a social engineering tactic that is used to persuade individuals to provide sensitive information. Malicious actors employ phishing techniques for a variety of reasons, including identity theft, access to proprietary information, transmission of malicious software to include ransomware, unauthorized remote access, and initiation of unauthorized financial transactions [50]. The most common form of phishing is the **phishing email** which usually attempts to appeal to a recipient's fear, duty, obligation, curiosity, or greed [51].

In late January 2020, Coronavirus-themed Emotet spam campaigns were reported, primarily targeting Japanese entities [52,53]. From January to April 2020, Interpol detected about 907,000 spam messages tied to COVID-19 [54]. During April 2020, Google reportedly blocked more than 18 million malware and phishing emails related to COVID-19 and in addition to more than 240 million COVID-related daily spam messages [55].

Consequently, and as a final methodological step, a cybersecurity culture assessment campaign was sketched aiming to post-evaluate the health domain's workforce familiarity with phishing email techniques in specific. Recent research shows a statistically significant positive correlation between workload and the probability of health care staff opening a phishing email [28]. Therefore, we decided to create a phishing quiz, instead of a simple questionnaire, including several different phishing emails. Its duration needed to be short to ensure the commitment and concentration of the participants given their extremely heavy workload and resulting fatigue.

A phishing simulation exercise–where the participants would receive a phishing email without prior knowledge, containing a link they should not click on-could have been a more realistic approach towards evaluating the actual workforce behavior given the concurrent circumstances. Yet, such an approach was rejected by the collaborating IT experts after extensive discussions. One of the main reasons was that such an evaluation exercise would suggest a significant effort in altering the configuration of the existing security solutions in place to allow those "phishing" emails to reach their targeted participants. Moreover, participants needed to be informed and consent to become part of this security evaluation campaign. Due to the psychologically and emotionally demanding period of the COVID-19 pandemic, it was agreed that most people would willingly take a short quiz initiated on-demand and in their time of choice rather than accept to be evaluated via a simulation test performed over a specific period of time. The latter would significantly increase the evaluation stress and, therefore, decrease the participation rate.

Phishing emails that were either blocked by the deployed antispam solutions or communicated to the IT departments by the healthcare recipients and processed accordingly based on the applied security protocols have been gathered by SPHINX security experts and collaboratively examined for similarities and differences. After a number of evaluation sessions, they concluded with the five emails presented in Table 1.

The specific survey targeted hospitals' workforce during the COVID-19 crisis. A significant percentage of the IT staff, technicians and administrative clerks exercised teleworking due to the COVID-19 restrictions opposite to the medical, nursing and laboratory personnel that had no such alternative. Therefore, our main goal was to evaluate the familiarity of non-medical personnel with phishing email techniques and assess their readiness while in teleworking conditions and following previous cybersecurity training and familiarity campaigns (Table 2).

Table 1. Emails Used in The Evaluation Campaign.

ID	Description	Phishing	Legit
Email I	X Bank asking recipients to protect their accounts by following a specific hyperlink.	✓	
Email II	Unknown sender blackmailing recipients asking for ransom in Bitcoin in order not to reveal personal videos recorded via their hacked workstation cameras.	✓	
Email III	Y Bank asking recipients to protect their accounts by following a specific hyperlink.	✓	
Email IV	An email supposedly sent by the IT department asking for account verification to avoid inactivation.	✓	
Email V	An email related to the Ministry of Internal Affairs deriving from the repository of public expenditures.		✓

Table 2. Groups of Users Participating in The Evaluation Campaign.

	IT	Technicians	Clerks
Institution A	group01 (user01–user03)		
Institution B	group02 (user04–user06)	group03 (user07–user09)	group04 (user10–user23)
Institution C	group05 (user24–user28)	group06 (user29–user36)	group07 (user37–user50)

IT: employees working in the information technology department; technicians: employees working in the electro-mechanical and biomedical departments; clerks: employees working in the accounting, finance, and procurement departments.

A special invitation email was sent to the selected participants providing a connection link and appropriate authentication credentials. Each participant was able to complete only once the phishing quiz, with no time limitations, and had to provide an answer to each one of the emails included in the campaign. Both the invitation email and the phishing quiz were localized, ensuring proximity, and lifting language barriers usually introduced to such evaluations.

The campaign was available for participation for almost a month, starting from 26 April 2021 and ending on 28 May 2021. During that period, all 50 invited participants completed the phishing quiz anonymously, thus, achieving 100% participation rate. Participation rate varied based on the hospitals' patient capacity concluding to a 54% from Institution A, 40% from Institution B and 6% from Institution C. More specifically, 56% of the participants were clerks, 22% were IT professionals, and 22% were technicians (as presented in Figure 2).

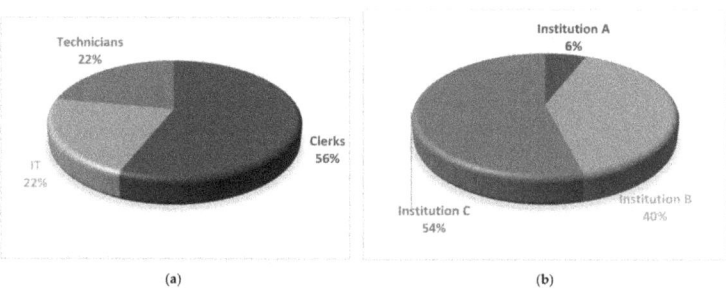

Figure 2. Campaign General Participation Information: (a) Expertise, (b) Healthcare Institution.

4. Detailed Assessment Results

4.1. Cybersecurity Awareness Webinar Results Analysis

Immediately after the conclusion of the cybersecurity awareness webinar, participants were asked to complete a questionnaire (presented in Appendix A) voluntarily and anonymously. Based on its results Table 3, 56.7% of the participants were aged between 40–49 years old, while 43.3% were female. Moreover, 56.7% held an MSc, while 80.0% had more than ten years of working experience in the field of healthcare IT. Around 70.0% were employed in hospitals, and 33.3% held managerial positions, while 36.7% worked for healthcare institutions that employ more than 1201 healthcare professionals.

Table 3. Demographics of Workshop Participants That Answered the Questionnaire.

Category	Participants
Total	$n = 30$ (100%)
Gender	
Male	17 (56.7%)
Female	13 (43.3%)
Age	
20–29	2 (6.7%)
30–39	6 (20.0%)
40–49	17 (56.7%)
50–59	5 (16.7%)
Education	
Secondary Education	2 (6.7%)
Bachelor's degree	7 (23.3%)
MSc	17 (56.7%)
PhD	4 (13.3%)
Years of Experience	
0–5	5 (16.7%)
6-10	1 (3.3%)
> 10	24 (80.0 %)
Position	
ICT staff	12 (40.0%)
ICT manager	10 (33.3%)
ICT director	3 (10.0%)
Other	5 (16.7%)
Organization	
Hospital	21 (70.0%)
Health Authority	3 (10.0%)
Other	6 (20.0%)
Number of Employees in your Organization	
<100	4 (13.3%)
100–300	2 (6.7%)
301–600	7 (23.3%)
601–1000	3 (10.0%)
1001–1200	3 (10.0%)
>1201	11 (36.7%)

ICT: Internet and Communication Technologies.

Figure 3 presents the questionnaire results associated with information security and policies. More specifically, 90% responded correctly that Health Insurance Portability and Accountability Act (HIPAA) [56] and ISO/IEC 27799 (Health informatics—Information security management in health using ISO/IEC 27002) [57] standards are those they should be aware of, while the rest of the participants (10%) answered incorrectly that COBIT and ITIL or PCI/DSS and SOX should be taken into consideration. Furthermore, in the question related to the resources' allocation towards the discovery of cybersecurity events, 77% replied correctly that resources should be exclusively allocated to this task, while 23% considered that it would be better to allocate these resources elsewhere or that resources should be allocated based on the availability of an IT team. A total of 67% of the responders correctly stated that a vulnerability management plan that includes, among others, scanning for patch levels, functions, ports, protocols, and services could support risk assessment in comparison to 33% that replied negatively or were unaware. Only 37% replied correctly that the assessment scale for the impact and the likelihood could not only vary between the values one and ten, while 63% replied either positively or ignorant.

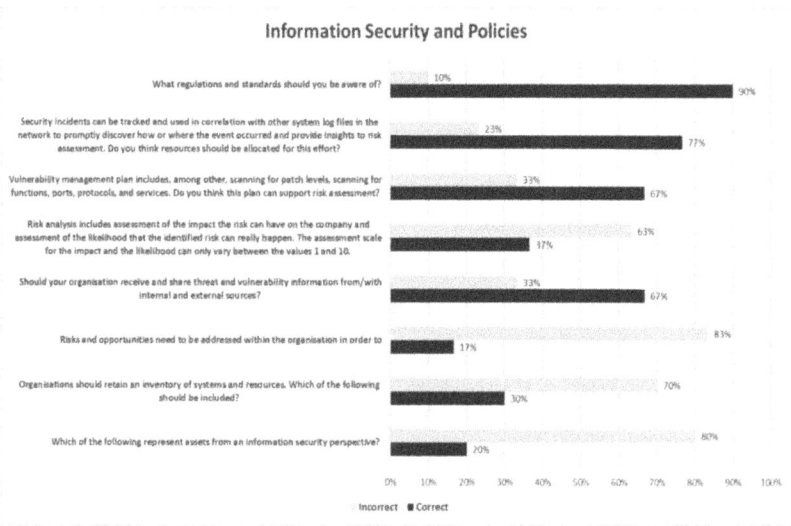

Figure 3. Evaluation of the Information Security and Policy Comprehension.

Around 67% answered correctly that it was necessary for their organization to receive and share threat and vulnerability information from/with internal and external sources. Regarding the multiple answers question about the necessity to address risk and opportunities within their organization, only 17% responded that it was required to both prevent and reduce undesired effects and achieve continual improvement. The rest—83%, answered either partially or in combination with other alternatives. Only 30% replied correctly that every organization asset should be encompassed in the inventory of systems and resources, while 70% replied partially correctly to the question. Finally, 20% replied correctly that people, software, and paper-based information represented assets from an information security perspective. The rest—80%, responded only partially correctly or considered that unauthorized modification or low awareness of information security could be assets too.

Figure 4 collectively presents answers to questions associated with network security and data management. More specifically, this part of the questionnaire revealed that 53% of the participants prefer a standard password expiration policy at regular intervals, while 47% stated they prefer to change the default passwords and, thereafter, not asking end-users to change their passwords. A total of 83% of the responders considered that a centralized administration of virus control, such as distribution of signature updates, reporting, policy enforcement and vendor management, was important to their daily IT operations because it helped them do their work faster and real-time monitor their assets. On the other hand, 17% replied that they had manually installed antivirus software to their assets and consequently did not consider this an important security policy. The vast majority (87%)

recognized a flat network topology as a vulnerable architecture. Furthermore, from a CIA perspective (confidentiality, integrity, availability), 90% replied that regular backups and restoration tests ensured availability and reduction of the recovery time in restoring a system to operational mode. On the other hand, 10% stated ignorant or that only backups were important for availability, reducing the risk of losing data. Further, 73% responded correctly that the concept of reducing the attack surface involved segmentation of network zones, blocking of activities associated with vulnerabilities and combating malicious code. In addition, 27% replied partially correct by selecting only one from the aforementioned actions.

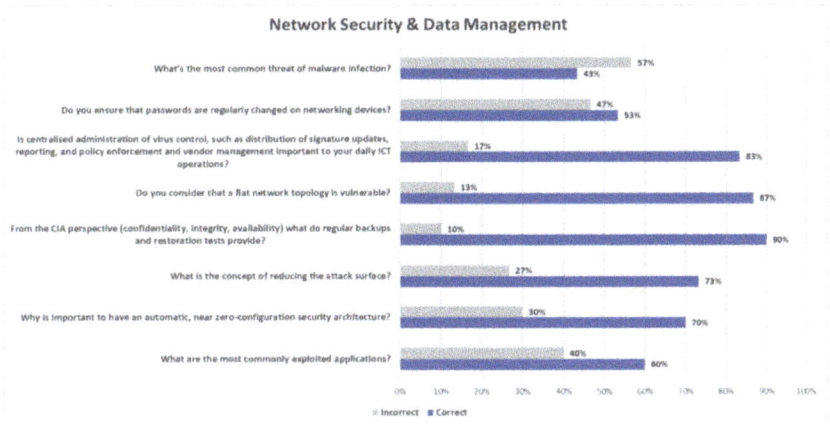

Figure 4. Evaluation of the Comprehension of Network Security and Data Management.

Furthermore, 70% answered that it was important to have an automatic, near zero-configuration security architecture because it reduced manual labor and human error, while 30% added incorrectly that it would also be cheaper and easier to implement. In addition, 60% replied correctly that the most commonly exploited application is the Office Suite, while the rest 40% reported either browsers, operating systems, JAVA or PDF files. Moreover, 43% stated correctly that Trojans were the most common threat of malware infection while the rest 57% answered adware, viruses, or potentially unwanted programs. When questioned if intrusion detection and intrusion prevention software was considered as one of the important components in edge security, 63% replied positively having active subscription while the rest 37% responded positively too without having an active subscription, considering though to procure it in the future.

4.2. Phishing Awareness Campaign Results Analysis

Based on the phishing quiz results, as presented in Figure 5, 1 out of 4 participants was able to distinguish a legit from a phishing email with a 100% success score. Only 10% of them did not manage to obtain a passing score since they only identified two out of five emails. Although such a score would be considered quite satisfying in many cases, the same does not apply to the cybersecurity reality where an organization is as strong as its weakest link.

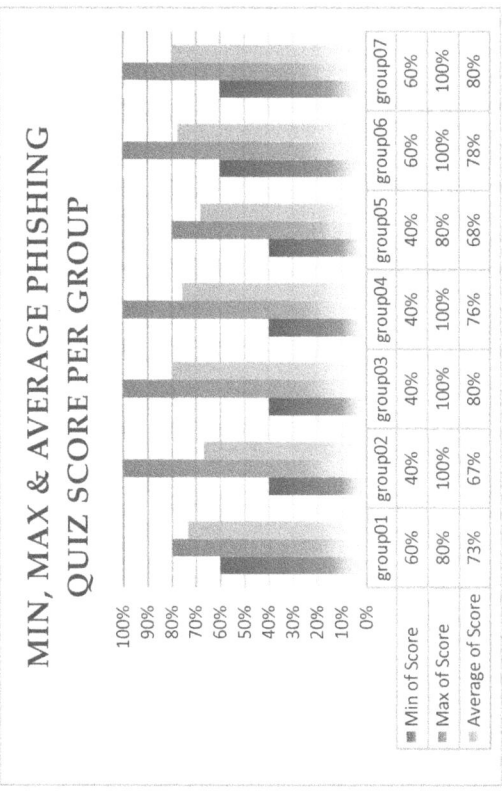

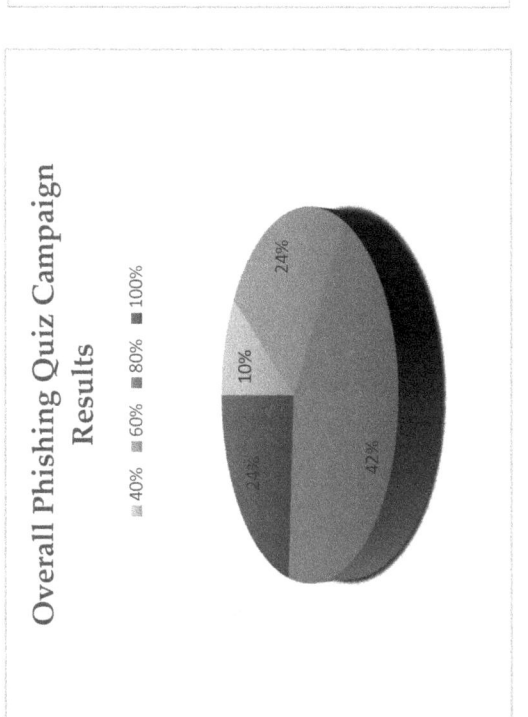

(a)

(b)

Figure 5. *Cont.*

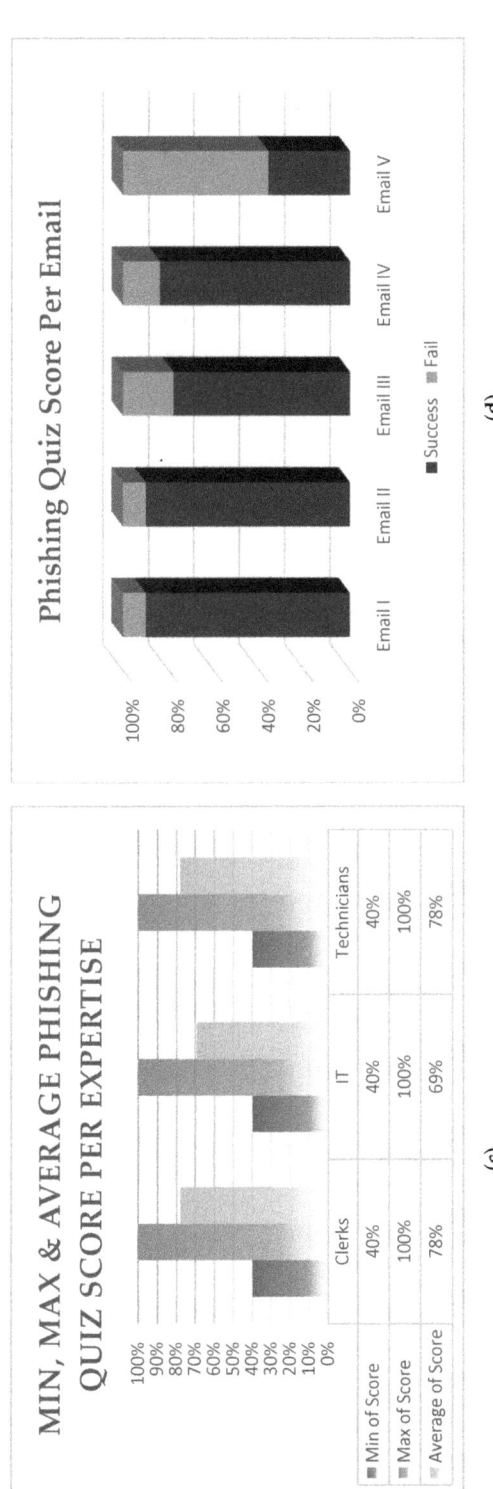

Figure 5. Campaign generic assessment results: (**a**) overall, (**b**) per group, (**c**) per expertise and (**d**) per email.

When examining the overall campaign's results from a group perspective, as depicted in Figure 5b, we notice that five out of seven groups managed to achieve a score higher than 70%. Probably, a disturbing observation, though, is that IT personnel appears to bear the lowest average in comparison with the rest of the groups, meaning the clerks and the technicians (Figure 5c). Due to the close correlation of the Information Technology and Information Security domains, a better cybersecurity awareness and phishing techniques' familiarity was expected of the IT experts.

Narrowing down to achievement scores per email, Emails I and II appear to have better phishing identification scores (higher than 80% by all participating groups), as presented in Figures 5d and 6. Interestingly, these two emails bear no similarities. The first one, as presented in Table 1, is related to a bank institution, containing an easily recognizable logo and seeking account verification by clicking on a hyperlinked text where a suspicious redirection is being hidden. The second one is quite long, containing only text and attempting to convince, using slang language, its recipients to pay an amount of ransom in Bitcoin in order not to reveal personal videos recorded via their hacked workstation cameras. Phishing techniques used in these two cases are quite different and usually aim at different target audiences. Email I have an appeal on a recipient's sense of duty and punctuality, whereas Email II on fear and uncertainty. Yet, hospital employees participating in this evaluation campaign managed in their majority to recognize both of them as not legit.

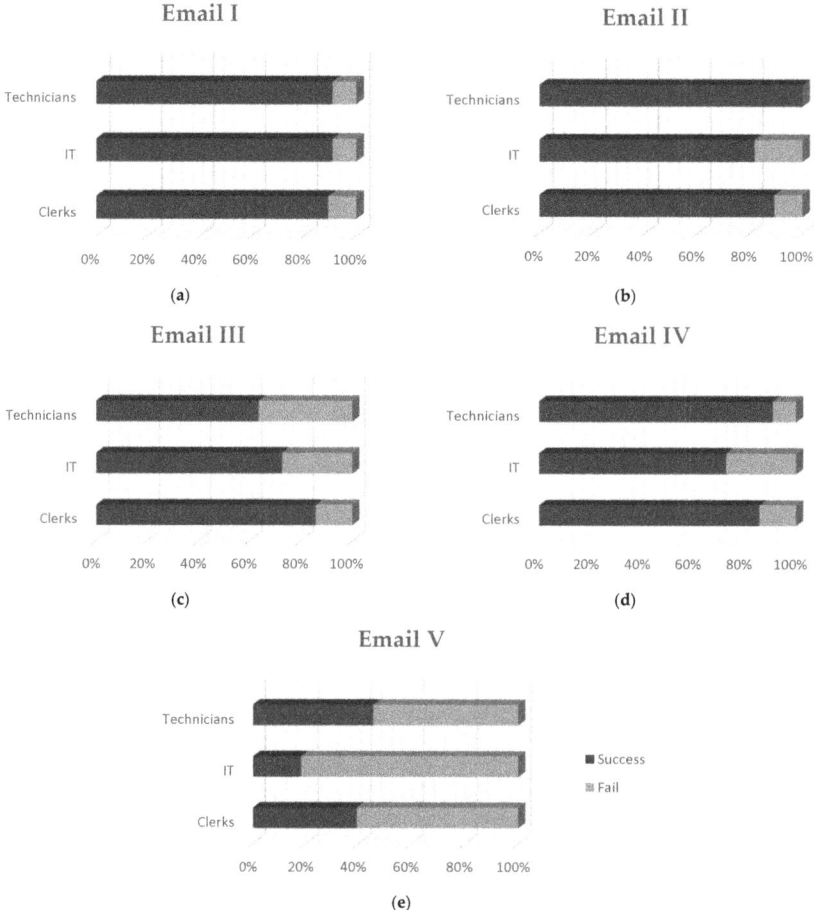

Figure 6. Campaign assessment results per expertise for: (**a**) email I, (**b**) email II, (**c**) email III, (**d**) email IV and (**e**) email V, of the phishing quiz.

One would expect that Email III would present similar results with Email I since, as presented in Table 1, they look alike. Email III is also related to a bank institution, containing its logo, seeking account verification by providing a hyperlink that is not hidden but instead is fully visible to its readers. Therefore, better results were anticipated since less effort was needed to locate the misleading redirection. Since it was the third entry in the phishing quiz, boredom and carelessness could be taking the lead from caution and reservedness explaining the degrading scores. However, such a conclusion would not agree with the results noticed for Email IV, as depicted in Figures 5d and 6, where scores are improved.

Last but not least, we notice that the majority of the participants (64%) failed to identify the only legit email included in the phishing quiz. The specific email was short (no more than 38 words), containing no images or logos, no special font formatting or email structures (e.g., tables). The word "here" was used to provide a hidden hyperlink (could be previewed when the user hovered over the word with the mouse) which could be easily acknowledged that it redirects to the legit Ministry of Internal Affairs website. Even though the specific result could be attributed to the increased cautiousness of the users due to the special circumstances of the crisis and the nature of the assessment, it remains quite disturbing. Legit emails might be forwarded for security analysis, rejected, or even deleted without communicating their context to their recipients due to them being erroneously identified as phishing attempts.

5. Key Findings

The analysis of the webinar's questionnaire showed that the IT departments comprehended sufficiently concepts such as standards' application to their policies and the incorporation of iterative risk assessment of their assets among their operations. Additionally, they exhibited high familiarity with the various network topologies and advanced cybersecurity tools. However, more emphasis should be given to focused training programs targeting risk assessment and data asset identification. It is deduced that healthcare IT employees are highly aware of cybersecurity concepts and how to protect their network and information systems.

Summing up the results of the targeted post-assessment campaign on phishing, the most apparent and at the same time unexpected observation is that the lowest average score is attributed to the IT professionals. They were expected to be the most qualified of the respondents and the ones apt to guide and advise the hospitals' personnel on their actions with respect to suspicious emails. However, these results came after a series of Emotet spam campaigns that affected their hospitals. These events can have reasonably sensitized their awareness and hardened their judgment. Indeed, the lowest score emerges for Email V where only 18% of the IT personnel identified successfully that that was a legit email (Figure 6). Although the above reasoning could adequately justify this result, it cannot be considered an explanation where no action is required. Behavioral awareness in cybersecurity calls for the right decisions where legit emails will reach their recipients and enjoy appropriate handling, while phishing emails will be immediately detected and rejected. Therefore, the results suggest that there is still room for dedicated training programs that should first—but not exclusively—target the hospitals' IT departments for them to be able to offer a robust first security layer and provide the right advice when requested. Besides, the great success of phishing emails in deceiving can be attributed to the fact that phishers become smarter [58]. Therefore, even the tech-savvy people can be deceived, while regular training can certainly shield an organization, as previous works suggest [59,60].

Another observation is that there is no notable difference among the three groups of IT personnel, technicians, and clerks, as indicated by both their average scores and the individual analysis, which would constitute the one better prepared than the others. We see two explanations that can be given to that. Firstly, in general, people tend to have difficulty relating to such a theoretical problem, which they believe will not happen to them [61]. Therefore, when receiving a new email, they do not invest the time and effort to question its intentions. Secondly, more tech-savvy people tend to be overconfident in their ability over others to identify fraud and mal-intent, which usually turns to be a naive perception [61].

Finally, the analysis results yielded no noteworthy differences among the three Greek healthcare institutions participating in the analysis. As depicted in Figure 7, the encouraging finding is that the lowest scores appear for all three hospitals for Email V, the only legit email of the phishing quiz. However, this finding should not remain unaddressed for the reasons explained previously. In general, advancing phishing email filters [62] in a way that would ensure that only the bare minimum of phishing emails and only rarely will remain undetected and surpass the filter would well safeguard the hospitals and take the weight of increased awareness off the employees' shoulders. Experience has shown, though, that a perfect phishing email filtering mechanism could not exist, and the recipients' cybersecurity awareness is the key to phishers' failure.

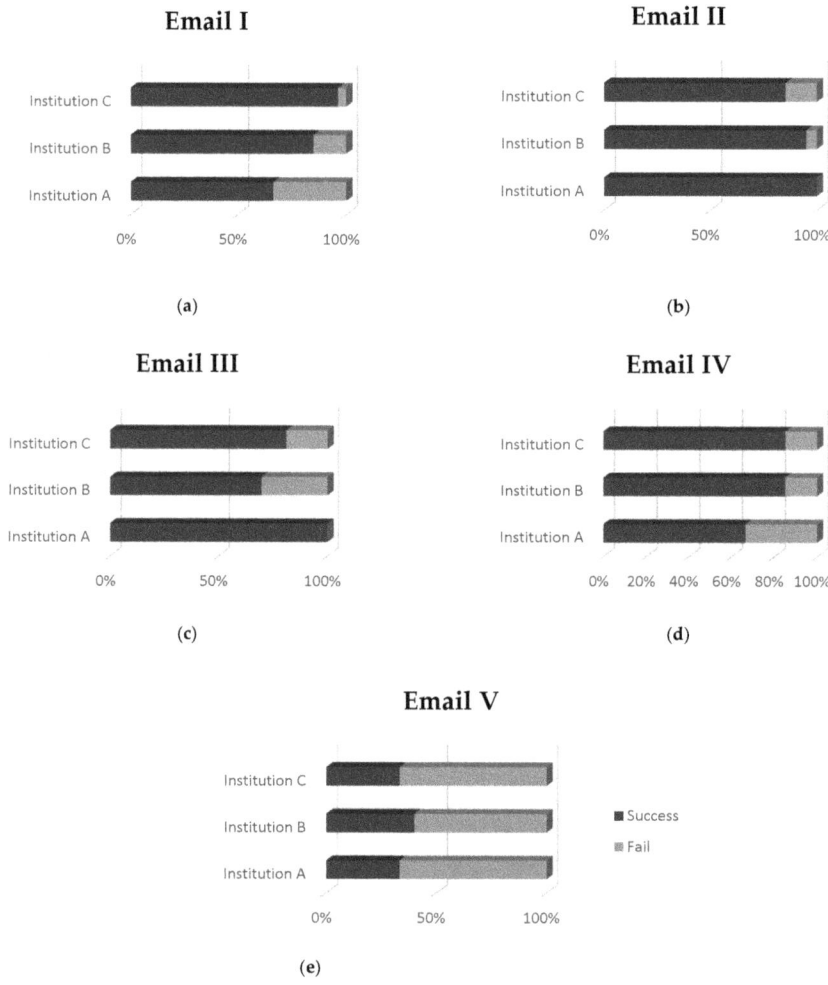

Figure 7. Campaign assessment results per hospital for: (**a**) email I, (**b**) email II, (**c**) email III, (**d**) email IV and (**e**) email V, of the phishing quiz.

6. Considerations and Limitations

The security awareness webinar and the post-evaluation phishing campaign were conducted during the COVID-19 crisis. Cyber-attacks against critical infrastructures were on the rise, while, on parallel, the health sector necessitated advanced cybersecurity protection mechanisms and enhanced security culture as this is introduced by an organization's human capital. In this context, we aimed at informing the hospitals' personnel regarding concurrent cybersecurity risks and mitigation strategies against them. We then evaluated their cybersecurity resilience using both a simplified questionnaire and a phishing campaign. The prioritization of the phishing quiz campaign against the other alternatives provided by the Cybersecurity Culture Framework presented in Section 2.1 was set by the IT and security experts of the participating hospitals, giving their alarming frequency. A phishing simulation exercise, which could also serve the same purpose, was rejected, after careful consideration, due to the extra effort required by the IT and security personnel to properly configure and by-pass the anti-spam solutions in place. Concerns related to ensuring a high participation rate without further disrupting or stressing participants were also in favor of the phishing quiz approach.

Due to COVID-19 and the profoundly heavy schedule of the medical staff, we decided not to engage them at this stage, which, of course, restricted the extent of our analysis and the application scope and generalizability of its findings. Our next steps involve engaging a fair sample of the medical staff of these three hospitals in the campaign when conditions permit it. This will allow a complete understanding of the hospitals' readiness concerning phishing attacks since staff from all key roles of the hospitals' operation will have been engaged.

Another limitation is the fact that the campaign was restricted in Greece; thus, not making possible the comparison of the cybersecurity culture in the health sector among countries in the EU or even globally. Furthermore, the selection of five emails (four of them not being legitimate) for the phishing quiz that the participants had to take might be considered small and not adequate for assessing one person and his security behavior. However, the engagement of a satisfactory number of the hospitals' staff in the campaign and their focus during the quiz's completion were the top priorities, susceptible to non-satisfaction if an enlarged, more complex quiz had been given. In parallel, these five emails were proven enough to highlight potential gaps and weaknesses in Greek hospitals' security culture and pinpoint new training routes.

7. Conclusions and Future Work

The current manuscript aimed to explore cybersecurity culture of the hospitals' personnel during the COVID-19 pandemic. A questionnaire examined participants' knowledge and familiarity with information security concepts, policies, procedures, and practices, while a phishing campaign focused on their attitude and behavior towards phishing techniques; probably the most disturbing security issue faced during the COVID-19 crisis. The assessment's design was based on a robust methodology, which is part of a broader context, the Cybersecurity Culture Framework presented in Section 2.1. Three Greek hospitals participated in the evaluation campaign with staff members belonging to one of the following three groups: IT professionals, technicians, and clerks.

In that view and given the previously identified considerations concerning the current work, our next steps involve extending the analysis in three levels: (a) participants' involvement and role in the hospital, (b) the examined security dimensions of the cybersecurity culture framework, and (c) the geographical coverage. Two new cybersecurity culture assessment campaigns are now planned, aiming after the first and second levels, respectively. In particular, the first campaign aims to continue the current phishing campaign involving more staff members, focusing on the medical staff, to allow a full overview of the participating hospitals' readiness concerning phishing attacks. The second campaign aims to involve and examine more security dimensions of the cybersecurity culture framework through an effective combination of questionnaires, tests, simulations, and serious games targeted to the background and needs of the health sector. This campaign will focus on selected personnel with key roles with respect to security in the participating hospitals. The extension of these campaigns to more countries will follow the completion of the objectives mentioned above.

Author Contributions: Conceptualization, A.G., A.M.-P. and F.G.; methodology, A.G., A.M.-P., F.G., E.S., A.T., K.G. and G.D.; software, A.G. and A.M.-P.; validation, F.G., E.S., A.T., K.G. and G.D.; formal analysis, A.G., A.M.-P. and F.G.; resources, A.M.-P., C.N., L.L.R. and D.A.; writing—original draft preparation, A.G., A.M.-P. and F.G.; writing—review and editing, A.G., A.M.-P. and F.G.; visualization, A.G., A.M.-P. and F.G.; supervision, A.M.-P., C.N., L.L.R. and D.A.; project administration, A.M.-P., C.N., L.L.R. and D.A.; funding acquisition, L.L.R. and D.A. All authors have read and agreed to the published version of the manuscript.

Funding: This research was funded by the European Union's Horizon 2020 Research and Innovation Programme, Grant Number 832907. Moreover, this work was funded by the SPHINX project that has received funding from the European Union's Horizon 2020 Research and Innovation Programme under Grant Agreement No. 826183 on Digital Society, Trust and Cyber Security E-Health, Well-being and Ageing.

Institutional Review Board Statement: Not applicable.

Informed Consent Statement: Not applicable.

Data Availability Statement: The data presented in this study are available on request from the corresponding author.

Acknowledgments: This project has received funding from the European Union's Horizon 2020 Research and Innovation Programme under Grant Agreements Nos. 832907 and 826183.

Conflicts of Interest: The authors declare no conflict of interest.

Appendix A

General Characteristics-Demographics

1. Country

    (Free Text)

2. Age

    20–29 ☐ 30–39 ☐ 40–49 ☐ 50–59 ☐ 60 + ☐

3. Gender

    Male ☐ Female ☐

4. Education

Secondary Education	☐
Vocational training Institution	☐
Bachelor's Degree	☐
MSc	☐
PhD	☐

5. Position

ICT director	☐
ICT manager	☐
ICT personnel	☐
Other	☐

6. Years of experience

6–10	☐
more than 10	☐

7. Organization

Hospital	☐
Clinic	☐
Health Authority	☐
National	☐
Regional	☐
Local	☐
Other	☐

8. Number of Employees in your Organization

Employees <100	☐
Employees 100–300	☐
Employees 301–600	☐
Employees 601–1000	☐
Employees 1001–1200	☐
Employees > 1201	☐

Information Security and Policies

9. Which of the following represent assets from an information security perspective?

People	☐
Unauthorized modification	☐
Software	☐
Low awareness of information security	☐
Paper-based information	☐

10. Organizations should retain an inventory of systems and resources. Which of the following should be included?

Every device, including computers, tablets, routers, printers, servers, and phones, on the network	☐
Only important network resources	☐
Information regarding connection types and data types	☐
Only network resources for which there is available information	☐
Information regarding the departments with access to systems, and their vendors	☐

11. Risks and opportunities need to be addressed within the organization in order to:

Demonstrate IT team readiness	☐
Prevent or reduce undesired effects	☐
Achieve continual improvement	☐

12. Ensure all employees are aware of the risks and opportunities ☐ Should your organization receive and share threat and vulnerability information from/with internal and external sources?

Yes	☐
No	☐
Don't Know	☐

13. Risk analysis includes assessment of the impact the risk can have on the company and assessment of the likelihood that the identified risk can really happen. The assessment scale for the impact and the likelihood can only vary between the values 1 and 10.

Yes	☐
No	☐
Don't Know	☐

14. Vulnerability management plan includes, among other, scanning for patch levels, scanning for functions, ports, protocols, and services. Do you think this plan can support risk assessment?

Yes	☐
No	☐
Don't Know	☐

15. Security incidents can be tracked and used in correlation with other system log files in the network to promptly discover how or where the event occurred and provide insights to risk assessment. Do you think resources should be allocated for this effort?

Yes, resources should be allocated exclusively for this purpose	☐
Yes, resources should be allocated based on the availability of ICT team	☐
No, it is better to allocate these resources elsewhere	☐
Don't Know	☐

16. What regulations and standards should you be aware of?

HIPAA and ISO/IEC 27799	☐
PCI/DSS and SOX	☐
COBIT and ITIL	☐

Network Security & Data Management

17. What's the most common threat of malware infection (select only one from the following)?

Trojans	☐
Potentially Unwanted Programs	☐
Viruses	☐
Adware	☐
Worms	☐

18. Do you consider Intrusion Detection / Intrusion Prevention Software as one of the important components in the edge security?–

Yes, and our department uses it with active subscription	☐
Yes, but our subscription has expired	☐
Yes, and we consider purchasing in the future	☐
No, it is not important	☐
Don't Know	☐

19. What are the most commonly exploited applications (select only one from the following)?

Operating systems, Win/Linux/MacOS	☐
Mobile Operating Systems, Android/IOS	☐
Browsers	☐
Office Suite	☐
Java	☐
Flash	☐
PDF	☐

20. From the CIA perspective (confidentiality, integrity, availability) what do regular backups and restoration tests provide?

Ensure availability and reduce the recovery time to restore a system back to operational mode	☐
Only Backups are important for availability, since they reduce the risk of losing all your data	☐
Don't Know	☐

21. Do you consider that a flat network topology is vulnerable?

22. Is centralized administration of virus control, such as distribution of signature updates, reporting, and policy enforcement and vendor management important to your daily ICT operations?

- No, and it is used to easily administrate the network ☐
- Yes, because once a node is breached it has access to every other one on the same network ☐
- Don't Know ☐

22. Is centralized administration of virus control, such as distribution of signature updates, reporting, and policy enforcement and vendor management important to your daily ICT operations?

- No, as soon as we have manually installed antivirus software to our assets ☐
- Yes, because it helps to do our work faster and real-time monitor our assets ☐
- Don't Know ☐

23. Do you ensure that passwords are regularly changed on networking devices?

- No, as soon as we have changed the default passwords ☐
- Yes, and we do this twice per year ☐
- Don't Know ☐

24. What is the concept of reducing the attack surface?

- Segment network zones ☐
- Block activities associated with vulnerabilities and combat malicious code ☐
- All of the above ☐

25. Why is important to have an automatic, near zero-configuration security architecture

- It reduces manual labor and human error ☐
- It will be cheaper and easier to implement ☐
- All of the above ☐

References

1. Velavan, T.P.; Meyer, C.G. The COVID-19 epidemic. *Trop. Med. Int. Health* **2020**, *25*, 278–280. [CrossRef] [PubMed]
2. Hui, D.S.; I Azhar, E.; Madani, T.A.; Ntoumi, F.; Kock, R.; Dar, O.; Ippolito, G.; Mchugh, T.D.; Memish, Z.A.; Drosten, C.; et al. The continuing 2019-nCoV epidemic threat of novel coronaviruses to global health—The latest 2019 novel coronavirus outbreak in Wuhan, China. *Int. J. Infect. Dis.* **2020**, *91*, 264–266. [CrossRef] [PubMed]
3. World Health Organization. In *WHO Director-General's Opening Remarks at the Media Briefing on COVID-19*; WHO: Geneva, Switzerland, 2020.
4. World Health Organization. WHO Coronavirus (COVID-19) Dashboard. Available online: https://covid19.who.int/ (accessed on 21 September 2021).
5. Talamàs, E. The Great Shutdown: Challenges and Opportunities. *Forbes*. 14 May 2020. Available online: https://www.forbes.com/sites/iese/2020/05/14/the-great-shutdown-challenges-and-opportunities/#60eaf6e86f12. (accessed on 7 July 2020).
6. Wolf, M. The World Economy is Now Collapsing. *Financial Times*. 14 April 2020. Available online: https://www.ft.com/content/d5f05b5c-7db8-11ea-8fdb-7ec06edeef84. (accessed on 1 July 2020).
7. International Labour Organization (ILO). *ILO Monitor:COVID-19 and the World of Work*, 2nd ed.; ILO: Geneva, Switzerland, 2020.
8. Gopinath, G. The Great Lockdown: Worst Economic Downturn Since the Great Depression. *IMFBlog*. 14 April 2020. Available online: https://blogs.imf.org/2020/04/14/the-great-lockdown-worst-economic-downturn-since-the-great-depression/ (accessed on 7 July 2020).
9. Bick, A.; Blandin, A.; Mertens, K. *Work from Home Before and after the Covid-19 Outbreak*; CEPR: San Antonio, TX, USA, 2020.
10. Dingel, J.I.; Neiman, B. How many jobs can be done at home? *J. Public Econ.* **2020**, *189*, 104235. [CrossRef]
11. INTERPOL. *COVID-19 Cyberthreats*; 2020; Available online: https://www.interpol.int/en/Crimes/Cybercrime/COVID-19-cyberthreats. (accessed on 7 July 2020).
12. Blanco, A.G. The Impact of COVID-19 on the Spread of Cybercrime. *BBVA*. 27 April 2020. Available online: https://www.bbva.com/en/the-impact-of-covid-19-on-the-spread-of-cybercrime/ (accessed on 7 July 2020).
13. Monster Cloud. Top Cyber Security Experts Report: 4000 Cyber Attacks a Day Since COVID-19 Pandemic. *PR Newswire*. 11 August 2020. Available online: https://www.prnewswire.com/news-releases/top-cyber-security-experts-report-4-000-cyber-attacks-a-day-since-covid-19-pandemic-301110157.html. (accessed on 17 June 2021).

14. He, Y.; Aliyu, A.; Evans, M.; Luo, C. Health Care Cybersecurity Challenges and Solutions Under the Climate of COVID-19: Scoping Review. *J. Med. Internet Res.* **2021**, *23*, e21747. [CrossRef]
15. Kim, L.J.D. Cybersecurity and related challenges during the COVID-19 pandemic. *Nursing* **2021**, *51*, 17–20. [CrossRef] [PubMed]
16. Lallie, H.S.; Shepherd, L.A.; Nurse, J.R.; Erola, A.; Epiphaniou, G.; Maple, C.; Bellekens, X. Cyber security in the age of COVID-19: A timeline and analysis of cyber-crime and cyber-attacks during the pandemic. *Comput. Secur.* **2021**, *105*, 102248. [CrossRef]
17. Stubbs, J.; Bing, C. Exclusive: Iran-Linked Hackers Recently Targeted Coronavirus Drugmaker Gilead—Sources. *REUTERS*. 8 May 2020. Available online: https://www.reuters.com/article/us-healthcare-coronavirus-gilead-iran-ex-idUSKBN22K2EV (accessed on 17 June 2021).
18. Stein, S.; Jacobs, J. Cyber-Attack Hits, U.S. Health Agency Amid Covid-19 Outbreak. *Bloomberg*. 16 March 2020. Available online: https://www.bloomberg.com/news/articles/2020-03-16/u-s-health-agency-suffers-cyber-attack-during-covid-19-response (accessed on 17 June 2021).
19. Cimpanu, C. Hackers Preparing to Launch Ransomware Attacks against Hospitals Arrested in Romania. *ZDNet*. 15 May 2020. Available online: https://www.zdnet.com/article/hackers-preparing-to-launch-ransomware-attacks-against-hospitals-arrested-in-romania/ (accessed on 17 June 2021).
20. INTERPOL. Cybercriminals Targeting Critical Healthcare Institutions with Ransomware. *INTERPOL*. 04 April 2020. Available online: https://www.interpol.int/en/News-and-Events/News/2020/Cybercriminals-targeting-critical-healthcare-institutions-with-ransomware/. (accessed on 17 June 2021).
21. National Cyber Security Center. Cyber Warning Issued for Key Healthcare Organisations in UK and USA. In *National Cyber Security Center*; 05 May 2020. Available online: https://www.ncsc.gov.uk/news/warning-issued-uk-usa-healthcare-organisations (accessed on 17 June 2021).
22. Giansanti, D. Cybersecurity and the Digital-Health: The Challenge of This Millennium. *Healthcare* **2021**, *9*, 62. [CrossRef]
23. Jalali, M.S.; Russell, B.; Razak, S.; Gordon, W.J. EARS to cyber incidents in health care. *J. Am. Med. Inform. Assoc.* **2019**, *26*, 81–90. [CrossRef] [PubMed]
24. Coventry, L.; Branley, D. Cybersecurity in healthcare: A narrative review of trends, threats and ways forward. *Maturitas* **2018**, *113*, 48–52. [CrossRef]
25. Argaw, S.T.; Troncoso-Pastoriza, J.R.; Lacey, D.; Florin, M.-V.; Calcavecchia, F.; Anderson, D.; Burleson, W.; Vogel, J.-M.; O'Leary, C.; Eshaya-Chauvin, B.; et al. Cybersecurity of Hospitals: Discussing the challenges and working towards mitigating the risks. *BMC Med. Inform. Decis. Mak.* **2020**, *20*, 146. [CrossRef] [PubMed]
26. Boddy, A.; Hurst, W.; Mackay, M.; El Rhalibi, A. A study into data analysis and visualisation to increase the cyber-resilience of healthcare infrastructures. In Proceedings of the 1st International Conference on Internet of Things and Machine Learning, New York, NY, USA, 17–18 October 2017. [CrossRef]
27. Gordon, W.J.; Wright, A.; Aiyagari, R.; Corbo, L.; Glynn, R.J.; Kadakia, J.; Kufahl, J.; Mazzone, C.; Noga, J.; Parkulo, M.; et al. Assessment of Employee Susceptibility to Phishing Attacks at US Health Care Institutions. *JAMA Netw. Open* **2019**, *2*, e190393. [CrossRef] [PubMed]
28. Jalali, M.S.; Bruckes, M.; Westmattelmann, D.; Schewe, G. Why Employees (Still) Click on Phishing Links: Investigation in Hospitals. *J. Med. Internet Res.* **2020**, *1*, e16775. [CrossRef] [PubMed]
29. Gebrasilase, T.; Lessa, L.F. Information Security Culture in Public Hospitals: The Case of Hawassa Referral Hospital. *Afr. J. Inf. Syst.* **2011**, *3*, 1.
30. Landolt, S.; Hirschel, J.; Schlienger, T.; Businger, W.; Zbinden, A.M. Assessing and Comparing Information Security in Swiss Hospitals. *Interact. J. Med. Res.* **2012**, *2*, e11. [CrossRef] [PubMed]
31. Luethi, M.; Knolmayer, G.F. Security in Health Information Systems: An Exploratory Comparison of U.S. and Swiss Hospitals. In Proceedings of the 42nd Hawaii International Conference on System Sciences, Washington, DC, USA, 5–8 January 2009.
32. Ferrag, M.A.; Maglaras, L.; Moschoyiannis, S.; Janicke, H. Deep learning for cyber security intrusion detection: Approaches, datasets, and comparative study. *J. Inf. Secur. Appl.* **2020**, *50*, 102419. [CrossRef]
33. European Union Agency for Cybersecurity. COVID19-ENISA. Available online: https://www.enisa.europa.eu/topics/wfh-covid19 (accessed on 18 June 2021).
34. Lambert, M.; Louiset, J.-L.; Sidibe, M.-J. Telework Successfully During (and after) the COVID-19 Pandemic. *ISACA*. 5 May 2020. Available online: https://www.isaca.org/resources/news-and-trends/isaca-now-blog/2020/telework-successfully-during-and-after-the-covid-19-pandemic (accessed on 18 June 2021).
35. Alzahrani, A. Coronavirus Social Engineering Attacks: Issues and Recommendations. *Int. J. Adv. Comput. Sci. Appl.* **2020**, *11*, 5. [CrossRef]
36. CYBERAWARE4HEALTH: Cybersecurity Awareness in Healthcare Employees. *SPHINX H2020 Project A Uni-versal Cyber Security Toolkit for Health-Care Industry Project*. 16 December 2020. Available online: https://sphinx-project.eu/cyberaware4health/. (accessed on 26 July 2021).
37. Energy Shield: 2019. Available online: https://energy-shield.eu/ (accessed on 25 March 2020).
38. Georgiadou, A.; Mouzakitis, S.; Bounas, K.; Askounis, D. A Cyber-Security Culture Framework for Assessing Organization Readiness. *J. Comput. Inf. Syst.* **2020**, 1–11. [CrossRef]
39. Georgiadou, A.; Mouzakitis, S.; Askounis, D. Assessing MITRE ATT&CK Risk Using a Cyber-Security Culture Framework. *Sensors* **2021**, *21*, 3267. [CrossRef] [PubMed]

40. Georgiadou, A.; Mouzakitis, S.; Askounis, D. Detecting Insider Threat via a Cyber-Security Culture Framework. *J. Comput. Inf. Syst.* **2021**. [CrossRef]
41. Georgiadou, A.; Mouzakitis, S.; Askounis, D. Designing a Cyber-security Culture Assessment Survey Targeting Critical Infrastructures During Covid-19 Crisis. *Int. J. Netw. Secur. Its Appl.* **2021**, *13*, 33–50. [CrossRef]
42. Georgiadou, A.; Mouzakitis, S.; Askounis, D. Working from home during COVID 19 crisis: A cyber security culture assessment survey. *Secur. J.* **2021**. [CrossRef]
43. SPHINX Project EU. SPHINX Project EU. *SPHINX*. 1 January 2019. Available online: https://sphinx-project.eu/. (accessed on 19 June 2021).
44. D7.1—Pilot plans including evaluation framework. *SPHINX H2020 Project a Universal Cyber Security Toolkit for Health-Care Industry*. 31 June 2021. Available online: https://zenodo.org/record/3935794. (accessed on 26 July 2021).
45. The European Parliament and the Council of the European Union. 2018 Reform of EU Data Protection Rule. Official Journal of the European Union. 25 May 2018. Available online: https://gdpr-info.eu/ (accessed on 26 March 2020).
46. ISO/IEC. *ISO/IEC 27001. Information Security Management*; International Organization for Standardization (ISO): Geneva, Switzerland, 2015.
47. The European Parliament and the Council of the European Union. EUR-Lex- 32016L1148-EN-EUR-Lex. 6 July 2016. Available online: https://eur-lex.europa.eu/eli/dir/2016/1148/oj. (accessed on 26 March 2020).
48. Panhellenic Scientific Association for Health Informatics. Available online: https://www.hsshi.gr/. (accessed on 29 July 2021).
49. HIMSS. HIMSS Healthcare Cybersecurity Survey. *HIMSS*. 16 November 2020. Available online: https://www.himss.org/resources/himss-healthcare-cybersecurity-survey (accessed on 22 June 2021).
50. Gordon, W.J.; Wright, A.; Glynn, R.J.; Kadakia, J.; Mazzone, C.; Leinbach, E.; Landman, A. Evaluation of a man-datory phishing training program for high-risk employees at a US healthcare system. *J. Am. Med. Inform. Assoc.* **2019**, *26*, 547–552. [CrossRef] [PubMed]
51. Akbar, N. Analysing Persuasion Principles in Phishing Emails. Master's Thesis, University of Twente, Enschede, The Netherlands, October 2014.
52. Walter, J. Threat Intel | Cyber Attacks Leveraging the COVID-19/CoronaVirus Pandemic. *SentinelLABS*. 4 September 2020. Available online: https://labs.sentinelone.com/threat-intel-update-cyber-attacks-leveraging-the-covid-19-coronavirus-pandemic/ (accessed on 22 June 2021).
53. TREND Micro. Emotet Uses Coronavirus Scare in Latest Campaign, Targets Japan. *TREND Micro*. 31 January 2020. Available online: https://www.trendmicro.com/vinfo/mx/security/news/cybercrime-and-digital-threats/emotet-uses-coronavirus-scare-in-latest-campaign-targets-japan (accessed on 22 June 2021).
54. Davis, J. COVID-19 Impact on Ransomware, Threats, Healthcare Cybersecurity. *Health IT Security*. 04 August 2020. Available online: https://healthitsecurity.com/news/covid-19-impact-on-ransomware-threats-healthcare-cybersecurity (accessed on 22 June 2021).
55. Kumaran, N.; Lugani, S. Protecting businesses against cyber threats during COVID-19 and beyond. *Google Cloud*. 16 April 2020. Available online: https://cloud.google.com/blog/products/identity-security/protecting-against-cyber-threats-during-covid-19-and-beyond (accessed on 22 June 2021).
56. U.S. Department of Health and Human Services. Health Insurance Portability and Accountability Act of 1996 | ASPE. *ASPE-Office of the Assistant Secretary for Planning and Evaluation*, 20 August 1996. Available online: https://aspe.hhs.gov/reports/health-insurance-portability-accountability-act-1996 (accessed on 25 August 2021).
57. ISO/IEC. *ISO 27799:2016 Health informatics—Information Security Management in Health Using ISO/IEC 27002*; ISO: Geneva, Switzerland, 2016.
58. Jagatic, T.N.; Johnson, N.; Jakobsson, M.; Menczer, F. Social Phishing. *Commun. ACM* **2007**, *50*, 94–100. [CrossRef]
59. Miranda, M.J.A. Enhancing cybersecurity awareness training: A comprehensive phishing exercise approach. *Int. Manag. Rev.* **2018**, *14*, 5–10.
60. Jampen, D.; Gür, G.; Sutter, T.; Tellenbach, B. Don't click: Towards an effective anti-phishing training. A comparative literature review. *Hum.-Cent. Comput. Inf. Sci.* **2020**, *10*, 1–41. [CrossRef]
61. Kumaraguru, P.; Rhee, Y.; Acquisti, A.; Cranor, L.F.; Hong, J.; Nunge, E. Protecting people from phishing: The design and evaluation of an embedded training email system. In Proceedings of the CHI '07: Proceedings of the SIGCHI Conference on Human Factors in Computing Systems, San Jose, CA, USA, 28 April–3 May 2007.
62. Almomani, A.; Gupta, B.B.; Atawneh, S.; Meulenberg, A.; Almomani, E. A Survey of Phishing Email Filtering Techniques. *IEEE Commun. Surv. Tutor.* **2013**, *15*, 2070–2090. [CrossRef]

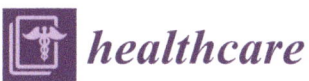

Article

Privacy-Preserving Authentication Protocol for Wireless Body Area Networks in Healthcare Applications

Hyunho Ryu and Hyunsung Kim *

School of Computer Science, Kyungil University, Gyeongsan-si 38428, Korea; ryoofamily0430@gmail.com
* Correspondence: kim@kiu.ac.kr

Abstract: Mobile healthcare service has become increasingly popular thanks to the significant advances in the wireless body area networks (WBANs). It helps medical professionals to collect patient's healthcare data remotely and provides remote medical diagnosis. Since the health data are privacy-related, they should provide services with privacy-preserving, which should consider security and privacy at the same time. Recently, some lightweight patient healthcare authentication protocols were proposed for WBANs. However, we observed that they are vulnerable to tracing attacks because the patient uses the same identifier in each session, which could leak privacy-related information on the patient. To defeat the weakness, this paper proposes a privacy-preserving authentication protocol for WBANs in healthcare service. The proposed protocol is only based on one-way hash function and with exclusive-or operation, which are lightweight operations than asymmetric cryptosystem operations. We performed two rigorous formal security proofs based on BAN logic and ProVerif tool. Furthermore, comparison results with the relevant protocols show that the proposed protocol achieves more privacy and security features than the other protocols and has suitable efficiency in computational and communicational concerns.

Keywords: healthcare service; body area network; privacy; authentication; security protocol

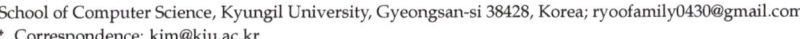

Citation: Ryu, H.; Kim, H. Privacy-Preserving Authentication Protocol for Wireless Body Area Networks in Healthcare Applications. *Healthcare* **2021**, *9*, 1114. https://doi.org/10.3390/healthcare9091114

Academic Editors: Daniele Giansanti and Tin-Chih Toly Chen

Received: 13 July 2021
Accepted: 24 August 2021
Published: 28 August 2021

Publisher's Note: MDPI stays neutral with regard to jurisdictional claims in published maps and institutional affiliations.

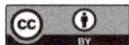

Copyright: © 2021 by the authors. Licensee MDPI, Basel, Switzerland. This article is an open access article distributed under the terms and conditions of the Creative Commons Attribution (CC BY) license (https://creativecommons.org/licenses/by/4.0/).

1. Introduction

Advances in mobile networking for Internet of Things (IoT) are powering the fourth industrial revolution. It connects physical things with digital worlds and allows for better collaboration and access across network participants, application services and people [1–5]. Wireless sensor network (WSN) technology is an essential component of IoT because it consists of a collection of sensors connected wirelessly. In the diverse kinds of WSNs, wireless body area network (WBAN) is a highly suitable communication network for medical IoT devices [6–9]. Healthcare services based on WBAN could provide remote mechanisms to monitor and collect patient's health data. The distance between patients and professional doctor can affect health status [10–13]. However, locational inequality in the medical system such as lower hospital and professional doctor is a problem that exists in almost all countries [14,15]. However, the remote healthcare system can be helpful for this problem. Especially, the remote healthcare system is beneficial for chronic diseases such as diabetes, heart failure, and chronic obstructive pulmonary disease [16]. And chronic diseases are an increasingly important concern for remote healthcare systems [17]. Because the remote healthcare system can check a patient's health status anytime and anywhere. In addition, since the patient's health status is checked in real-time, it has the advantage of able to cope quickly and the doctor can early diagnosis if the patient's health status become emergency [18,19]. Additionally, remote healthcare monitoring allows people to continue to stay at home rather than in expensive healthcare facilities such as hospitals or nursing homes [20,21].

However, privacy and security play key roles in protecting these data during data collection and transmission since remote healthcare service is vulnerable to various attacks [22–29]. If any attacker successfully launches the attacks, unintended functions may be performed via WBAN and these can cause a life threat to the patient. Therefore, it is imperative to devise authentication and key establishment protocols for securing remote healthcare applications.

There have been many authentication protocols for WBANs in healthcare applications [30–41]. Especially, the first anonymous authentication protocol based on smartcards was proposed by Zhu et al., which provides authentication with one round message communication but keeps user anonymity [30]. However, Lee et al. showed that Zhu et al.'s protocol cannot provide perfect user anonymity and backward secrecy and proposed an enhanced protocol [31]. Zhu et al.'s protocol and Lee et al.'s protocol were based on hash operations, a symmetric key cryptography and exclusive-or operations. Memon et al. proposed an anonymous authentication protocol for location-based services, which is based on elliptic curve cryptography (ECC) [32]. Soon after Reddy et al. showed vulnerabilities of Memon et al.'s protocol focused on key compromised impersonation attack, insider attack and insecure password changing phase and a problem of imperfect mutual authentication. Reddy et al. also proposed a two-factor authentication protocol based on ECC and smartcards [33]. Memon et al.'s protocol and Reddy et al.'s protocol are depending on asymmetric key cryptography, especially ECC. For the telecare medicine information system, Khatoon et al. and Ostad-Sharif et al. separately proposed authentication and key agreement protocol based on ECC [34,35]. By adopting a fuzzy extractor for the identification of patients using biometrics, Khatoon et al.'s protocol purposed to provide secure and privacy-preserving of the patient, bilinear pairing-based, unlinkable, mutual authentication and key agreement [34]. Ostad-Sharif et al. designed an anonymous and unlinkable authentication and key agreement protocol to provide perfect forward secrecy, which provided the formal security analysis using simulation tool AVISPA result [35]. Apart from the research efforts, Ali et al. proposed an authentication and access control protocol for securing wireless healthcare WSNs [36]. Ali et al.'s protocol is based on ECC and bilinear pairing and is proven to be secure based on AVISPA tool and Burrows–Abadi–Needham (BAN) logic [37].

Primitives based on ECC or bilinear pairing have computational overhead than any other cryptographic primitives and thereby they are heavily weighted on WBANs. To cope with the overhead, Khan et al. proposed an anonymous biometric-based authentication protocol using chaotic maps [38]. To use biometrics in the protocol, Khan et al. hired the Chebyshev chaotic map and hash function, which is a lightweight authentication cryptographic primitives. Aman et al. proposed a lightweight authentication protocol over WBANs, which are based on physical unclonable functions (PUFs) [39]. Aman et al.'s protocol is based on hash functions and exclusive-or operations. Even if two protocols from Khan et al. and Aman et al. provide operational efficiency, PUF assumption is a big burden to WBANs environment. Xu et al. proposed a lightweight anonymous authentication and key agreement protocol for WBANs without using the chaotic map nor PUFs [40]. Their protocol is only based on a hash function and exclusive-or operations and has an advantage in operational cost. However, Alzahrani et al. showed that Xu et al.'s protocol is vulnerable against replay attacks and key compromise impersonation attacks and suffers from the offline identity-guessing attack [41]. Furthermore, they proposed an improved protocol for WBANs in healthcare applications. Even though Alzahrani et al.'s protocol provides a lightweight computational overhead with various advantages on security and privacy concerns, we found that Alzahrani et al.'s protocol does not provide unlinkability of patients because it uses the same identifier of access point in each session.

The contributions of this paper are as follows:

(1) A new privacy-preserving authentication protocol for WBANs in remote healthcare applications is devised. In the protocol, an entity could protect privacy and security with a session key establishment for secure communication.

(2) The proposed protocol utilizes lightweight operations, which are based on the hash function and exclusive-or operation. This makes the protocol suitable for WBANs in remote healthcare applications.

(3) The formal security proof in BAN logic [37] demonstrates that the proposed protocol supports privacy and security. The formal security verification with ProVerif tool [42] shows that the proposed protocol can withstand both passive and active attacks. The informal analysis of its privacy and security is presented to verify the robustness of the proposed protocol against the well-known attacks.

(4) Efficiency analysis is done based on the complexity analysis of computation and communication overheads. The results show that the proposed protocol has a little overhead than the existing protocols.

The remainder of this paper is structured as follows. Section 2 summarizes the preliminaries of the research focused on healthcare system configuration, CK threat model and design goals. Section 3 gives a detailed description of the proposed privacy-preserving authentication protocol for remote healthcare applications. Section 4 demonstrates the formal, semi-formal and informal privacy and security results of the proposed protocol. Section 5 shows performance results focused on computation and communication. Section 6 provides discussion of importance of this research with future works. Section 7 concludes the work.

2. Preliminaries

In the digital age, hospitals and health service providers have pursued innovations for rich healthcare services. WBAN technology allows patients to be treated always even in remote areas and enables doctors to diagnose diseases and treat patients in medical institutions. And its technology can help anyone to easily access medical information [43]. It also serves to reduce patient anxiety by providing easy access to current medical information such as coronavirus disease 2019 (COVID-19). This section briefly reviews a system configuration for the target remote healthcare service and the design goals of the proposed protocol.

2.1. System Configuration

The target remote healthcare service is based on WBAN for patients. As shown in Figure 1, there are three main entities, which are a patient (PT) with some sensor nodes (SNs) on WBAN, access point (AP) and hub node (HN) as a server of the remote healthcare system. Especially, a system administrator (SA) is required for the system set-up but HN could do this role instead if it is necessary. The roles of each entity are defined as follows:

- SA: It sets up system parameters and registers participants by deploying important secret values in the memory of each party.
- HN: It has a very important role as the central server for the healthcare service, which collects and keeps a database of electronic health records (EHRs) for the registered PTs. In addition to this, it works also as a registration center for all network participants and issues SNs and APs for PTs. Furthermore, it works as an authentication server to check the authenticity of system entities.
- AP: AP works as a communication gateway from SN to HN and vice versa via wireless communication link. Thereby, it does not perform any validation of messages. It is assumed that an AP belongs to a specific PT only.
- SN: Some SNs are deployed on a PT, as notated as 1, 2, 3, 4 and 5 in the left part of Figure 1, to form a WBAN by HN or SA, which do the role of collecting EHR data of the PT and transmitting them to HN. An SN has sensors to check the purposed health status such as body temperature, blood pressure, electrocardiogram and so on. It needs to consider EHR privacy because the healthcare service is data sensitive.
- PT: PT is a subject of the remote healthcare service. Normally, PT does not take part in the network communication directly but subscribes the service to SA or HN. Then, SA or HN issues some SNs and an AP of the PT for the service.
- Doctor: Doctors make the diagnosis based on PT's EHRs by accessing HN. Doctors need to regularly check the health status of PTs and provide proper medical treatments via on-line.

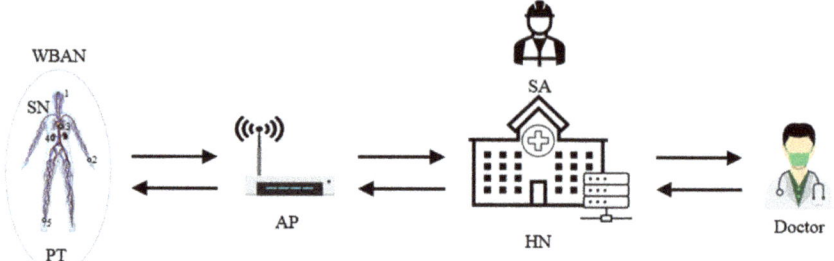

Figure 1. System configuration for remote healthcare service.

2.2. CK Threat Model

This subsection describes the widely accepted and well-known Canetti and Krawczyk (CK) threat model, which defines the ability of an adversary and is one of the foundations for formal privacy and security analysis on cryptographic protocol [44,45]. In the CK model, the adversary can fully control the communication links by listening to, altering, deciding on and injecting into the transferring information. Apart from these basic adversarial capabilities, in this model, it is assumed that the adversary can obtain secret information stored in the parties' memories via explicit attacks. As a result, the security of an authentication protocol should guarantee that the leakage of private values, such as session ephemeral secrets, would have the least possible influence on the security of other sessions and other private credentials of the communicating entities.

2.3. Design Goals

The healthcare system should provide privacy and security at the same time [46,47]. Normally, only anonymity is considered to provide privacy of PT in some other protocols in [40,41]. However, we also need to further consider unlinkability as another important privacy feature. To design a new authentication protocol for the remote healthcare service based on the CK threat model, the following five security properties and two privacy requirements are considered in this paper.

[SP1] Mutual authentication: To allow only authorized PT to get the medical services provided by HN, mutual authentication between SN and HN is required.

[SP2] Session key agreement: After a successful process of mutual authentication, further EHR data communications between SN and HN should be encrypted based on the session key to achieve confidentiality and integrity.

[SP3] Message freshness: Each entity in the system needs to check message freshness to cope with various attacks. It could be supported either by using timestamp or random nonce.

[SP4] Perfect forward secrecy: It could assure that the security of the system will not be compromised even if long-term secrets used in the protocol are compromised.

[SP5] Attack resistance: Due to the open environment in the remote healthcare service, the transmitted messages among network entities may be intercepted, modified and replayed by the adversary. Therefore, the proposed authentication protocol should be able to withstand various attacks, such as replay attack, impersonation attack, man-in-the-middle attack and known session-specific temporary information attack.

[PP1] Anonymity: Anonymity is an important privacy feature in the remote healthcare service. To protect the identity privacy of PT, the proposed protocol should guarantee that no one can get the PT's identity from the intercepted messages on the public channels.

[PP2] Unlinkability: Unlinkability is another important privacy feature in the remote healthcare service, which guarantees that the adversary cannot distinguish whether these different session's messages are related or not. The cryptographic protocol should not only guarantee the PT's anonymity but also provide unlinkability between sessions.

3. Proposed Authentication Protocol

In this section, a privacy-preserving authentication protocol for WBANs in healthcare service is proposed. The proposed protocol uses only the hash function with exclusive-or operations to provide the design goals. We assume that all the participants are synchronized on time using any proper scheme and a maximum transmission delay Δt is agreed on mutually. The proposed protocol consists of four phases, i.e., initialization phase, registration phase, authentication phase and identity modification phase. First of all, the initialization phase sets up a security building block for the overall network. PT possessed with SN and AP is a target for the registration phase to either SA or HN. The authentication phase is for the basic security service to check whether the entity is legal or not and is also to set up a session key for further secure communications. The identity modification phase is used when PT wants to change SN's identity for privacy reasons. Table 1 defines the symbols and their meanings used in this paper.

Table 1. Notations.

Notation	Descriptions
SA	System administrator
HN	Healthcare central server
PT	Patient
SN	Sensor node
AP	Access point
ID_{SN}	Identity of SN
ID_{AP}	Identity of AP
Y_{SN}	Pseudonym identity of SN
PID_{AP}	Pseudonym identity of AP
KS_{HN}	Long-term master key of HN
K_S	Established session key
T_{i_j}	i-th timestamp of an entity j
S_{i_j}	i-th random number of an entity j
a_{SN}, na_{SN}, q	Random numbers
HC_i	Hash chain value of SN
$h()$	Secure one-way hash function
$\|\|$	Concatenation operation
$\oplus$	Exclusive-or operation
Δt	Allowed transmission delay

3.1. Initialization Phase

For the system initialization, SA performs the following steps.

Step 1. SA selects a long-term master key KS_{HN} for HN.
Step 2. SA stores KS_{HN} in the memory of HN.

3.2. Registration Phase

When a PT wants to subscribe to a remote healthcare service, HN performs the following steps after issuing SN and AP for PT as shown in Figure 2. All parameters are established by HN for WBANs over a secure channel.

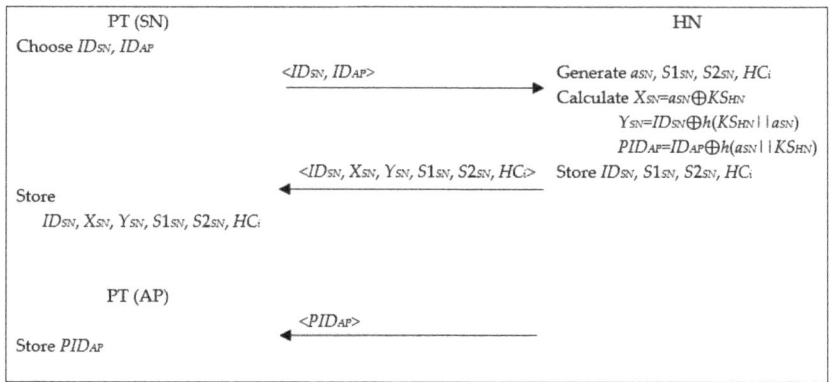

Figure 2. Registration phase.

Step 1. PT chooses two identities ID_{SN} and ID_{AP} for SN and AP, respectively, and sends them to HN. After receiving the information, HN generates four random numbers $a_{SN}, S1_{SN}, S2_{SN}$ and HC_i for SN, forms a set <$ID_{SN}, S1_{SN}, S2_{SN}, HC_i$> and stores it in the memory.

Step 2. After that, HN calculates $X_{SN} = a_{SN} \oplus KS_{HN}$, $Y_{SN} = ID_{SN} \oplus h(KS_{HN} || a_{SN})$ and $PID_{AP} = ID_{AP} \oplus h(a_{SN} || KS_{HN})$, composes a set <$ID_{SN}, X_{SN}, Y_{SN}, S1_{SN}, S2_{SN}, HC_i$> and stores it in the memory of SN. They are used for authenticity check of PT.

Step 3. HN stores PID_{AP} in the memory of AP.

3.3. Authentication Phase

When a PT wants to use the subscribed remote healthcare service, PT with SN and AP needs to use this phase to log-in HN as shown in Figure 3. SN does whole roles of PT periodically to send the predefined sensed EHR data to HN via AP. This phase has two purposes, mutual authentication and session key agreement. Timestamp in each message is used to provide message freshness, which is used to cope with the replay attack. The detailed steps are as follows:

Step 1. SN gets the current timestamp $T1_{SN}$, calculates a message authentication code $RID_S = (ID_{SN} || X_{SN} || Y_{SN} || S2_{SN} || HC_i || T1_{SN})$ and composes a message {$X_{SN}, Y_{SN}, RID_S, T1_{SN}$} to submit to AP.

Step 2. When AP receives the message, it adds a session dependent pseudo identity PID_{AP} to the message {$X_{SN}, Y_{SN}, RID_S, T1_{SN}, PID_{AP}$} and sends the message to HN.

Step 3. When HN receives the message, it gets the current timestamp $T1_{HN}$ and verifies the freshness of the message by validating $T1_{HN} - T1_{SN} \leq \Delta t$ where Δt is the allowed transmission delay of the network. If it does not hold, HN treats this message as a replay attack and aborts the session. Otherwise, HN calculates $a_{SN}' = X_{SN} \oplus KS_{HN}$ and $ID_{AP}' = PID_{AP} \oplus h(a_{SN}' || KS_{HN})$. After that, HN calculates $ID_{SN}' = Y_{SN} \oplus h(KS_{HN} || a_{SN}')$ and compares it with ID_{SN} stored in its memory. Only if the verification is successful, HN calculates $RID_S' = h(ID_{SN}' || X_{SN} || Y_{SN} || S2_{SN} || HC_i || T1_{SN})$ using the parameters in its repository. Finally, HN checks whether RID_S' is equal to RID_S or not.

Step 4. Only after all verifications are successful, HN could believe the authenticity of SN and AP and forms a reply message with two options, one is to be authenticated to SN and AP and another is to update the authentication parameters for the next authentication for SN and AP, respectively. For this, HN gets the current timestamp $T2_{HN}$, generates two random numbers q and na_{SN}, and calculates $X_{SN}' = na_{SN} \oplus KS_{HN}$, $Y_{SN}' = ID_{SN}' \oplus h(KS_{HN} || na_{SN})$, $NPID_{AP} = ID_{AP}' \oplus h(na_{SN} || KS_{HN})$, $j = ID_{SN}' \oplus Y_{SN} \oplus X_{SN}$, $r = q \oplus j$, $g = h(q || j || S2_{SN})$, $Z_{AP} = h(PID_{AP} || NPID_{AP} || ID_{AP}')$,

$NX_{SN} = X_{SN}' \oplus g$, $NY_{SN} = Y_{SN}' \oplus g$, $C_{SN} = h(q \mid\mid ID_{SN}' \mid\mid j \mid\mid X_{SN}' \mid\mid Y_{SN}' \mid\mid T2_{HN})$ and $K_S = h(q \mid\mid S1_{SN} \mid\mid S2_{SN} \mid\mid HC_i)$. After that, HN overwrites $S1_{SN}$ into $S2_{SN}$ and changes $S2_{SN}$ with K_S in its memory, which are used for the next authentication for privacy provision. And then, HN calculates $HC_i' = h(HC_i)$ and replaces it to HC_i as $HC_i = HC_i'$, which is for updating the session key parameter. After that, HN composes a message $\{r, NX_{SN}, NY_{SN}, C_{SN}, T2_{HN}, NPID_{AP}, Z_{AP}\}$ and sends it to AP.

Step 5. After receiving the message, AP checks the freshness of message by calculating $Z_{AP}' = h(PID_{AP} \mid\mid NPID_{AP} \mid\mid ID_{AP})$ and verifying whether Z_{AP}' is the same as Z_{AP} in the message or not. Only if the verification is successful, AP overwrites $NPID_{AP}$ into PID_{AP} in its memory. After that, AP drops $NPID_{AP}$ and Z_{AP} from the message and sends the reformed message $\{r, NX_{SN}, NY_{SN}, C_{SN}, T2_{HN}\}$ to SN.

Step 6. When SN receives the message, it gets the current timestamp $T2_{SN}$ and verifies the freshness of the message by validating $T2_{SN} - T2_{HN} \leq \Delta t$. If it is not successful, SN aborts the session, which is treated as a replay attack. Otherwise, it calculates $j' = ID_{SN} \oplus Y_{SN} \oplus X_{SN}$, $q' = r \oplus j'$, $g' = h(q \mid\mid j' \mid\mid S2_{SN})$, $X_{SN}'' = NX_{SN} \oplus g'$, $Y_{SN}'' = NY_{SN} \oplus g'$ and $C_{SN}' = h(q' \mid\mid ID_{SN} \mid\mid j' \mid\mid X_{SN}'' \mid\mid Y_{SN}'' \mid\mid T2_{HN})$ and validates C_{SN}' by comparing it with C_{SN} in the message. It aborts the session if the validation fails. Otherwise, SN implicitly accept the authenticity of HN and calculates a session key $K_S' = h(q' \mid\mid S1_{SN} \mid\mid S2_{SN} \mid\mid HC_i)$ and overwrite $S1_{SN}$ into $S2_{SN}$ and changes $S2_{SN}$ with K_S. SN replaces the two parameters, X_{SN}'' and Y_{SN}'' into X_{SN} and Y_{SN}, respectively, which are the next authentication parameters. Finally, SN calculates $HC_i' = h(HC_i)$ and replaces it to HC_i as $HC_i = HC_i'$, which is for updating the session key parameter.

3.4. Identity Modification Phase

Whenever a PT wants to change his (or her) identity, this phase should be performed. To change identity of PT, SN sends the identity modification request to HN. Then HN provides identity modification parameter only after the successful authentication. The phase is performed as follows:

Step 1. SN sets the current timestamp $T1_{SN}$, selects a new identity ID_{SN}^{NEW}, calculates $NID_{SN} = ID_{SN}^{NEW} \oplus S2_{SN}$ and $RID_S = h(ID_{SN} \mid\mid X_{SN} \mid\mid Y_{SN} \mid\mid S2_{SN} \mid\mid NID_{SN} \mid\mid HC_i \mid\mid T1_{SN})$, composes a message $\{X_{SN}, Y_{SN}, RID_S, T1_{SN}, NID_{SN}\}$ and submits it to AP.

Step 2. When AP receives the message, it adds PID_{AP} to the message $\{X_{SN}, Y_{SN}, RID_S, T1_{SN}, NID_{SN}, PID_{AP}\}$ and sends the message to HN.

Step 3. When HN receives the message, it sets the current timestamp $T1_{HN}$. And HN validates the freshness of the message by verifying $T1_{HN} - T1_{SN} \leq \Delta t$. If T_{SN} is not fresh, HN aborts the session. Otherwise, HN calculates authentication parameters $a_{SN}' = X_{SN} \oplus KS_{HN}$ and $ID_{AP}' = PID_{AP} \oplus h(a_{SN}' \mid\mid KS_{HN})$. After that, HN calculates $ID_{SN}' = Y_{SN} \oplus h(KS_{HN} \mid\mid a_{SN}')$ and compares it with ID_{SN} stored in its memory. Only if the verification is successful, HN calculates $RID_S' = h(ID_{SN}' \mid\mid X_{SN} \mid\mid Y_{SN} \mid\mid S2_{SN} \mid\mid NID_{SN} \mid\mid HC_i \mid\mid T1_{SN})$ using the parameters in its repository. Finally, HN checks whether RID_S' is equal to RID_S.

Step 4. Only after all verifications are successful, HN withdraws the new identity from SN by computing $ID_{SN}^{NEW'} = NID_{SN} \oplus S2_{SN}$. After that, HN generates current timestamp $T2_{HN}$ and random numbers q and calculates the new identity related authentication parameters $Y_{SN}' = ID_{SN}^{NEW'} \oplus h(KS_{HN} \mid\mid a_{SN}')$, $j = ID_{SN} \oplus Y_{SN} \oplus X_{SN}$, $r = q \oplus j$, $g = h(q \mid\mid j \mid\mid S2_{SN})$, $NY_{SN} = Y_{SN}' \oplus g$ and $C_{SN} = h(q \mid\mid ID_{SN} \mid\mid j \mid\mid Y_{SN}' \mid\mid T2_{HN})$. Then HN overwrites $ID_{SN}^{NEW'}$ into ID_{SN} in its memory. Next HN composes a message $\{r, NY_{SN}, C_{SN}, T2_{HN}\}$ and sends it to AP.

Step 5. After receiving the message, AP sends the message $\{r, NY_{SN}, C_{SN}, T2_{HN}\}$ to SN.

Step 6. When SN receives the message, it sets the current timestamp $T2_{SN}$. And SN validates the freshness of the message by verifying $T2_{SN} - T2_{HN} \leq \Delta t$. If $T2_{HN}$ is not fresh, SN aborts the session. Otherwise, SN calculates $j' = ID_{SN} \oplus Y_{SN} \oplus X_{SN}$, $q' = r \oplus j'$, $g' = h(q \mid\mid j' \mid\mid S2_{SN})$, $Y_{SN}'' = NY_{SN} \oplus g'$ and $C_{SN}' = h(q' \mid\mid ID_{SN} \mid\mid j' \mid\mid Y_{SN}'' \mid\mid$

$T2_{HN}$), which are withdrawing the new identity related authentication parameters. After that, SN validates $C_{SN}{'}$ by comparing it with C_{SN} in the message. It aborts the session if the validation fails. Otherwise, SN replaces Y_{SN} with $Y_{SN}{''}$ in its memory.

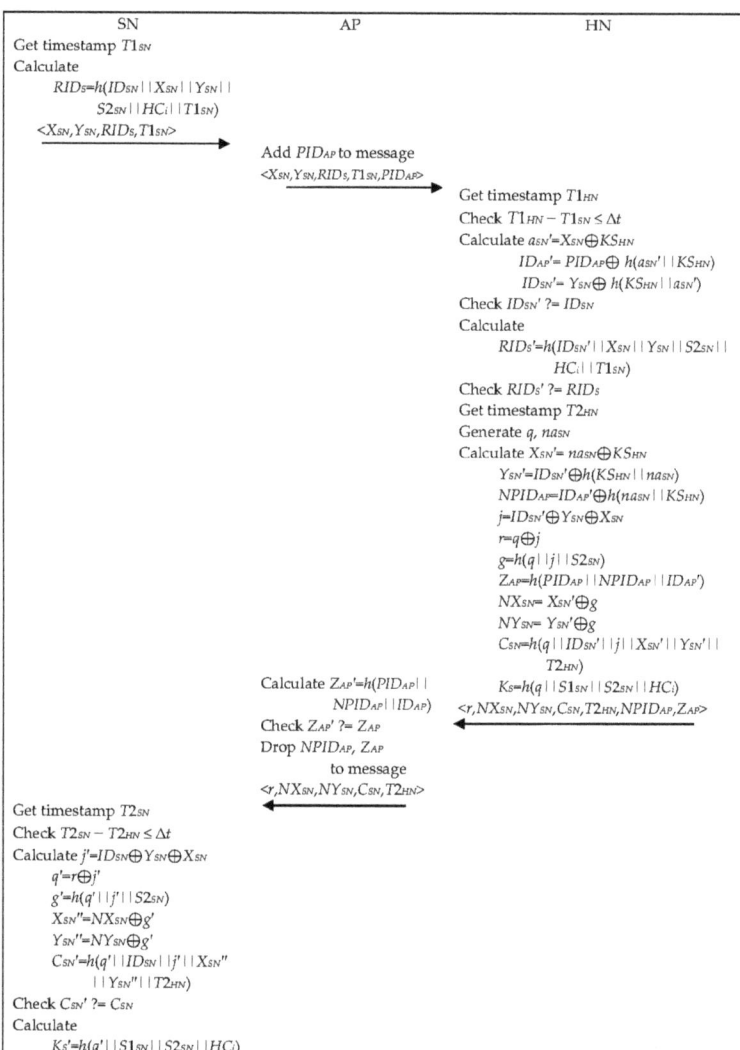

Figure 3. Authentication phase.

4. Security and Privacy Results

This section provides security analysis of the proposed protocol by using BAN logic and ProVerif tool based on the CK threat model [37,42]. Then, we demonstrate that the proposed protocol can achieve higher privacy and security features than the other related protocols.

4.1. BAN Logic Result

In this subsection, we analyze the security of the proposed protocol based on BAN logic. BAN logic is a widely adopted major formal method of valuation of any authentication protocol. BAN logic analyses using axioms to verify message origin, message freshness and faithful of the origin of the message [37]. The notations in formal security analysis for BAN logic are listed as follows:

- $Q| \equiv X$: Principal Q believes the statement X.
- $\#(X)$: Formula X is fresh.
- $Q| \Longrightarrow X$: Principal Q has jurisdiction over the statement X.
- $Q \triangleleft X$: Principal Q sees the statement X.
- $Q|\sim X$: Principal Q once said the statement X.
- (X, Y): Formula X or Y is one part of the formula (X, Y).
- $\langle P \rangle_Q$: Formula P combined with the formula Q.
- $Q \overset{SK}{\leftrightarrow} R$: Principal Q and R may use the shared session key, SK to communicate among each other. SK is good, in that any principal except Q and R will never discover it.

In addition, we use the following BAN logic rules to prove that the proposed protocol provides a secure mutual authentication between SN, AP and HN:

- Message-meaning rule: $\frac{R|\equiv R \overset{Y}{\leftrightarrow} S,\ R \triangleleft <X>_Y}{R|\equiv S|\sim X}$
- Nonce-verification rule: $\frac{R|\equiv \#(X),\ R|\equiv S|\sim X}{R|\equiv S|\equiv X}$
- Jurisdiction rule: $\frac{R|\equiv S|\Longrightarrow X,\ R|\equiv S|\equiv X}{R|\equiv X}$
- Freshness rule: $\frac{R|\equiv \#(X)}{R|\equiv \#(X,Y)}$

To show how the proposed protocol provide secure mutual authentication between SN and HN, we need to achieve the following goals:

Goal 1: $HN| \equiv (HN \overset{Ks}{\leftrightarrow} SN)$
Goal 2: $SN| \equiv (SN \overset{Ks}{\leftrightarrow} HN)$
Goal 3: $HN| \equiv SN| \equiv (SN \overset{Ks}{\leftrightarrow} HN)$
Goal 4: $SN| \equiv HN| \equiv (HN \overset{Ks}{\leftrightarrow} SN)$

Idealized form: The arrangement of the transmitted messages between *SN*, *AP* and *HN* in the proposed protocol to the idealized forms is as follows:

Message 1. SN → AP: $<X_{SN}>_{KSHN}$, $<Y_{SN}>_{KSHN}$, $<RIDs>_{KSHN}$, $T1_{SN}$
Message 2. AP → HN: $<X_{SN}>_{KSHN}$, $<Y_{SN}>_{KSHN}$, $<RIDs>_{KSHN}$, $T1_{SN}$, $<PID_{AP}>_{KSHN}$
Message 3. HN → AP: $<r>_{KSHN}$, $<NX_{SN}>_{KSHN}$, $<NY_{SN}>_{KSHN}$, $<C_{SN}>_{KSHN}$, $<NPID_{AP}>_{KSHN}$, $<Z_{AP}>_{KSHN}$, $T2_{HN}$
Message 4. AP → SN: $<r>_{KSHN}$, $<NX_{SN}>_{KSHN}$, $<NY_{SN}>_{KSHN}$, $<C_{SN}>_{KSHN}$, $T2_{HN}$

Assumptions: The following are the initial assumptions of the proposed protocol:
A1: $HN| \equiv \#(T1_{SN})$
A2: $HN| \equiv \#(T2_{SN})$
A3: $SN| \equiv \#(T1_{HN})$
A4: $SN| \equiv \#(T2_{HN})$
A5: $SN| \equiv HN \overset{X_{SN}}{\leftrightarrow} SN$
A6: $HN| \equiv HN \overset{X_{SN}}{\leftrightarrow} SN$
A7: $SN| \equiv HN \Longrightarrow HN \overset{X_{SN}}{\leftrightarrow} SN$
A8: $HN| \equiv SN \Longrightarrow HN \overset{X_{SN}}{\leftrightarrow} SN$

Proof. In the following, we prove the test goals in order to show the secure authentication using BAN logic rules and the assumptions. □

Based on Message 1, we could derive:
Step 1. $AP \triangleleft (<X_{SN}>_{KSHN}, <Y_{SN}>_{KSHN}, <RIDs>_{KSHN}, T1_{SN})$
Based on Step 1, AP adds $<PID_{AP}>_{KSHN}$ to the message and sends it to HN. Based on Message 2, we could derive:
Step 2. $HN \triangleleft (<X_{SN}>_{KSHN}, <Y_{SN}>_{KSHN}, <RIDs>_{KSHN}, T1_{SN}, <PID_{AP}>_{KSHN})$
According to assumption A6 and the message-meaning rule, we get:

Step 3. $HN|\equiv AP|\sim(<X_{SN}>_{KSHN}, <Y_{SN}>_{KSHN}, <RIDs>_{KSHN}, T1_{SN}, <PID_{AP}>_{KSHN})$
According to assumptions A1 and A2 and the freshness concatenation rule, we get:
Step 4. $HN|\equiv\#(<X_{SN}>_{KSHN}, <Y_{SN}>_{KSHN}, <RIDs>_{KSHN}, T1_{SN}, <PID_{AP}>_{KSHN})$
According to Steps 3 and 4 and the nonce verification rule, we get:
Step 5. $HN|\equiv SN|\equiv(<X_{SN}>_{KSHN}, <Y_{SN}>_{KSHN}, <RIDs>_{KSHN}, T1_{SN}, <PID_{AP}>_{KSHN})$
According to Step 5, assumption A6 and the believe rule, we get:
Step 6. $HN|\equiv SN|\equiv(HN\overset{KS_{HN}}{\leftrightarrow}SN)$
According to assumption A8 and the jurisdiction rule, we get:
Step 7. $HN|\equiv(HN\overset{KS_{HN}}{\leftrightarrow}SN)$
According to Steps 5, 6 and 7 and the nonce verification rule, we conclude:
Step 8. $HN|\equiv SN|\equiv(SN\overset{K_S}{\leftrightarrow}HN)$ **(Goal 3)**
According to assumption A8 and the jurisdiction rule, we get:
Step 9. $HN|\equiv(HN\overset{K_S}{\leftrightarrow}SN)$ **(Goal 1)**
Based on Message 3, we could derive:
Step 10. $AP\triangleleft(<r>_{KSHN}, <NX_{SN}>_{KSHN}, <NY_{SN}>_{KSHN}, <C_{SN}>_{KSHN}, <NPID_{AP}>_{KSHN}, <Z_{AP}>_{KSHN}, T2_{HN})$
According to the message meaning rule, we get:
Step 11. $AP|\equiv HN|\sim(<r>_{KSHN}, <NX_{SN}>_{KSHN}, <NY_{SN}>_{KSHN}, <C_{SN}>_{KSHN}, <NPID_{AP}>_{KSHN}, <Z_{AP}>_{KSHN}, T2_{HN})$
Based on Step 10, AP drops $<NPID_{AP}>_{KSHN}$ and $<Z_{AP}>_{KSHN}$ to the message and sends it to HN.
Based on Message 4, we derive:
Step 12. $SN\triangleleft(<r>_{KSHN}, <NX_{SN}>_{KSHN}, <NY_{SN}>_{KSHN}, <C_{SN}>_{KSHN}, T2_{HN})$
According to assumption A5 and the message-meaning rule, we get:
Step 13. $SN|\equiv AP|\sim(<r>_{KSHN}, <NX_{SN}>_{KSHN}, <NY_{SN}>_{KSHN}, <C_{SN}>_{KSHN}, T2_{HN})$
According to assumptions A3 and A4 and the freshness concatenation rule, we get:
Step 14. $SN|\equiv\#(<r>_{KSHN}, <NX_{SN}>_{KSHN}, <NY_{SN}>_{KSHN}, <C_{SN}>_{KSHN}, T2_{HN})$
According to Steps 12 and 13 and the nonce verification rule, we get:
Step 15. $SN|\equiv HN|\equiv(<r>_{KSHN}, <NX_{SN}>_{KSHN}, <NY_{SN}>_{KSHN}, <C_{SN}>_{KSHN}, T2_{HN})$
According to Step 14, assumption A5 and the believe rule, we get:
Step 16. $SN|\equiv HN|\equiv(HN\overset{KS_{HN}}{\leftrightarrow}SN)$
According to assumption A7 and the jurisdiction rule, we get:
Step 17. $SN|\equiv(HN\overset{KS_{HN}}{\leftrightarrow}SN)$
According to Steps 14, 15 and 16 and the nonce verification rule, we get:
Step 18. $SN|\equiv HN|\equiv(HN\overset{K_S}{\leftrightarrow}SN)$ **(Goal 4)**
According to assumption A7 and the jurisdiction rule, we get:
Step 19. $SN|\equiv(SN\overset{K_S}{\leftrightarrow}HN)$ **(Goal 2)**

According to Steps 9 and 19, the proposed authentication protocol successfully achieves the four goals. Both SN and HN could believe that they share the common session key $K_S = K_S' = h(q'||S1_{SN}||S2_{SN})$.

4.2. ProVerif Result

ProVerif is an automated tool for verifying security in cryptographic protocol [42]. It is supposed to be based on the CK threat model for security verification. ProVerif is a powerful tool that can verify all the possible attacks regarding mutual authentication. It also can prove safety of security properties for mutual authentication. For ProVerif analysis, we first define two channels ch1 and ch2 as public channels, among SN, AP and HN. In the ProVerif analysis, we used svalueA and svalueB to validate the session dependency. There are four events to check mutual authentication between SN and HN, which are SHbegin(entity), HSbegin(entity), SHend(entity) and HSend(entity). Session key security could be proved based on two queries, query attacker(svalueA) and query attacker(svalueB) based on the shared session key. For the basic operations, we defined Hash(bitstring) and XOR(bitstring, bitstring) for a one-way hash function and an exclusive-or operation, respectively. After defining processes of each entity, we performed a ProVerif demo for the entities of SN, AP and HN.

We have configured the ProVerif code as follows:

(*–The two public channel–*)
free ch1: channel.
free ch2: channel.
    (*–The basic type–*)
type entity.
type nonce.
type key.
    (*–Hash operation–*)
fun Hash(bitstring): bitstring.
    (*–XOR operation–*)
fun XOR(bitstring, bitstring): bitstring.
equation forall x: bitstring, y: bitstring;
XOR(XOR(x, y), y) = x.
    (*–Concat operation–*)
fun Con(bitstring, bitstring): bitstring.
fun Enc(bitstring,key): bitstring.
reduc forall x: bitstring, y: key;
Dec(Enc(x,y),y) = x.
    (*–Type convertion–*)
fun nontobit(nonce): bitstring [data,typeConverter].
fun bittokey(bitstring): key [data,typeConverter].
    (*–The basic variables–*)
free SN, AP, HN: entity. (*—three entities in the proposed protocol–*)
free T1SN: bitstring.
free T2HN: bitstring.
free S1SN: bitstring.
free S2SN: bitstring.
free HCi: bitstring.
free KSHN: bitstring[private]. (*—public key–*)
    (*–Authentication queries–*)
event SHbegin(entity).
event SHend(entity).
event HSbegin(entity).
event HSend(entity).
query t: entity; inj-event(SHend(t)) ==> inj-event(SHbegin(t)).
query t: entity; inj-event(HSend(t)) ==> inj-event(HSbegin(t)).
    (*–Queries–*)
free svalueA, svalueB: bitstring [private].
query attacker(svalueA);
attacker(svalueB).
    (*–SN–*)
let processSN(IDSN: bitstring, XSN: bitstring, YSN: bitstring) =
let (RIDs: bitstring) = Hash(Con(IDSN, Con(XSN, Con(YSN, Con(S2SN, Con(HCi,T1SN)))))) in
event HSbegin(HN);
    (*– SN > AP –*)
out(ch1, (XSN, YSN, RIDs, T1SN, true));
    (*– AP > SN –*)
in(ch1, (r: bitstring, NXSN: bitstring, NYSN: bitstring, CSN: bitstring));

```
let (xj: bitstring) = XOR(IDSN, XOR(YSN, XSN)) in
let (xq: bitstring) = XOR(r, xj) in
let (xg: bitstring) = Hash(Con(xq, Con(xj, S2SN))) in
let (xXSN: bitstring) = XOR(NXSN, xg) in
let (xYSN: bitstring) = XOR(NYSN, xg) in
let (xCSN: bitstring) = Hash(Con(xq, Con(IDSN, Con(xj, Con(xXSN, Con(xYSN, T2HN)))))) in
if xCSN = CSN then
let (xKs: bitstring) = Hash(Con(xq, Con(S1SN, Con(S2SN, HCi)))) in
event SHend(SN);
out(ch1, Enc(svalueA, bittokey(xKs))).
    (*–AP–*)
let processAP(IDAP: bitstring, PIDAP: bitstring) =
in(ch1, (XSN: bitstring, YSN: bitstring, RIDs: bitstring));
    (*– AP > HN –*)
out(ch2, (XSN, YSN, RIDs, T1SN, PIDAP, true));
    (*– HN > AP –*)
in(ch2, (r: bitstring, NXSN: bitstring, NYSN: bitstring, CSN: bitstring, NPIDAP: bitstring, ZAP: bitstring));
let (xZAP: bitstring) = Hash(Con(PIDAP, Con(NPIDAP, IDAP))) in
if xZAP = ZAP then
    (*– AP > SN –*)
out(ch1, (r, NXSN, NYSN, CSN, T2HN, true)).
    (*–HN–*)
let processHN(IDAP: bitstring, IDSN: bitstring) =
in(ch2, (XSN: bitstring, YSN: bitstring, RIDs: bitstring, PIDAP: bitstring));
let (a: bitstring) = XOR(XSN, KSHN) in
let (xIDAP: bitstring) = XOR(PIDAP,Hash(Con(a,KSHN))) in
let (xIDSN: bitstring) = XOR(YSN,Hash(Con(KSHN,a))) in
if xIDSN = IDSN then
let (xRIDs: bitstring) = Hash(Con(IDSN,Con(XSN,Con(YSN,Con(S2SN, Con(HCi, T1SN)))))) in
if xRIDs = RIDs then
event SHbegin(SN);
new q: nonce;
new nasn: nonce;
let (xXSN: bitstring) = XOR(nontobit(nasn),KSHN) in
let (xYSN: bitstring) = XOR(IDSN,Hash(Con(KSHN,nontobit(nasn)))) in
let (NPIDAP: bitstring) = XOR(IDAP,Hash(Con(nontobit(nasn),KSHN))) in
let (j: bitstring) = XOR(IDSN,XOR(YSN,XSN)) in
let (r: bitstring) = XOR(nontobit(q),j) in
let (g: bitstring) = Hash(Con(nontobit(q),Con(j,S2SN))) in
let (ZAP: bitstring) = Hash(Con(PIDAP,Con(NPIDAP,IDAP))) in
let (NXSN: bitstring) = XOR(xXSN,g) in
let (NYSN: bitstring) = XOR(xYSN,g) in
let (CSN: bitstring) = Hash(Con(nontobit(q), Con(IDSN, Con(j, Con(xXSN, Con(xYSN, T2HN)))))) in
let (Ks: bitstring) = Hash(Con(nontobit(q),Con(S1SN, Con(S2SN, HCi)))) in
    (*– HN > AP –*)
out(ch2, (r, NXSN, NYSN, CSN, T2HN, NPIDAP, ZAP, true));
event HSend(HN);
out(ch2, Enc(svalueB, bittokey(Ks))).
    (*–Start process–*)
process(
```

new XSN: bitstring;
new YSN: bitstring;
new PIDAP: bitstring;
new IDSN: bitstring;
new IDAP: bitstring;
(!processSN(IDSN, XSN, YSN)) |
(!processAP(IDAP, PIDAP)) |
(!processHN(IDAP, IDSN))
)

Figure 4 shows ProVerif result, which provides the successful security validation of the proposed protocol. From the result, we could find that "Query inj-event(SHend(t)) ==> inj-event(SHbegin(t)) is true." and "Query inj-event(HSend(t)) ==> inj-event(HSbegin(t)) is true." Those are to show mutual authentication property and replay attack resistance of the proposed protocol. After "Query not attacker (svalueA[]) is true." and "Query not attacker (svalueB[]) is true." show the anonymity of network participants and secrecy of the shared session key. It shows that the proposed protocol is properly performed by the tool without having any problems. As a result, we could conclude that the proposed protocol could establish a secure session key between SN and HN and the CK adversary could not discover the session key.

```
ProVerif text output:

Completing equations...
Completing equations...
-- Process 1-- Query inj-event(SHend(t)) ==> inj-event(SHbegin(t)) in process 1
Translating the process into Horn clauses...
Completing...
200 rules inserted. Base: 200 rules (32 with conclusion selected). Queue: 28 rules.
400 rules inserted. Base: 365 rules (32 with conclusion selected). Queue: 10 rules.
Starting query inj-event(SHend(t)) ==> inj-event(SHbegin(t))
RESULT inj-event(SHend(t)) ==> inj-event(SHbegin(t)) is true.
-- Query inj-event(HSend(t)) ==> inj-event(HSbegin(t)) in process 1
Translating the process into Horn clauses...
Completing...
200 rules inserted. Base: 200 rules (32 with conclusion selected). Queue: 24 rules.
Starting query inj-event(HSend(t)) ==> inj-event(HSbegin(t))
RESULT inj-event(HSend(t)) ==> inj-event(HSbegin(t)) is true.
-- Query not attacker(svalueA[]); not attacker(svalueB[]) in process 1
Translating the process into Horn clauses...
Completing...
200 rules inserted. Base: 198 rules (32 with conclusion selected). Queue: 20 rules.
Starting query not attacker(svalueA[])
RESULT not attacker(svalueA[]) is true.
Starting query not attacker(svalueB[])
RESULT not attacker(svalueB[]) is true.
--------
Verification summary:

Query inj-event(SHend(t)) ==> inj-event(SHbegin(t)) is true.

Query inj-event(HSend(t)) ==> inj-event(HSbegin(t)) is true.

Query not attacker(svalueA[]) is true.

Query not attacker(svalueB[]) is true.
--------
```

Figure 4. ProVerif result.

4.3. Informal Privacy and Security Analysis

As mentioned in [48], past research over the last thirty decades has told us that, a security proof is highly prone to be fallacious due to the adoption of an insufficient security model which fails to capture all the realistic capabilities of the adversary or due to a flawed or non-tight security reduction, and the field of provable security is a much an art as a science. While formal methods are often misused and reductionist security proofs are usually very intricate, turgid and prone to errors, particular care shall be given when conducting proof for an authentication protocol. To cope with the formal methods problems, this subsection is dedicated to present informal privacy and security analysis of the proposed protocol, which is focused on the privacy and security goals depicted in Section 2.3. For the CK threat model, we use the definition mentioned in Section 2.2. Table 2 shows the feature comparisons among the related protocols devised by Khatoon et al. in [34], Ostad-Sharif et al. in [35], Khan et al. in [38], Xu et al. in [40] and Alzahrani et al. in [41].

Table 2. Privacy and security feature comparison result.

Protocol \ Feature	Khatoon et al. [34]	Ostad-Sharif et al. [35]	Khan et al. [38]	Xu et al. [40]	Alzahrani et al. [41]	Proposed
SP1	O	O	O	O	O	O
SP2	O	O	O	O	O	O
SP3	O	O	O	O	O	O
SP4	O	O	X	X	X	O
SP5	X	X	X	X	X	O
PP1	O	O	O	X	O	O
PP2	O	O	O	X	X	O

SP1: mutual authentication, SP2: session key agreement, SP3: message freshness, SP4: perfect forward secrecy, SP5: attack resistance, PP1: anonymity, PP2: unlinkability.

[SP1] Mutual authentication: Authentication is performed between SN and HN mutually in the proposed protocol. Authentication is related to the messages from SN to HN and vice versa. SN needs to be authenticated by HN based on $\{X_{SN}, Y_{SN}, RID_S, T1_{SN}, PID_{AP}\}$, which is a message from SN to HN via AP. Only the legal SN could be authenticated by HN in the proposed protocol because a CK adversary needs to compute $RID_S = h(ID_{SN} || X_{SN} || Y_{SN} || S2_{SN} || T1_{SN})$, which needs knowledge on ID_{SN} and $S2_{SN}$ at the same time even if the adversary could get and use the previous session's X_{SN} and Y_{SN}. However, there is no way that the adversary could get them in the proposed protocol. HN needs to be authenticated by SN based on $\{r, NX_{SN}, NY_{SN}, C_{SN}, T2_{HN}\}$, which is a message from HN to SN via AP. Adversaries need to form a message, which could be validated by SN, especially C_{SN} validation that is related with knowledge of $q, ID_{SN}, j, X_{SN}', Y_{SN}'$ and $T2_{HN}$. However, the knowledge is related with KS_{HN}, which is the master key of HN. It means that the proposed protocol provides mutual authentication between SN and HN and there is no way that the adversary could succeed in the authentication process.

[SP2] Session key agreement: Session key is required to establish a secure channel between SN and HN to provide confidentiality on data. SN and HN agree on a session key $Ks = h(q || S1_{SN} || S2_{SN})$ after the successful authentication. There is no way that a CK adversary could get any information on Ks from the session messages $\{X_{SN}, Y_{SN}, RID_S, T1_{SN}\}, \{X_{SN}, Y_{SN}, RID_S, T1_{SN}, PID_{AP}\}, \{r, NX_{SN}, NY_{SN}, C_{SN}, T2_{HN}, NPID_{AP}, Z_{AP}\}$ and $\{r, NX_{SN}, NY_{SN}, C_{SN}, T2_{HN}\}$. The parameters of Ks are not exposed to any parameter in the messages. Especially, q is related to $r = q \oplus j$ but the adversary needs to know j to extract out the wanted value from r. However, the adversary could not get q from r due to the format of $j = ID_{SN} \oplus Y_{SN} \oplus X_{SN}$, which is related with the knowledge of KS_{HN}. Thereby, the proposed protocol provides a secure session key agreement only between SN and HN.

[SP3] Message freshness: There are two ways to provide message freshness in cryptographic protocol, which are based on challenge-response mechanism and timestamp mechanism. The proposed protocol uses a timestamp mechanism to cope with replay attacks because the network entity could be synchronized with a time when SA issues SN and AP for a PT during the registration phase. If a CK adversary wants to succeed in any attack against message freshness, the adversary needs to know and change timestamp-related values. From the session messages $\{X_{SN}, Y_{SN}, RID_S, T1_{SN}\}, \{X_{SN}, Y_{SN}, RID_S, T1_{SN}, PID_{AP}\}, \{r, NX_{SN}, NY_{SN}, C_{SN}, T2_{HN}, NPID_{AP}, Z_{AP}\}$ and $\{r, NX_{SN}, NY_{SN}, C_{SN}, T2_{HN}\}$, there are two integrity values $RID_S = h(ID_{SN} || X_{SN} || Y_{SN} || S2_{SN} || T1_{SN})$ and

$C_{SN} = h(q || ID_{SN} || j || X_{SN}' || Y_{SN}' || T2_{HN})$ that the adversary needs to compute. If the adversary gets a proper current timestamp $T1_{SN}'$, the adversary should compute two new values of $RID_S = h(ID_{SN} || X_{SN} || Y_{SN} || S2_{SN} || T1_{SN}')$ and $C_{SN} = h(q || ID_{SN} || j || X_{SN}' || Y_{SN}' || T1_{SN}')$. However, the two computations are impossible because the adversary needs to know the other parameters except $T1_{SN}'$ to compute RID_S and C_{SN}. Furthermore, each entity checks the freshness of the message using Δt each time they receive any message. So, the proposed protocol provides message freshness.

[SP4] Perfect forward secrecy: It is a very strong form of long-term security which guarantees that future disclosures of some long-term secret keys do not compromise past session keys [49]. It is widely accepted that the perfect forward secrecy can only be provided by asymmetric schemes. Nonetheless, there are a small number of existing symmetric-key protocols that provide secrecy [50–52]. The proposed protocol uses the dynamic authentication credential, which keeps evolving in sessions to achieve the perfect forward secrecy. In the proposed protocol, if an adversary has obtained the long-term key, K_{HN}, the adversary still cannot get the session key K_S. The reason is that after each successful session, the values HC_i, $S1_{SN}$ and $S2_{SN}$ will be updated by one-way hash function. Because of the one-wayness of the hash function, there is no way to get these values to compute the session key to the adversary. Therefore, the proposed protocol can provide perfect forward secrecy.

[SP5] Attack resistance: We could argue that any attack is successful if a CK adversary finds any mechanism to do various attacks, such as replay attack, impersonation attack and man-in-the-middle attack. Most of all, replay attack is tightly related with the message freshness. It means that any protocol with challenge-response or timestamp mechanism could cope with the attack. Messages in the proposed protocol are together with timestamp as the form of $T1_{SN}$ and $T2_{HN}$, respectively. Thereby, the proposed protocol is strong against replay attack. Impersonation attack is the second one we need to consider, which has a relationship with mutual authentication. As we mentioned in the mutual authentication, the adversary needs to form the first message $\{X_{SN}, Y_{SN}, RID_S, T1_{SN}\}$ to disguise as SN and the third message $\{r, NX_{SN}, NY_{SN}, C_{SN}, T2_{HN}, NPID_{AP}, Z_{AP}\}$ to masquerade as HN, respectively. However, they are related to the knowledge of KS_{HN}. So, the proposed protocol could cope with impersonation attacks. Man-in-the-middle attack is similar to an active eavesdropping in which the adversary makes independent connections with the network entities and relays messages between them to make them believe they are communicating directly to each other but in fact, the entire communication is controlled by the adversary. It is quite related to mutual authentication and confidentiality of parameters in the messages. Since we mentioned the mutual authentication provision from the proposed protocol, we will only consider confidentiality of the messages. There are only possibilities on knowing secret key-related information to legally registered SNs and HN but not any others. In the CK model, it is required that the generated session key from the protocol should not be compromised even in the case of ephemeral secrets leakage. In the proposed protocol, the ephemeral secrets are a_{SN} and q. Having access to these two, the adversary also needs to know both $S1_{SN}$ and $S2_{SN}$ to compute the session key K_S. Since only SN and HN know the values, the proposed protocol can withstand this attack. That is why any adversary could not get any useful information even if the adversary could tap into the communication link among SN, AP and HN. Thereby, the proposed protocol provides attack resilience. Finally, known session-specific temporary information attack should be considered in the protocol, which has an assumption that an adversary could get the ephemeral random number q to get the session key K_S since the attacker has no way to compute the long-term key KS_{HN} and one-time hash chain value HC_i. Moreover, the messages transmitted in the public channel are unhelpful to compute the session key K_S. Therefore, the proposed protocol has the ability to prevent the session-specific temporary information attack.

[PP1] Anonymity: Anonymity is defined as "the state of being not identifiable within a system." Anonymity from a CK adversary's perspective means that the adversary cannot identify any entity within a system. In security protocol, it is necessary to check identity-related information in messages transmitted among system entities to consider anonymity. There are Y_{SN}, RID_S, NY_{SN} and C_{SN}, for ID_{SN} and PID_{AP}, $NPID_{AP}$ and Z_{AP} for ID_{SN}, respectively, in the messages, which has a relationship with the identity factor. Adversaries do not have any method to identify any entity from the parameters in the proposed protocol. To do so, the adversary needs to have knowledge of KS_{HN}, which is not feasible. As a result, the proposed protocol provides anonymity.

[PP2] Unlinkability: It has a meaning after a system with anonymity has been defined and the entities interested in linking by a CK adversary have been characterized. Unlinkability of two or more sessions of interest from the adversary's perspective means that within the system, the adversary cannot distinguish whether they are related or not. As we discussed on anonymity, session linkability is related to the identifier and the message freshness of session message parameters. Each parameter in the session messages has a relationship with the session-dependent random numbers of a_{SN}, $S1_{SN}$, $S2_{SN}$, q and na_{SN} and timestamps of $T1_{SN}$ and $T2_{HN}$ in the proposed protocol. It means that the proposed protocol uses session-dependent parameters to form messages to cope with unlinkability. So, the proposed protocol provides unlinkability.

As shown in Table 2, the proposed protocol satisfies all the security and privacy properties as we set our protocol design goal in Section 2.3. However, Khatoon et al.'s protocol does not provide SP5, especially against the known-session-specific temporary information attack as mentioned in [53]. Thereby, the adversary could compute the session key SK in Khatoon et al.'s protocol based on the session-specific temporary information, T_i, R_i, T_s and R_s, which are parameters to compute SK and are exposed on the public communication channel. As stated above, the attacker can compute L_s. Ostad-Sharif et al.'s protocol is weak against the denial-of-service attack, the password guessing attack and the stolen verifier attack [54]. So, Ostad-Sharif et al.'s protocol does not provide SP5 also. Furthermore, Khan et al.'s protocol has security weakness against the user impersonation attack, which is related to SP5 again [55]. Xu et al.'s protocol does not provide the replay attack since an attacker could configure a valid request by merging two session parameters by intercepting contents of the previous session and the current session parameters [41]. Alzahrani et al.'s protocol has a security weakness against the known-session-specific temporary information attack because it does not provide SP4 also. Furthermore, Xu et al.'s protocol and Alzahrani et al.'s protocol do not provide PP2 especially. In addition to this, Xu et al.'s protocol is not secure against the replay attack and the impersonation attack and does not provide PP1 due to the offline identity guessing attack feasibility [41].

5. Performance Results

In this section, we provide performance analysis focused on computation and communication overheads by providing comparisons with the related protocols in [34,35,38,40,41]. A dataset is developed to produce further testing and enhancements instead of spending a considerable amount of time, money and effort for data collection. 10 users were tested in the proposed protocol run for a total of 10 times. The experiment of the protocols was performed over ARM Microcontrollers MCU Mainstream Arm Cortex-M4 running on MCU 170 MHz with 128 KB of flash memory.

5.1. Computation Result

There are four phases in the proposed protocol, which are initialization phase, registration phase, authentication phase and identity modification phase. We will concentrate on the computation requirements of the authentication phase only from the proposed protocol because the phase is the most frequently used one. To facilitate computation analysis, we define the computational requirements of a one-way hash function as T_h, a symmetric key encryption and decryption as T_{sym}, an elliptic curve cryptosystem as T_{ecc} and a bilinear pairing operation as T_{bp}, respectively, but do not consider the overhead of the exclusive-or operations, which require a comparatively quite low overhead than any other operations. Table 3 shows the computational overhead comparison among the related protocols.

Table 3. Computation cost comparison result.

Entity \ Protocol	Khatoon et al. [34]	Ostad-Sharif et al. [35]	Khan et al. [38]	Xu et al. [40]	Alzahrani et al. [41]	Proposed
SN	$5T_h + 1T_{bp} + 1T_{sym} + 3T_{ecc}$	$7T_h + 2T_{ecc}$	$7T_h$	$4T_h$	$4T_h$	$4T_h$
AP	-	-	-	-	-	$1T_h$
HN	$4T_h + 1T_{bp} + 1T_{sym} + 2T_{ecc}$	$7T_h + 2T_{sym} + 2T_{ecc}$	$4T_h$	$6T_h$	$6T_h$	$9T_h$
Total	$9T_h + 2T_{bp} + 2T_{sym} + 5T_{ecc}$	$14T_h + 2T_{sym} + 4T_{ecc}$	$11T_h$	$10T_h$	$10T_h$	$14T_h$

From the experiment, we acquired the required time for T_h, T_{sym}, T_{ecc} and T_{bp}, which are approximately 0.08 ms, 0.14 ms, 4.31 ms and 14.48 ms, respectively. The proposed protocol requires 14 hash operations, which is a bit more expensive than the protocols in [38,40,41] but quite lower than the works in [34,35]. However, the protocols in [40,41] do not provide the privacy concerns as we discussed in Table 2. So, we could say that the computational overhead in the proposed protocol is for the sake of privacy-preserving. Especially, it is better to get less computational overhead on the patient side than the server side as the proposed protocol. However, Khan et al.'s protocol is opposite from the notion, which has a more burden to the patient's side. Figure 5 shows the performance comparisons among the related protocols.

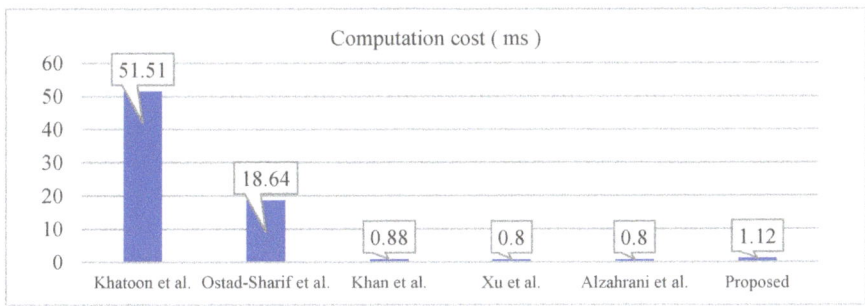

Figure 5. Computation cost comparison.

From Figure 5, we could know that the proposed protocol requires about 40% more computational overhead than the protocols in [38,40,41], which could be the overhead to provide unlinkability. However, the proposed protocol is relatively lightweight compared to the protocols in [34,35].

5.2. Communication Result

For the communication analysis, we assumed that the lengths of identity and random numbers are 128 bits each. However, we considered that the lengths for timestamp, hash function, symmetric key cryptosystem, elliptic curve cryptosystem and bilinear pairing are 32 bits, 160 bits, 128 bits, 256 bits and 256 bits, respectively. Table 4 shows a comparison for the communication cost among the related protocols.

Table 4. Communication cost comparison result.

Feature	Protocol	Khatoon et al. [34]	Ostad-Sharif et al. [35]	Khan et al. [38]	Xu et al. [40]	Alzahrani et al. [41]	Proposed
Message length	SN	832 bits	1408 bits	1120 bits	896 bits	896 bits	896 bits
	AP	-	-	-	1024 bits + 544 bits	1024 bits + 544 bits	1312 bits + 480 bits
	HN	640 bits	1120 bits	640 bits	672 bits	672 bits	1184 bits
	Total	1472 bits	2528 bits	1760 bits	3136 bits	3136 bits	3872 bits
Number of messages		2 messages	2 messages	2 messages	4 messages	4 messages	4 messages

Protocols of Khatoon et al., Ostad-Sharif et al. and Khan et al. require 2 messages with 1472 bits, 2528 bits and 1760 bits, respectively. However, protocols of Xu et al., Alzahrani et al. and the proposed one need 4 messages of 3136 bits, 3136 bits and 3872 bits, respectively. The first three protocols in Table 4 do not involve any intermediate entity between two end parties for the communication. That is why the communication requirements are less than those four other protocols. In addition to this, the proposed protocol requires about 700 bits more than Xu et al.'s protocol and Alzahrani et al.'s protocol due to the session-dependent dynamic identifier distribution to entities in the system. As shown in Figure 6, in contrast with the computational overhead, the proposed protocol requires the heaviest communicational overhead due to the usage of AP in between SN and HN, which is different from the other protocols.

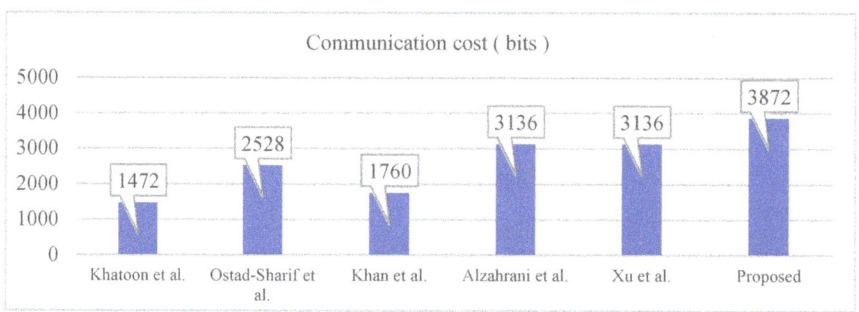

Figure 6. Communication cost comparison.

6. Discussion

This section discusses challenges and solutions on the authentication protocol for WBAN based healthcare applications. After that, we will provide some future work.

6.1. Challenges and Soluitons

Healthcare systems can provide an opportunity to meet the needs of individuals or households facing health difficulties. However, the healthcare system has an obligation to protect the privacy of patients [56]. And all participants in healthcare such as professionals of medical industries, always must be provide privacy with health data. Furthermore, healthcare professionals and medical industries around the globe are urged to fight against various security and privacy attacks on the healthcare system. WBAN based healthcare application shares some common functionalities with a typical computer network as it is a special type of network and also exhibits several unique characteristics that are specific to it. WBAN based healthcare application requires to guarantee security, privacy, data integrity and confidentiality of patient's EHR at all times. Towards the design of efficient cryptographic solution, there are more challenges in the WBANs than wired networks. They are the wireless nature of communication, resource inadequacy on SNs and very large and dense networks. Authentication is considered as the basic security building block for any systems, which is a process by which the identity of a node in a network is verified and guarantees that the data or the control messages originate from an authenticated source. So, we will address some challenges and solutions for the authentication protocol.

The first challenge is to provide security in healthcare services that use the public network. Authentication protocol based on the public network is vulnerable against various attacks such as replay attack, impersonation attack and man-in-the-middle attack. The security issues could be overcome by utilizing various cryptographic primitives including asymmetric key cryptography, symmetric key cryptography, hash function and so on. Recently, researchers have been developing lightweight protocols, such as hash-based protocol and symmetric key cryptography-based protocol, to achieve feasibility on WBANs. Furthermore, designing authentication protocols with PUFs could help to resolve the security issues.

The second challenge is to preserve the privacy of network entities. Patient personal information is one of the most sensitive data in message transmission over the public network. The privacy issues could be dealt with by utilizing session-dependent information such as a one-time pseudonym for only the session usage. Recently, researchers have been deploying unidirectional hash chain values. A hash value from the chain is used only once and authentication protocol based on the value could provide unlinkability between sessions. In addition, cryptographic researchers should collaborate with healthcare professionals and medical industry workers to adopt and recognize various target field requirements from different backgrounds and aspects.

6.2. Future Work

In short, the proposed authentication protocol tries to generalize the process of mutual authentication and session key agreement for WBANs in healthcare applications. The proposed protocol takes full lightweight advantage of one-way hash function and exclusive-or operation to establish better security and privacy in solving authentication and session key establishment issues. In our future work, we aim to implement the proposed protocol in a real hospital environment with a big EHR database. We will focus on conducting experiments by optimizing patient side operational and communicational overhead of the proposed protocol to achieve better WBAN feasibility in terms of improved security and privacy. In addition, we will deploy a real-time adaptive artificial intelligence model on categorizing and analyzing EHR data to provide much richer patient healthcare services. Artificial intelligence can bring numerous benefits to the evolving of the healthcare industry. Based on artificial intelligence software, certain symptoms can be detected before the obvious symptoms of diseases such as lung cancer appear [57]. In addition, in the case of learned artificial intelligence, it can reduce the possibility of a doctor's misdiagnosis, to reducing patient anxiety [58]. Moreover, this research work will motivate researchers to pay more attention to security and privacy and explore the combination of other technologies, such as multimedia, robots and smart cities, to provide more convenient healthcare services to patients.

7. Conclusions

In this paper, we proposed a privacy-preserving authentication protocol for WBANs in healthcare applications. First of all, we set our design goals focused on 5 security properties and 2 privacy requirements, which are mutual authentication, session key agreement, message freshness, perfect forward secrecy, attack resistance, anonymity and unlinkability. To satisfy those features, we designed a new authentication protocol based on only two simple and lightweight operations, hash and exclusive-or. Especially, to provide 2 privacy requirements, the proposed protocol uses session-dependent pseudo identifiers for SN and AP. The formal and informal privacy and security analyses demonstrate the resistance of the proposed protocol against all sorts of privacy and security attacks. Especially, the privacy and security features of the proposed protocol are formally verified and validated based on BAN logic and ProVerif simulation tool. Performance analysis showed that the proposed protocol has a reasonable overhead compared to the related previous protocols but still lightweight. We need to note that privacy-preserving is an important feature in healthcare service because healthcare information is sensitive. Nobody wants to expose their EHR-related information to others.

Author Contributions: Conceptualization, H.K.; methodology, H.K.; software, H.R.; validation, H.K. and H.R.; formal analysis, H.K.; writing—review and editing, H.R.; supervision, H.K.; project administration, H.K.; funding acquisition, H.K. All authors have read and agreed to the published version of the manuscript.

Funding: This research was funded by Basic Science Research Program through the National Research Foundation of Korea (NRF) funded by the Ministry of Education (NRF-2017R1D1A1B04032598).

Institutional Review Board Statement: Not applicable.

Informed Consent Statement: Not applicable.

Data Availability Statement: Data could be downloaded with the following URL at https://github.com/hs-kim-andre/healthcare.git, accessed on 26 August 2021.

Conflicts of Interest: The authors declare that there are no conflicts of interest regarding the publication of this paper.

References

1. Dua, A.; Kumar, N.; Das, A.K.; Susilo, W. Secure Message Communication Protocol among Vehicles in Smart City. *IEEE Trans. Veh. Technol.* **2018**, *127*, 4359–4373. [CrossRef]
2. Roy, S.; Chatterjee, S.; Das, A.K.; Chappopadhyay, S.; Kumar, N.; Vasilakos, A.V. On the Design of Provably Secure Lightweight Remote User Authentication Scheme for Mobile Cloud Computing Services. *IEEE Access* **2017**, *5*, 25808–25825. [CrossRef]
3. Bali, R.S.; Kumar, N.S. Secure clustering for efficient data dissemination in vehicular cyber-physical systems. *Future Gener. Comput. Syst.* **2016**, *56*, 476–492. [CrossRef]
4. Li, X.; Liu, T.; Obaidat, M.S.; Wu, F.; Vijayakumar, P.; Kumar, N. A Lightweight Privacy-Preserving Authentication Protocol for VANETs. *IEEE Syst. J.* **2020**, *14*, 3547–3557. [CrossRef]
5. Vijayakumar, P.; Azees, M.; Chang, V.; Deborah, J.; Balusamy, B. Computationally efficient privacy preserving authentication and key distribution techniques for vehicular ad hoc networks. *Clust. Comput.* **2017**, *20*, 2439–2450. [CrossRef]
6. Pradhan, B.; Bhattacharyya, S.; Pal, K. IoT-Based Applications in Healthcare Devices. *J. Helathcare Eng.* **2021**, *2021*, 6632599.
7. Paek, J.; Gaglione, O.; Gnawali, O.; Vieira, M.A.M.; Hao, S. Advances in Mobile Networking for IoT Leading the 4th industrial Revolution. *Mob. Inf. Syst.* **2018**, *2018*, 8176158. [CrossRef]
8. Malik, N.N.; Alosaimi, W.; Uddin, M.I.; Alouffi, B.; Alyami, H. Wireless Sensor Network Applications in Healthcare and Precision Agriculture. *J. Healthc. Eng.* **2020**, *2020*, 8836613. [CrossRef]
9. Cho, S.; Kim, H. Secure Authenticated Key Agreement for Telecare Health Services using Ubiquitous IoT. *Int. J. Adv. Electron. Comput. Sci.* **2019**, *6*, 28–32.
10. Zhang, N.; Ning, W.; Xie, T.; Liu, J.; He, R.; Zhu, B.; Mao, Y. Spatial Disparities in Access to Healthcare Professionals in Sichuan: Evidence from County-Level Data. *Healthcare* **2021**, *9*, 1053. [CrossRef]
11. Park, B.; Lee, H. Healthcare Safety Nets during the COVID-19 Pandemic Based on Double Diamond Model: A Concept Analysis. *Healthcare* **2021**, *9*, 1014. [CrossRef]
12. McDonald, Y.J.; Goldberg, D.W.; Scarinci, I.C.; Castle, P.E.; Cuzick, J.; Robertson, M.; Wheeler, C.M. Health Service Accessibility and Risk in Cervical Cancer Prevention: Comparing Rural Versus Nonrural Residence in New Mexico: Health Service Accessibility. *J. Rural. Health* **2017**, *33*, 382–392. [CrossRef] [PubMed]
13. Kaluski, D.N.; Stojanovski, K.; McWeeney, G.; Paunovic, E.; Ostlin, P.; Licari, L.; Jakab, Z. Health insurance and accessibility to health services among Roma in settlements in Belgrade, Serbia—The journey from data to policy making. *Health Policy Plan.* **2015**, *30*, 976–984. [CrossRef] [PubMed]
14. Ganann, R.; Sword, W.; Newbold, K.B.; Thabane, L.; Armour, L.; Kint, B. Influences on mental health and health services accessibility in immigrant women with post-partum depression: An interpretive descriptive study. *J. Psychiatr. Ment. Health Nurs.* **2020**, *27*, 87–96. [CrossRef] [PubMed]
15. Cookson, R.; Propper, C.; Asaria, M.; Raine, R. Socio-Economic Inequalities in Health Care in England. *Fisc. Stud.* **2016**, *37*, 371–403. [CrossRef]
16. Bisio, I.; Lavagetto, F.; Marchese, M.; Sciarrone, A. A smartphone-centric platform for remote health monitoring of heart failure. *Int. J. Commun. Syst.* **2015**, *28*, 1753–1771. [CrossRef]
17. Kalid, N.; Zaidan, A.A.; Zaidan, B.B.; Salman, O.H.; Hashim, M.; Albahri, O.S.; Albahri, A.S. Based on Real Time Remote Health Monitoring Systems: A New Approach for Prioritization "Large Scales Data" Patients with Chronic Heart Diseases Using Body Sensors and Communication Technology. *J. Med Syst.* **2018**, *42*, 1–37. [CrossRef]

18. Wang, P.; Tsao, L.; Chen, Y.; Lo, Y.; Sun, H. "Hesitating and Puzzling": The Experiences and Decision Process of Acute Ischemic Stroke Patients with Prehospital Delay after the Onset of Symptoms. *Healthcare* **2021**, *9*, 1061. [CrossRef]
19. Rahman, M.Z.U.; Karthik, G.V.S.; Fathima, S.Y.; Lay-Ekuakille, A. An efficient cardiac signal enhancement using time–frequency realization of leaky adaptive noise cancelers for remote health monitoring systems. *Measurement* **2013**, *46*, 3815–3835. [CrossRef]
20. Majumder, S.; Mondal, T.; Deen, M.J. Wearable Sensors for Remote Health Monitoring. *Sensors* **2017**, *17*, 130. [CrossRef]
21. Gu, D.; Humbatova, G.; Xie, Y.; Yang, X.; Zolotarev, O.; Zhang, G. Different Roles of Telehealth and Telemedicine on Medical Tourism: An Empirical Study from Azerbaijan. *Healthcare* **2021**, *9*, 1073. [CrossRef]
22. Al-Janabi, S.; Al-Shourbaji, I.; Shojafar, M.; Shamshirband, S. Survey of main challenges (security and privacy) in wireless body area networks for healthcare applications. *Egypt. Inform. J.* **2017**, *18*, 113–122. [CrossRef]
23. Liu, Q.; Mkongwa, K.G.; Zhang, C. Performance issues in wireless body area networks for the healthcare application: A survey and future prospects. *SN Appl. Sci.* **2021**, *3*, 1–19. [CrossRef]
24. Formica, D.; Schena, E. Smart Sensors for Healthcare and Medical Applications. *Sensors* **2021**, *21*, 543. [CrossRef] [PubMed]
25. Tovino, S.A. Privacy and Security Issues with Mobile Health Research Applications. *J. Law Med. Ethics* **2019**, *47*, 154–158.
26. Kim, H. Research Issues on Data Centric Security and Privacy Model for Intelligent Internet of Things based Healthcare. *ICSES Trans. Comput. Netw. Commun.* **2019**, *5*, 1–3. [CrossRef]
27. Kim, H. Data Centric Security and Privacy Research Issues for Intelligent Internet of Things. *ICSES Interdisiplinary Trans. Cloud Comput. IoT Big Data* **2017**, *1*, 1–2.
28. Vijayakumar, P.; Chang, V.; Deborah, L.J.; Balusamy, B.; Shynu, P.G. Computationally efficient privacy preserving anonymous mutual and batch authentication schemes for vehicular ad hoc networks. *Future Gener. Comput. Syst.* **2018**, *78*, 943–955. [CrossRef]
29. Vora, J.; Italiya, P.; Tanwar, S.; Tyagi, S.; Kumar, N.; Obaidat, M.S.; Hsiao, K.-F. Ensuring Privacy and Security in E-Health Records. In Proceedings of the 2018 International Conferecne on Computer, Information and Telecommunication Systems, Colmar, France, 11–13 July 2018.
30. Zhu, J.; Ma, J. A new authentication scheme with anonymity for wireless environments. *IEEE Trans. Consum. Electron.* **2004**, *50*, 231–235.
31. Lee, C.C.; Hwang, M.S.; Liao, I.E. Security enhancement on a new authentication scheme with anonymity for wireless environments. *IEEE Trans. Ind. Electron.* **2006**, *53*, 1683–1687. [CrossRef]
32. Memon, I.; Hussain, I.; Akhtar, R.; Chen, G. Enhanced Privacy and Authentication: An Efficient and Secure Anonymous Communication for Location Based Service Using Asymmetric Cryptography Scheme. *Wirel. Pers. Commun.* **2015**, *84*, 1487–1508. [CrossRef]
33. Reddy, A.G.; Das, A.K.; Yoon, E.J.; Yoo, K.Y. A Secure Anonymous Authentication Protocol for Mobile Services on Elliptic Curve Cryptography. *IEEE Access* **2016**, *4*, 4394–4407. [CrossRef]
34. Khatoon, S.; Rahman, S.M.M.; Alrubaian, M.; Alamri, A. Privacy-Preserved, Provable Secure, Mutually Authenticated Key Agreement Protocol for Healthcare in a Smart City Environment. *IEEE Access* **2019**, *7*, 47962–47971. [CrossRef]
35. Ostad-Sharif, A.; Abbasinezhad-Mood, D.; Kikooghadam, M. An enhanced anonymous and unlinkable user authentication and key agreement protocol for TMIS by utilization of ECC. *Int. J. Commun. Syst.* **2019**, *32*, e3913. [CrossRef]
36. Ali, Z.; Ghani, A.; Khan, I.; Chaudhry, S.A.; Islam, H.; Giri, D. A robust authentication and access control protocol for securing wireless healthcare sensor networks. *J. Inf. Secur. Appl.* **2020**, *52*. [CrossRef]
37. Burrows, M.; Abadi, M.; Needham, R. A logic of authentication. *R. Soc. Lond. Math. Phys. Eng. Sci.* **1989**, *426*, 233–271.
38. Khan, I.; Chaudhry, S.A.; Sher, M.; Khan, J.I.; Khan, M.K. An anonymous and provably secure biometric-based authentication scheme using chaotic maps for accessing medical drop box data. *J. Supercomput.* **2018**, *74*, 3685–3703. [CrossRef]
39. Aman, M.N.; Chua, K.C.; Sikdar, B. A light-weight mutual authentication protocol for IoT systems. In Proceedings of the 2017 IEEE Global Communications Conference, Singapore, 4–18 December 2017.
40. Xu, Z.; Xu, C.; Chen, H.; Yang, F. A lightweight anonymous mutual authentication and key agreement scheme for WBAN. *Concurr. Comput. Pract. Exp.* **2019**, *31*, e5295. [CrossRef]
41. Alzahrani, B.A.; Irshad, A.; Albeshri, A.; Alsubhi, K. A Provably Secure and Lightweight Patient-Healthcare Authentication Protocol in Wireless Body Area Networks. *Wirel. Pers. Commun.* **2021**, *117*, 47–69. [CrossRef]
42. Blanchet, B. Automatic Verification of Security Protocols in the Symbolic Model: The Verifier ProVerif. *Lect. Notes Comput. Sci.* **2013**, *8604*, 54–87.
43. Liu, B.; Han, B.; Zheng, H.; Liu, H.; Zhao, T.; Wan, Y.; Cui, F. Who Is the Most Vulnerable to Anxiety at the Beginning of the COVID-19 Outbreak in China? A Cross-Sectional Nationwide Survey. *Healthcare* **2021**, *9*, 970. [CrossRef]
44. Canetti, R.; Krawczyk, H. Analysis of Key-Exchange Protocols and Their Use for Building Secure Channels. In Proceedings of the EUROCRYPT 2001, Innsbruck, Austria, 6–10 May 2001; Springer: Berlin/Heidelberg, Germany, 2001; pp. 453–474.
45. Sarr, A.P.; Elbaz-Vincent, P.; Bajard, J.-C. A New Security Model for Authenticated Key Agreement. In Proceedings of the Security and Cryptography for Networks, Amalfi, Italy, 13–15 September 2010; Springer: Berlin/Heidelberg, Germany, 2010; pp. 219–234.
46. Xu, Z.; Luo, M.; Kumar, N.; Vijayakumar, P.; Li, L. Privacy-Protection Scheme Based on Sanitizable Signature for Smart Mobile Medical Scenarios. *Wirel. Commun. Mob. Comput.* **2020**, *2020*, 8877405. [CrossRef]
47. Klumpp, M.; Hintze, M.; Immonen, M.; Ródenas-Rigla, F.; Pilati, F.; Aparicio-Martínez, F.; Çelebi, D.; Liebig, T.; Jirstrand, M.; Urbann, O.; et al. Artificial Intelligence for Hospital Health Care: Application Cases and Answers to Challenges in European Hospitals. *Healthcare* **2021**, *9*, 961. [CrossRef]

48. Wang, D.; He, D.; Wang, P.; Chu, C. Anonymous Two-Factor Authentication in Distributed Systems: Certain Goals Are Beyond Attainment. *IEEE Trans. Dependable Secur. Comput.* **2015**, *12*, 428–442. [CrossRef]
49. Avoine, G.; Canard, S.; Ferreira, L. Symmetric-kay Authenticated Key Exchange (SAKE) with Perfect Forward Secrecy. In Proceedings of the CT-RSA, San Francisco, CA, USA, 24–28 February 2020; Springer: Cham, Switzerland, 2020; pp. 24–28.
50. Bellare, M.; Yee, B.B. Forward-security in private-key cryptography. In Proceedings of the CT-RSA, San Francisco, CA, USA, 13–17 April 2003; Springer: Berlin/Heidelberg, Germany, 2003; pp. 1–18.
51. Brier, E.; Peyrin, T. A forward-secure symmetric-key derivation protocol—How to improve classical DUKPT. In Proceedings of the ASIACRYPT, Singapore, 5–9 December 2010; Springer: Berlin/Heidelberg, Germany, 2010; pp. 250–257.
52. Abdalla, M.; Bellare, M. Increasing the lifetime of a key: A comparative analysis of the security of re-keying techniques. In Proceedings of the ASIACRYPT, Kyoto, Japan, 3–7 December 2000; Springer: Berlin/Heidelberg, Germany, 2000; pp. 546–559.
53. Nikooghadam, M.; Admintoosi, H. Cryptanalysis of Khatoon et al.'s ECC-based Authentication Protocol for Healthcare System. *arXiv* **2019**, arXiv:190608424N.
54. Li, W.; Wang, P. Two-factor authentication in industrial Internet-of_things: Attacks, evaluation and new construction. *Future Gener. Comput.* **2019**, *101*, 694–708. [CrossRef]
55. Babamir, F.; Kirci, M. Dynamic digest based authentication for client–server systems using biometric verification. *Future Gener. Comput. Syst.* **2019**, *101*, 112–126. [CrossRef]
56. Kaplan, B. How Should Health Data Be Used? Privacy, Secondary Use, and Big Data Sales. *Camb. Q. Healthc. Ethics* **2016**, *25*, 312–329. [CrossRef]
57. Richens, J.G.; Lee, C.M.I. Improving the accuracy of medical diagnosis with causal machine learning. *Nat. Commun.* **2021**, *12*, 3923. [CrossRef]
58. How AI Technologies Accelerate Progress in Medical Diagnosis. Available online: https://roboticsandautomationnews.com/2020/03/09/how-ai-technologies-accelerate-progress-in-medical-diagnosis/31184/ (accessed on 26 August 2021).

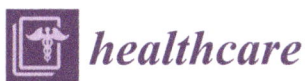

Article

Adolescents, Ambivalent Sexism and Social Networks, a Conditioning Factor in the Healthcare of Women

Jose Luis Gil Bermejo [1,*], Cinta Martos Sánchez [1,2], Octavio Vázquez Aguado [1] and E. Begoña García-Navarro [2,3]

[1] Department of Sociology, Social Work and Public Health, University of Huelva, 21004 Huelva, Spain; cmartos@dstso.uhu.es (C.M.S.); octavio@dstso.uhu.es (O.V.A.)
[2] Research Group "Estudios Sociales e Intervención Social", University of Huelva, 21004 Huelva, Spain; esperanza.garcia@denf.uhu.es
[3] Department of Nursing, University of Huelva, 21004 Huelva, Spain
* Correspondence: gestalt.jose@gmail.com, Tel.: +34-622-050-928

Abstract: Even though gender equality being present in the social and political sphere, we still encounter aspects that are characteristic of sexism. Such aspects impact upon gender inequality and different types of violence towards women. The present article aims to examine the behaviour of adolescents from Huelva with regards to ambivalent sexism towards women on social networks and their influence on health. Furthermore, we seek to uncover adolescent's perceptions with regards to gender differences in the use of social networks, the relationship between sexism and women's emotional well-being was observed. The study sample was formed by young people aged between 14 and 16 years who were residing in rural and urban zones in the south of Spain. A mixed methods approach was taken. At a quantitative level, a sample of 400 young people was recruited. These were administered a questionnaire about sexism which was composed of two scales and has been validated at a national and international level. At a qualitative level, the study counted on 33 young people who participated in in-depth discussions via interviews and discussion groups. The results showed that sexism emerges in adolescence in the analysed sample from the south of Spain. This favoured a digital gender gap and was reinforced through social networks such as Instagram and Snapchat. Rising awareness and a critical view of the aforementioned sexism was shown on the behalf of females, particularly those from urban backgrounds.

Keywords: sexism; social networks; adolescence; digital gender gap; emotional well-being

1. Introduction

In a postmodern society, such as today's, gender equality is seemingly addressed by public authorities and assumed to exist in society in general [1–3]. Steps towards gender equality and women's freedom have supposedly challenged the hegemony of the patriarchal system [4]. Yet, we maintain the belief that gender inequality still persists to a large extent and often manifests itself as recurrent violence towards women [5]. Unfortunately, such violence is being observed at increasingly younger ages, even being seen within the adolescent population [6]. This reality motivated us to conduct the present research.

Sexism is a complex construct that forms a part of the gender differentiation between males and females. It has especially negative repercussions for females and for anyone who moves away from the dominant hegemonic masculinity [7]. Sexism in itself, houses a set of beliefs regarding respect for established gender roles. It has very negative mental health repercussions for women and perpetuates their subordination to men [8–10]. A nuance of this can be explored through the concept of ambivalent sexism [8], which is composed of masculine dominance and represented through hostility and interdependence. From this perspective, ambivalent sexism has two components, namely, hostile sexism and benevolent sexism [8,9,11]. Hostile sexism concerns a gender ideology that is directly discriminatory and violent towards women. It has three fundamental factors. The first is male paternalism towards females in the sense of dominance due to the belief that women are the weaker sex relative to men. The second factor pertains to a competitive gender differentiation in which the belief is held that women cannot take responsibility over important issues, such as those that are economic or social in nature, in the same way that men can. The final factor concerns heterosexual hostility and assumes that women present a danger and a manipulative force to men [12]. On the other hand, we find that which is denominated benevolent sexism. This ideology involves subtle gender discrimination and is characterised by the following factors: Paternalism, complementary gender differentiation and cisgender heteronormative intimacy. The former is manifested in this type of sexism from the standpoint of protection, whilst the second factor refers to positive characteristics which complement the man and, equally, mark gender differences in a supposedly logical way. The latter, cisgender heteronormative intimacy comes from the belief that a man is incomplete without a woman [8,10].

During adolescence, we can observe that ambivalent sexism is transmitted through social networks. This occurs in a number of ways [13], for instance in writing via hashtags, likes, videogames, music and images, in addition to through expressive instrumentalised means, above all through mobile phones [14]. In the adolescent population, this type of sexism, through social networks, takes on special characteristics with regards to the rapid and direct dissemination of material, which quickly becomes viral in adolescent groups [15]. On the other hand, the anonymity offered by social networks means they can be used to promote more violent forms of sexism towards women [16,17]. The tendency towards audio visual preferences amongst younger people as a form of expression on social networks, for instance through photographs or videos [18–20], shows that females present such images in a more sexualised way. This occurs in virtual daily practices such as that known as sexting [21–23] and reflects sexism against women and the risk posed by this type of practice. Worryingly, such practices are increasingly more common on social networks, especially amongst women [24]. For this reason, it is important to deepen the knowledge of this worrying and current issue that especially affects the emotional state and healthcare of younger women [25]. The aim of the present work was to observe the way in which ambivalent sexism manifests itself through social networks in both men and women, a situation that has been shown to particularly affect the emotional health of women. Furthermore, we sought to examine its impact within a 14- to 16-year-old population from the region of Huelva given that this is an important age for determining the future state of the adult population and this geographical region is characterised by both urban and rural areas which have very different social realities.

The present study contributes to the examination of gender theory in relation to women's mental health through an analysis of the relationship of variables related with sexism and social networks. The gender theory perspective leads us to gender inequality in adolescence, expressed through sexism and social networks, since these issues have an impact on the emotional wellbeing of people, especially women. The key contribution of the present research is, therefore, its implications when it comes to addressing inequality between men and women [9,13,15].

2. Method

In order to respond to the proposed objectives, the present work took a quantitative and qualitative methodological approach which was fed by a pluralist methodological approach. It was accompanied by data and information triangulation [26]. This will enable us to better approach subtle issues regarding ambivalent sexism and gender differences [27,28]. Research met the requisite ethical conditions by obtaining informed written consent from minors' legal guardians.

2.1. Participants

A sample of 400 students aged between 14 and 16 years was selected from public educational centres in the province of Huelva. All participants were compulsory secondary education (ESO) students and came from 7 public educational centres. Students were classified as coming from rural (>5000 inhabitants) or urban (<5000 inhabitants) settings. The average age of participants was 15.01 years (SD = 0.82). Non-random sampling was performed in consideration of the study categories that is was necessary to represent. In other words, participants were selected to represent males (n = 200) and females (n = 200), whilst also equally representing all ages between 14 and 16 years, and rural and urban geographic regions (see Table 1). Survey data was only included from fully completed surveys with incompletes surveys being discarding.

With regards to the qualitative analysis, the sample was formed of three discussion groups. Of these, one was formed by 7 males, another was formed by 8 females and the third was a mixed group of 10 individuals. In addition to this, 8 in-depth interviews were conducted with four females and four males. Interview participants were different to those who attended discussion groups. Overall, qualitative analysis included a total of 33 individuals from urban and rural settings.

Table 1. Sample: Age, sex and geographical location.

Categories	Geographical Location		Total
	Urban	Rural	
14 years	100	32	132
15 years	96	38	134
16 years	85	49	134
Men	144	56	200
Women	137	63	200

Source: Developed by the author.

2.2. Instruments

Two types of rating scales on ambivalent sexism were administered. Some sociodemographic data were also collected, alongside to questions about social networks. The scales are described below.

The ambivalent sexism inventory, ASI, developed by Glick and Fiske [8] in the reduced Spanish version of Rodríguez, Lameiras and Carrera [29]. with hostile (traditional) and benevolent sexist attitudes (positive affective tone) towards women are measured. All items have a 6-point response format (from 1 "totally disagree" to 6 "totally agree"). Higher scores indicate higher level of sexism towards women. The present study obtained a Cronbach reliability alpha of 0.81 for hostile sexism (HS) and 0.76 for benevolent sexism (BS). The inventory of ambivalent sexism consists of 11 items and is intended for the general population.

The Detected Sexism in Adolescent scale (DSA), the most updated version [30], validated in its smallest version [31]. This scale measures in their items' hostile sexism and benevolent sexism (ambivalent sexism). The articles were answered on a 6-point Likert scale, with options running from 1 (totally disagree) to 6 (totally agree). The 10-item scale is intended for the adolescent population and measures ambivalent sexism. Two scales of ambivalent sexism were required in order to measure the hostile and benevolent aspects of sexism. This is important in order to be able to later link ambivalent sexism with social networks and their subsequent impact on women's emotional health.

In addition to including sociodemographic data for the instruments, we added two questions in relation to social networks in order to be analyzed with the previous scales. The first is, which networks are most commonly used? This question was posed with multiple response options being provided, specifically, the following alternatives were given: Whatsapp, Twitter, Facebook, Youtube, Tuenti, Instagram, SnapChat, blogs and other social networks. Whatsapp was included although it is not really a social network because we consider that this instant messaging application increasingly possesses characteristics that are fitting of a social network at its broadest communication level (through groups, distribution lists and 24 h states). The second question strives to uncover the reasons for which these networks are used. As with the former question, response options allowed various responses to be given, including: to gossip about others, talk with my partner (where relevant), communicate with my family, for school use and learning, to meet others, to hook up and to talk with friends/people I already know.

Qualitative analysis produced the following preliminary categories: differentiated use of social networks, references to the type of social networks and reasons for their use and attributes associated with the identification of either of the genders. Different categories underlying ambivalent sexism emerged during the interviews and discussion groups. Such themes arose following reflection.

2.3. Procedure

An observational design was developed, which was descriptive and cross-sectional in nature. The sample was selected through non-random convenience sampling. This was made possible sue to the ease of access granted by the participating educational centres in the province of Huelva. When selecting educational centres, the number of inhabitants in the locality was taken as a reference. Urban and rural settings were defined as having more or less than 5000 inhabitants, respectively. We selected a total of 7 public educational centres, with 4 coming from urban settings and 3 from rural settings. Once access was granted by the centre, a date and time was agreed upon to complete questionnaires. We then sent informed consent forms to the educational centres for legal guardians to sign on behalf of the students. The educational levels examined corresponded to the 3rd and 4th years of ESO. On the day on which questionnaires were completed in the classroom, discussion groups and interviews were organised with the students who voluntarily agreed to participate in one of the two slots. Volunteers were recruited until sex, age and geographical location groups were all well represented.

Qualitative analysis techniques were carried out the following week. Two team members participated in the interviews with the aim of minimizing bias resulting from not having physical contact between agents. One researcher proceeded to conduct the interview whilst the other took over the technical aspects and took fieldnotes.

2.4. Data Analysis

Quantitative data analysis was conducted using the statistical analysis program SPSS (IBM Statistics v.25). Comparative analysis was conducted of basic variables (n = 400). The variables explored were ambivalent sexism, use of social networks and sex. The main dependent variable was sexism and Chi-square analysis was performed.

Qualitative analysis was performed based on discourse analysis, considering emergent discourse from both discussion groups and interviews. This was conducted using the qualitative data handling program ATLAS. Ti. V.8. The categories that resulted from this analysis were as follows: differentiated use of social networks, references to the type of social networks and reasons for their use, and attributes associated with the identification of either of the genders. Next, the categories and sub-categories to emerge from quantitative analysis following the aforementioned techniques are detailed (see Table 2).

During data collection, informed consent was received from informants and confidentiality and anonymity were maintained throughout. Prior to study start, participants were informed about the study objectives and the bioethical principles of the Helsinki declaration were respected. In addition, data obtained from the various discourses comply with current regulations regarding the protection of personal data.

Table 2. Categories and subcategories to emerge from the study according to different techniques.

Dimension	Categories	Subcategories	Interviews	Discussion Groups
Ambivalent sexism on social networks	Differentiated use of social networks between males and females	Stereotyped image given of women	x	x
		Social networks used	x	x
	Benevolent sexism on social networks	Feminine stereotypes	x	x
		Chivalry		x
	Hostile sexism on social networks	Stigmatisation towards women if they don't conform with feminine stereotypes		x
	Geographic setting	Rural (control)		x
		Urban (critical view)		x

Source: elaborated by the authors in relation to data obtained through qualitative analysis.

3. Results

Next, we describe outcomes, giving detailed information on the extent of associations between the two used scales (ASI and DSA) in the adolescent population. It is worth mentioning that both scales measure ambivalent sexism but according to the different categories of hostile and benevolent sexism. The present study considers sexism in general when referring to ambivalent sexism. Outcomes presented in the following tables pertain to sexism and use of specific social networks (Instagram, Snapchat, YouTube/Blogs).

With regards to the study objectives, the existing relationship was analysed between the two ambivalent sexism scales employed and the social networks Instagram and Snapchat. Two scales were used that pertained to ambivalent sexism in adolescents (DSA) and ambivalent sexism in the general population (ASI), with these scales being significantly correlated ($p < 0.001$). Mean scores of the two scales are classified as sexist or otherwise with 57.6% of adolescents reporting scores corresponding to sexism. Chi-squared outcomes showed no significant differences between males and females.

A relationship was observed between sexism and Instagram use, with a significant relationship ($p < 0.05$) emerging on both scales, although a particularly strong relationship emerged for 8 items of the DSA scale and 3 items of the ASI scale (see Table 3).

If we move on to the social network Snapchat, we find more relationships between the variables, with these associations also showing a higher significance level (see Table 4). With regards to the DSA scale, for 7 of the sexist beliefs a positive association was found between confirmation of sexism and using Snapchat, with the same outcome for young people who used the social network and stated sexist beliefs. With regards to the ASI scale, more relationships emerged in relation with Snapchat than with Instagram, with significant relationships emerging with 10 sexist beliefs in the case of the latter.

Table 3. Relationship between the social network Instagram and sexism.

Variables	% of Young People Who Present with Sexism and Use Instagram	Chi-Squared Value
Instagram and 'patient woman' **	82.5%	10.1
Instagram and 'tender woman' ***	82.7%	14.48
Instagram and 'accommodating woman' ***	84.6%	16.52
Instagram and 'sympathetic woman' ***	83.5%	13.1
Instagram and 'fragile woman' **	84.5	11.38
Instagram and 'forgiving woman' **	81.7%	5.73
Instagram and 'woman at home' **	81.1%	4.57
Instagram and 'women suffering' **	82.3%	7.02
Instagram and 'women as a complement' **	88.4%	6.44
Instagram and 'loved and protected woman' **	81%	6.12
Instagram and 'man without woman' **	81.9%	8.51

Note: ** $p < 0.05$, *** $p < 0.001$; degrees of freedom = 1, DSA scale (gray), ASI scale (dark gray). Source: Developed by the authors.

Table 4. Relationship between the social network Snapchat and sexism.

Variables	% of Young People Who Present with Sexism and Use Snapchat	Chi-Squared Value
Snapchat and 'tender woman' ***	72.8%	24.1
Snapchat and 'sympathetic woman' ***	73.4%	19.13
Snapchat and 'women raise children' **	70.7%	10.16
Snapchat and 'forgiving woman' ***	72.3%	12.79
Snapchat and 'fragile woman' ***	47.1%	26.1
Snapchat and 'sensitive woman' **	69.2%	5.68
Snapchat and 'woman in the home' **	70.6%	7.99
Snapchat and 'women complement men' ***	70.6%	17.12
Snapchat and 'other heterosexual sex' **	69.3%	4.72
Snapchat and 'woman's purity' **	68.7%	4.27
Snapchat and 'loved woman' **	69.2%	6.67
Snapchat and 'love between man and woman' **	69.4%	8.93
Snapchat 'man without a woman' **	70.1%	8.66
Snapchat and 'women on a pedestal' **	69.9%	4.9
Snapchat and 'moral woman' **	68.8%	7.2
Snapchat and 'accommodating woman' ***	74.6%	22.35
Snapchat and 'patient woman' **	71.1%	11.41

Note: ** $p < 0.05$, *** $p < 0.001$; degrees of freedom = 1, DSA scale, (gray), ASI scale (dark gray). **Source**: Developed by the authors.

As we can see in Table 4, we observe that the use of other social networks, such as YouTube and blogs, was also related with sexist beliefs. In this case, aspects such as perceiving there to be greater compassion and suffering amongst women were related with the use of YouTube, whilst the idea that women should be put on a pedestal by men or that women have greater moral sensitivity was related with blog use. On the other hand, some results also pointed to the lack of associations. For instance, users of Tuenti did not demonstrate a large extent of sexism, whilst at the same time, those who did not present with sexist beliefs tended not to use Tuenti. Specifically, this relationship emerged with regards to beliefs around raising children, the fragility of women in respect to men and the idea that they should be rescued by men (see Table 5).

Table 5. Relationship between other social networks and sexism.

Variables	% of Young People Who Present with Sexism and Use YouTube/Blogs	Chi-Squared Value
YouTube and 'sympathetic woman' **	69.2%	4.27
YouTube and 'women suffering' **	68.2%	5.76
YouTube and 'women on a pedestal' **	67.6%	6.88
Blogs and 'moral woman' **	69.8%	4.53
Variables (Inverse Relationship)	% of Young People Who Do Not Present with Sexism and Do Not Use Tuenti	Chi-Squared value
Tuenti and 'women raise children' **	80.1%	8.41
Tuenti and 'fragile woman' **	77.2%	6.19
Tuenti and 'rescued woman' **	76%	5.74

Note: ** $p < 0.05$, *** $p < 0.001$; degrees of freedom = 1, DSA scale, (gray), ASI scale (dark gray). Source: Developed by the author.

Here we finish the presentation of the associations uncovered between data pertaining to social networks and sexist beliefs. Without a doubt, the two social networks with more visual impact such as Instagram and, especially, Snapchat, were the networks most strongly related with sexist beliefs when measured on either of the two utilized scales. We will now move onto the qualitative aspect in order to better understand the nuances present with regards to the relationship between sexism and social networks (see Table 6).

With regards to the discourse analysis (Transcription of categories: [UW16]: 16-year-old urban woman; [RM15]: 15-year-old rural man.), we will begin by addressing the relationship between sexism and sex.

Within women, we observe the way in which images of feminine ideals are promoted, not only with regards to attributes but also the sexist beliefs that seem to be acknowledged by women and act as coercive means to restrict behaviour within what is accepted by established norms.

- "Girls who look like boys are not viewed well, in fact they tell you that you are a lesbian, you've got to uphold a certain feminine image, you can be hooking up with another girl, but whilst you don't hold yourself like a guy there isn't any problem, nobody messes with you, if you always look good [UW15]".
- "It's not that we are better, more charming, more patient, what happens is that they label us in that way and if you don't abide by that even just a little they let you know [RW16]".
- "Here in the village the control is incredible, any situation, the way you dress or who you hang out with marks you and conditions you, for this reason you have to know really well what you are doing if you don't want to mess up [RW14]".

In the accounts given by females from rural settings social control emerged to a greater extent than it did in the accounts of urban females, where this theme emerged occasionally. Without a doubt, in settings with fewer inhabitants, such as in rural environments, there seems to be a greater indication that behaviour occurs outside of that which is normally accepted, in this waypromoting hostile sexism. In contrast, in urban areas there is a greater sense of criticism by females towards the recognition of hostile sexism through behaviour.

- "Yeah, but what do you do? On the one hand you have to be someone who waits on the man and lets him take decisions, and you're there as if you weren't, as if you didn't know what to do, stay or go, get out of the way, it's a pain, sometimes I can't

be bothered with it and I do what I like, and let them say that I'm losing my mind [UW14]".
- "For me, when its best for me I act one way and when it isn't I act another, I watch and act accordingly [UW14]".
- "I think that this doesn't happen in relationships between us, I don't feel like I have to play a role for them, you are more you, you've got to go outside of the norm a bit, if you don't you will stay in the last century [UW16]".

To another extent, in the discourse of males we see that "being a gentleman" is more associated with chivalry in males from rural areas. In this sense, it emerges as a form of masculine identity that is inherent to benevolent sexism.

- "Being attentive and a gentleman with girls is appreciated, as they give us attention and care for us better in a way that another person probably won't [RM14]".
- "The quality of a person is shown in the small details, and girls need affection and to be waited on, they like these things, we don't care so much about that, but for them it is important [RM16]".
- "I see my father do it and I don't see why it is wrong I don't know why it is criticized, it is being polite [RM14]".

Another dominant discourse to emerge amongst females, in this case amongst both rural and urban females, is the belief that women complement men. In this way, a heterosexual system of relationships and couples is promoted:

- "Without us they are lost, they don't know how to do anything, we have all the power [UW14]".
- "As hard as they try, with their buddies, going out, drinking with friends, wherever, they always come to find us afterwards, even if it is just to look good in front of the rest of their group, they need us [RW16]".
- "When they settle down later they come looking for you, deep down with us they share their most personal issues, we never leave them hanging, if they know how to behave [UW16]".

Another key aspect that we see in the discourse and represents a characteristic of benevolent sexism is the image of females. Stereotypes are associated to the female gender with regards to their behaviour, beauty and expression, and the way this is transmitted through social networks. In this sense, certain images are demanded by males and, resultantly, taken on by females:

- "I fix myself up as required, and when I do it I reap the rewards, I get myself out on social networks as best I can, with my selfies they don't confuse me with any old village lowlife [RW14]".
- "They should see you smile, we have to be ready and always prepared on the networks, to a high level [RW16]".
- "Women need a bit more loving on social networks, they are more tender, I definitely bear it in mind, obviously I like to see a beautiful girl and I will follow her on the networks [RM14]".
- "It seems crazy to me but I recognise that I log in and I look, I like to see beautiful girls, with good style doing selfies, if the photo is tacky I'm not interested [RM16]".

Table 6. Categories, subcategories and narratives associated with benevolent sexism in the adolescent population of Huelva (qualitative analysis).

Dimension	Categories	Subcategories	Relates
Sexism ambivalent on social networks	Differentiated social network use between males and females	Gender stereotyped images are stronger for females Use of social networks	— "Girls who look like boys are not looked well upon, they tell you that you are lesbian, you have to keep a certain feminine image, you can be hooking up with another girl but, whilst you don't present yourself like a guy there is no problem, nobody messes with you, if you look good in life [UW]". — "I fix myself up just enough, and when I do I reap the rewards, I put myself out online as well as I can, with my selfies they don't confuse me with any village lowlife [RW14]".
	Benevolent sexism on social networks	Feminine stereotypes Chivalry Heteronormativity	— "Being attentive and a gentleman with girls is appreciated, they give you attention and take care of you when another person probably wouldn't [RM14]". — "They [the guys] are lost without us, they don't know how to do anything, we have all the power [UW14]".
	Hostile sexism on social networks	Stigmatization towards women if they don't conform with feminine stereotypes	— "It's not that we are better, more charming, more patient, it's just that they give us that tag and as little as you don't conform with it they pull you up [RW16]".
	Geographic setting	Rural (control)	— "Control here in the town is incredible, whatever situation, way of dressing or who you go around with marks you and they condition you, for this you have to know well what you do if you don't want to mess up [RW14]".
		Urban (critical view)	— "I think that in the relationships between us this doesn't happen, I don't feel that I have to play a role for them [boys], you are more you, you have to break with the norm, if you don't you will stay in the past century [UW16]".

Source: Developed by the author.

4. Discussion

Various recent studies have verified ambivalent sexism to be a reality for Spanish youth [32–34]. In our study, males score higher in hostile sexism [35] despite its low social desirability [36].

Through the data obtained in the present research we identified equally high levels of sexism in both sexes. The qualitative nuance showed that females recognise sexism as a form of coercive social conditioning, which is manifested as behaving within accepted norms, a factor that generates hostile sexism [37].

In the same way as in the present research study, recent studies present a relationship between sexism in adolescents and social networks [38,39].

Another increasingly questioned aspect is the image of a chivalrous man, a characteristic that is framed within benevolent sexism. For women, this concept concerns education and is not associated with gender as they express not desiring to receive a different treatment simply for being women. For some men, this concept related to an identity pattern that pertains to how a man expresses interest in a woman in heteronormative relationships [40].

With regards to the examined differences in sexist beliefs between adolescents in rural and urban environments, outcomes did not reveal significant differences ($p > 0.495$). In contrast of this, the discourse analysis revealed that feelings of control in women are more important in the rural context as rural women explicitly referred to the risk they run by refusing to comply with accepted norms. Furthermore, chivalry was also observed to be an increasingly valued trait in the rural setting, especially for men. In some cases, it was even perceived as a model of masculinity to be followed within heterosexual couples by providing a way to act on romantic feelings [41].

The social networks found to be most strongly related with sexist beliefs were Instagram and Snapchat. Curiously, both encourage the use of photographs and videos. The influence of images, reflected by Instagram and Snapchat, shows us that the two social networks most related with sexism are characterised by various image-related features. These include a limited display time, almost instantaneous speed of content transmission and risk-taking in the exposure of images and text. The latter opens users up to an environment where one is observed and can act according to their free will without any restrictions [42].

With respect to photographs presented through *selfies* in females, these represent an image of a person who is alone in front of the camera and observes how the photo will look whilst they take it. In this way, individuals can present the image they wish to give within virtual settings. Furthermore, they later have the opportunity to fulfil idealized and sexualized desires, which are generally masculine [43,44]. This puts women in a situation in which they are more reliant on group self-esteem and this makes their mental health more vulnerable. Both numeric data and discourse showed us that sexism and social networks leads us to present and promote images of the ideal woman, especially, in relation to beauty ideals or formats of established femininity. Within this, we find ideals of sweetness, indulgence, sensuality, sexuality and many other attributes pertaining to how a woman should be. The image of women in social networks, given through photos and videos, is highly related with sexist beliefs. In such settings, women are once again particularly exposed as they are more vulnerable than men. Such settings can result in situations of harassment, blackmail and violence, in this way, opening up a new digital gender gap [45,46].

For the adolescents of Huelva, we can observe that social networks are not only associated with the digital gender gap. In fact, new and contrasting alternative performativity's are also emerging, which are more critical in nature and demonstrate disagreement with gender inequality in youth populations [47,48], all of this has repercussions on women's emotional distress, and their mental health has deteriorated to a great extent [49]

5. Conclusions

Results demonstrate that sexism remains an existing reality in adolescence, regardless of gender, with women being more aware of sexism and of the stigmatising factor women face when breaking free of norms and expected behaviours. In rural settings, this is manifested as a strong sense of control due to having to behave in accordance with sexist patterns in order to be socially accepted, a determinant of hostile sexism.

With regards to the heteronormative beliefs of establishing partnerships that are ideally between men and women, diverse sexist beliefs were upheld by both sexes, especially in rural settings. Another factor to be considered is that of chivalry, a characteristic of benevolent sexism. Whilst in men, this is occasionally established as a way of cementing identity, for example in the way a man expresses his love for a woman, this construct is increasingly less important within women and sometimes even criticised as an undesirable trait in men.

The social networks to most represent sexism were Instagram and Snapchat. This suggests that it is especially important for women to present themselves by sending images and videos with the aim of these becoming viral. Such acts respond to stereotyped feminine ideals, which revolve around ideas of dominant masculinity. This can be seen in the specific case of selfies that expose women to vulnerable situations in which their image is put at risk in a way that could seriously affect their self-esteem and emotional wellbeing and lead them to suffer gender-based violence. It is of great importance that future research continues to examine the way in which sexism occurs through specific social networks, photographs, videos, text, etc. Furthermore, we feel that it is important to investigate other non-heteronormative choices pertaining to relationships or desire, going beyond binary conceptions of sex or cisgender. The aim of this is to be able to be closer to the dynamic and changing reality currently lived by adolescents. On the other hand, the relationship between sexism in social networks greatly influences emotional well-being, especially among women, affecting their mental health.

In contrast of the digital gender gap related with existing sexism, we see that new standpoints, emerging masculinities, feminisms and forms of expression on social networks, show subjective, alternative, reflective and critical ways of thinking, which fall outside of the dominant behaviours or beliefs of youth.

Author Contributions: Conceptualization, J.L.G.B. and E.B.G.-N.; formal analysis, J.L.G.B. and E.B.G.-N.; research and analysis, C.M.S., O.V.A., J.L.G.B. and E.B.G.-N.; writing and preparation of the first draft, J.L.G.B. and E.B.G.-N.; drafting J.L.G.B. and E.B.G.-N. All authors have read and agreed to the published version of the manuscript.

Funding: This research received no external funding.

Institutional Review Board Statement: During data collection, informed consent was received from informants, and confidentiality and anonymity were maintained throughout. Prior to study start, participants were informed about the study objectives, and the bioethical principles of the Helsinki declaration were respected. The code of ethical approval 183-N/2020 PEIBA, the research ethics committee of the ministry of health Government of Andalusia, Spain.

Informed Consent Statement: Informed consent was obtained from all subjects involved in the study.

Data Availability Statement: The data is held by the research team and will not be published due to data protection law, but can be consulted on request.

Conflicts of Interest: The authors declare no conflict of interest.

References

1. León, M. Igualdad de género y seguridad social. *Pap. De Econ. Esp.* **2019**, *161*, 85–99.
2. Megías, P.E. Mujeres y Universidad: Situación actual y algunas propuestas para el cambio. *Educ. Law Rev.* **2019**, *20*. [CrossRef]
3. Salazar, A.L.F. Mecanismos de promoción de la igualdad de género en organismos electorales. *Rev. De Derecho Elect.* **2018**, *26*, 63–85.
4. Martínez, J.L.; Leiva, C.L.B. *Patriarcado y Capitalismo: Feminismo, Clase y Diversidad*; Akal: Madrid, España, 2019; ISBN 9788446048329.
5. Mimbrero, C.; Pallares, S.; Cantera, L.M. Competences of gender equality: Training for equality between women and men in organizations. *Athenea Digit.* **2017**, *17*, 265–286. [CrossRef]
6. Martín, A.; Pazos, M.; Montilla, M.V.C.; Romero, C. Una modalidad actual de violencia de género en parejas de jóvenes: Las redes sociales. *Education XX1* **2016**, *19*, 405–429. [CrossRef]
7. Hammond, M.D.; Milojev, P.; Huang, Y.; Sibley, C.G. Benevolent sexism and hostile sexism across the ages. *Social Psychol. Personal. Sci.* **2018**, *9*, 863–874. [CrossRef]
8. Glick, P.; Fiske, S.T. The Ambivalent Sexism Inventory: Differentiating hostile and benevolent sexism. *J. Personal. Soc. Psychol.* **1996**, *70*, 491–512. [CrossRef]
9. Glick, P.; Fiske, S.T. Ambivalent sexism. *Adv. Exp. Soc. Psychol.* **2001**, *33*, 115–188. [CrossRef]

10. Moya, M. *Actitudes sexistas y nuevas formas de sexismo. En Psicología y Género*; Barberá, E., Martínez, I., Eds.; Pearson Educación: Madrid, España, 2004; pp. 271–294.
11. Expósito, F.; Herrera, M.C.; Moya, M.; Glick, P. Don't rock the boat: Women's benevolent sexism predicts fears of marital violence. *Psychol. Women Q.* 2010, *34*, 36–42. [CrossRef]
12. Cross, E.J.; Overall, N.C.; Low, R.S.; McNulty, J.K. An interdependence account of sexism and power: Men's hostile sexism, biased perceptions of low power, and relationship aggression. *J. Personal. Soc. Psychol.* 2019, *117*, 338–363. [CrossRef]
13. Chatzakou, D.; Kourtellis, N.; Blackburn, J.; De Cristofaro, E.; Stringhini, G.; Vakali, A. Measuring #GamerGate: A tale of hate, sexism, and bullying. In Proceedings of the 26th International Conference on World Wide Web Companion, Perth, Australia, 3–7 April 2017; Barret, R., Ed.; Association for Computing Machinery: Perth, Australia, 2017; pp. 1285–1290. [CrossRef]
14. Bosson, J.K.; Kuchynka, S.L.; Parrott, D.J.; Swan, S.C.; Schramm, A.T. Injunctive norms, sexism, and misogyny network activation among men. *Psychol. Men Masc.* 2020, *21*, 124–138. [CrossRef]
15. Fox, J.; Cruz, C.; Lee, J.Y. Perpetuating online sexism offline: Anonymity, interactivity, and the effects of sexist hashtags on social media. *Comput. Hum. Behav.* 2015, *52*, 436–442. [CrossRef]
16. Finneman, T.; Jenkins, J. Sexism on the set: Gendered expectations of TV broadcasters in a social media world. *J. Broadcast. Electron. Media* 2018, *62*, 479–494. [CrossRef]
17. Butkowski, C.P.; Dixon, T.L.; Weeks, K.R.; Smith, M.A. Quantifying the feminine self (ie): Gender display and social media feedback in young women's Instagram selfies. *New Media Soc.* 2020, *22*, 817–837. [CrossRef]
18. Abbott, W.; Donaghey, J.; Hare, J.; Hopkins, P. An Instagram is worth a thousand words: An industry panel and audience Q&A. *Libr. Hi Tech News* 2013, *30*, 1–6. [CrossRef]
19. Ting, H.; Wong, W.; De Run, S.; Choo, S. Beliefs about the Use of Instagram: An Exploratory Study. *Int. J. Bus. Innov.* 2015, *2*, 15–31.
20. Oropesa, M.P.; Sánchez, X.C. Motivaciones sociales y psicológicas para usar Instagram. *Commun. Pap.* 2016, *5*, 27–36.
21. Rice, C.; Watson, E. Girls and sexting: The missing story of sexual subjectivity in a sexualized and digitally-mediated world. In *Learning Bodies*; Coffey, J., Budgeon, S., Cahill, H., Eds.; Springer: Singapore, 2016; pp. 141–156. [CrossRef]
22. Ševčíková, A. Girls' and boys' experience with teen sexting in early and late adolescence. *J. Adolesc.* 2016, *51*, 156–162. [CrossRef]
23. García-Gómez, A. Teen girls and sexual agency: Exploring the intrapersonal and intergroup dimensions of sexting. *Media Cult. Soc.* 2017, *39*, 391–407. [CrossRef]
24. Renold, E.; Ringrose, J. Selfies, relfies and phallic tagging: Posthuman participations in teen digital sexuality assemblages. *Educ. Philos. Theory* 2017, *49*, 1066–1079. [CrossRef]
25. Borrell, C.; Artazcoz, L.; Gil-González, D.; Pérez, K.; Pérez, G.; Vives-Cases, C.; Rohlfs, I. Determinants of Perceived Sexism and Their Role on the Association of Sexism with Mental Health. *Women Health* 2011, *51*, 583–603. [CrossRef]
26. Flick, U. *An Introduction to Qualitative Research*, 6th ed.; SAGE Publications: London, UK, 2018; ISBN 9781526445643.
27. Westbrook, L.; Saperstein, A. New categories are not enough: Rethinking the measurement of sex and gender in social surveys. *Gend. Soc.* 2015, *29*, 534–560. [CrossRef]
28. Lafrance, M.N.; Stetl, M.; Bullock, K. "I'm not gonna fake it": University women's accounts of resisting the normative practice of faking orgasm. *Psychol. Women Q.* 2017, *41*, 210–222. [CrossRef]
29. Rodríguez, Y.; Lameiras, M.; Carrera, M. Validación de la versión reducida de las escalas ASI y AMI en una muestra de estudiantes españoles. *Psicogente* 2009, *12*, 284–295.
30. Luzón, J.M.; Ramos, E.; Recio, P.; de la Peña, E.M. *Proyecto Detecta Andalucía. Factores de Riesgo y de Protección en la Prevención Contra la Violencia de Género en la Pareja*; Instituto Andaluz de la Mujer: Sevilla, España, 2011.
31. Recio, P.; Cuadrado, I.; Ramos, E. Propiedades psicométricas de la escala de detección de sexismo en adolescentes (DSA). *Psicothema* 2007, *19*, 522–528.
32. García, V.; Lana, A.; Fernández, A.; Bringas, C.; Rodríguez, L.; Rodríguez, F.J. Actitudes sexistas y reconocimiento del maltrato en parejas jóvenes. *Aten. Prim.* 2018, *50*, 398–405. [CrossRef]
33. Leaper, C.; Brown, C.S. Sexism in childhood and adolescence: Recent trends and advances in research. *Child Dev. Perspect.* 2018, *12*, 10–15. [CrossRef]
34. Hornos, M.J.D.; Núñez, M.T.S. Adolescencia, sexismo e inteligencia emocional. Claves para prevenir actitudes sexistas. *Rev. INFAD De Psicol. Int. J. Dev. Educ. Psychol.* 2019, *1*, 157–172. [CrossRef]
35. Lameiras, M.; Rodríguez, Y. Evaluación del sexismo moderno en adolescentes. *Rev. De Psicol. Soc.* 2002, *17*, 119–127. [CrossRef]
36. León, C.M.; Aizpurúa, E. ¿Persisten las actitudes sexistas en los estudiantes universitarios? Un análisis de su prevalencia, predictores y diferencias de género. *Education XX1* 2019, *23*, 275–296. [CrossRef]
37. Radke, H.R.; Hornsey, M.J.; Barlow, F.K. Barriers to women engaging in collective action to overcome sexism. *Am. Psychol.* 2016, *71*, 863–874. [CrossRef]
38. Charteris, J.; Gregory, S.; Masters, Y. 'Snapchat', youth subjectivities and sexuality: Disappearing media and the discourse of youth innocence. *Gend. Educ.* 2018, *30*, 205–221. [CrossRef]
39. Frenda, S.; Ghanem, B.; Montes-y-Gómez, M.; Rosso, P. Online Hate Speech against Women: Automatic Identification of Misogyny and Sexism on Twitter. *J. Intell. Fuzzy Syst.* 2019, *36*, 4743–4752. [CrossRef]
40. Villanueva, J.; Hernández, C.I.; Monter, N.S. Amor romántico entre estudiantes universitarios (hombres y mujeres), una mirada desde la perspectiva de género. *La Ventana Rev. De Estud. De Género* 2019, *6*, 218–247. [CrossRef]

41. Sicilia, A.S.; Serra, J.C. Discurso amoroso adolescente: Análisis del repertorio del amor romántico en el programa chicos y chicas. *Athenea Digit. Rev. De Pensam. E Investig. Soc.* **2019**, *19*, 12. [CrossRef]
42. Handyside, S.; Ringrose, J. Snapchat memory and youth digital sexual cultures: Mediated temporality, duration and affect. *J. Gend. Stud.* **2017**, *26*, 347–360. [CrossRef]
43. Senft, T.M.; Baym, N.K. Selfies introduction~ What does the selfie say? Investigating a global phenomenon. *Int. J. Commun.* **2015**, *9*, 19.
44. García, A. From selfies to sexting: Tween girls, intimacy, and subjectivities. *Girlhood Stud.* **2018**, *11*, 43–58. [CrossRef]
45. Reed, L.A.; Tolman, R.M.; Ward, L.M. Gender matters: Experiences and consequences of digital dating abuse victimization in adolescent dating relationships. *J. Adolesc.* **2017**, *59*, 79–89. [CrossRef]
46. Kusz, J.; Bouchard, M. Nymphet or Lolita? A Gender Analysis of Online Child Pornography Websites. *Deviant Behav.* **2019**, *41*, 805–813. [CrossRef]
47. Mendes, K.; Ringrose, J.; Keller, J. *Digital Feminist Activism: Girls and Women Fight Back against Rape Culture*; Oxford University Press: New York, NY, USA, 2019. [CrossRef]
48. Bonavitta, P.; Presman, C.; Becerra, J.E.C. Ciberfeminismo. Viejas luchas, nuevas estrategias: El escrache virtual como herramienta de acción y resistencia. *Anagramas Rumbos Y Sentidos De La Comun.* **2020**, *18*, 159–180. [CrossRef]
49. Borgogna, N.C.; Aita, S.L. Are sexist beliefs related to mental health problems? *Soc. Sci. J.* **2020**, *51*, 1–15. [CrossRef]

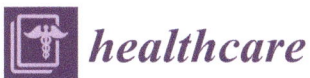

Article

Health-ID: A Blockchain-Based Decentralized Identity Management for Remote Healthcare

Ibrahim Tariq Javed [1,*], Fares Alharbi [2], Badr Bellaj [3], Tiziana Margaria [1,4], Noel Crespi [3] and Kashif Naseer Qureshi [5]

1 Lero-Science Foundation Ireland Research Centre for Software, University of Limerick, V94 T9PX Limerick, Ireland; tiziana.margaria@ul.ie
2 Computer Science Department, Shaqra University, Shaqra 15526, Saudi Arabia; faalhrbi@su.edu.sa
3 Institut Mines-Télécom, Télécom SudParis, CEDEX, 91011 Evry, France; badr.bellaj@telecom-sudparis.eu (B.B.); noel.crespi@mines-telecom.fr (N.C.)
4 The Health Research Institute (HRI), University of Limerick, V94 T9PX Limerick, Ireland
5 Department of Computer Science, Bahria University, Islamabad 44000, Pakistan; knaseer.buic@bahria.edu.pk
* Correspondence: Ibrahimtariq.javed@lero.ie

Citation: Javed, I.T.; Alharbi, F.; Bellaj, B.; Margaria, T.; Crespi, N.; Qureshi, K.N. Health-ID: A Blockchain-Based Decentralized Identity Management for Remote Healthcare. *Healthcare* **2021**, *9*, 712. https://doi.org/10.3390/healthcare9060712

Academic Editor: Daniele Giansanti

Received: 24 April 2021
Accepted: 5 June 2021
Published: 10 June 2021

Publisher's Note: MDPI stays neutral with regard to jurisdictional claims in published maps and institutional affiliations.

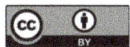

Copyright: © 2021 by the authors. Licensee MDPI, Basel, Switzerland. This article is an open access article distributed under the terms and conditions of the Creative Commons Attribution (CC BY) license (https://creativecommons.org/licenses/by/4.0/).

Abstract: COVID-19 has made eHealth an imperative. The pandemic has been a true catalyst for remote eHealth solutions such as teleHealth. Telehealth facilitates care, diagnoses, and treatment remotely, making them more efficient, accessible, and economical. However, they have a centralized identity management system that restricts the interoperability of patient and healthcare provider identification. Thus, creating silos of users that are unable to authenticate themselves beyond their eHealth application's domain. Furthermore, the consumers of remote eHealth applications are forced to trust their service providers completely. They cannot check whether their eHealth service providers adhere to the regulations to ensure the security and privacy of their identity information. Therefore, we present a blockchain-based decentralized identity management system that allows patients and healthcare providers to identify and authenticate themselves transparently and securely across different eHealth domains. Patients and healthcare providers are uniquely identified by their health identifiers (healthIDs). The identity attributes are attested by a healthcare regulator, indexed on the blockchain, and stored by the identity owner. We implemented smart contracts on an Ethereum consortium blockchain to facilities identification and authentication procedures. We further analyze the performance using different metrics, including transaction gas cost, transaction per second, number of blocks lost, and block propagation time. Parameters including block-time, gas-limit, and sealers are adjusted to achieve the optimal performance of our consortium blockchain.

Keywords: digital identity; decentralized identity; identity management; healthcare; blockchain; smart contract; Ethereum

1. Introduction

Since SARS-CoV-2 (COVID-19) emerged, the demand for eHealth has gone viral. The novel coronavirus has swept across communities forcing a new normal that requires social distancing. Governments strongly suggest enforcing medical distancing to minimize physical contact between patients and healthcare providers. As a result, hospitals and other healthcare organizations have rapidly adopted digital alternatives to deliver healthcare services. Telehealth applications facilitate clinical benefits for patients such as consultation, diagnoses, treatment, and prevention from a distance overcoming the geographical barrier. They can also support non-clinical services for healthcare providers, such as training, meetings, and education [1]. Furthermore, eHealth applications also provide real-time health monitoring using various devices and sensors [2]. In 2020, remote healthcare applications shifted from a previously slow adoption rate to a record pace of uptake. The searches for online consultations have sky rocketed by 350%. Whereas in 2021, the global eHealth market is expected to witness a 37.1% increase [3]. It is further predicted to rise to USD 310.09 billion by 2027, according to Data Bridge Market Research [4].

Healthcare organizations' rapid transition to digital—where medical records and online services are the norms—has created new challenges in securing access to sensitive patient data and clinical applications. This, combined with evolving compliance regulations, drives a need for technologies that enhance security while maintaining a superior level of healthcare service and enabling healthcare professionals to securely and seamlessly access patient information and applications at all times in compliance with regulatory requirements. However, meeting regulatory demands and demonstrating compliance can be challenging with centralized legacy identity management (IdM) solutions. Failure to comply can result in substantial fines and reputation damage. Furthermore, the proliferation of healthcare organization data breaches [5], which put lives at risk, make centralized legacy identity management (IdM) solutions less desirable.

The centralized IdM creates silos of users restricting inter-operable identification between different applications [6]. For each application, the consumer has to identify and authenticate themselves separately. A user identified in one domain cannot verify itself to a user present in another domain. Moreover, the web-based IdM allows users to create self-asserted profiles without performing any identity proofing. Therefore, identity theft is becoming common on web applications to commit scams and frauds [7,8]. Furthermore, centralized IdM has several weaknesses in ensuring data security and privacy [9]. In a centralized IdM, the identity owner must completely trust their service provider, thus having no or limited control over their identity. Users are unable to control the type of data collected and shared during the identification and authentication process. There remains no way for a consumer to check whether the security and privacy regulations are being followed by their service provider [10]. Moreover, centralized IdM remains more prone to hacking and data breaches, which may lead to susceptible data disclosure for eHealth applications [11]. In centralized IdM, the data of users are stored, updated, and managed through centralized databases. Centralized databases are high-value targets for different security attacks, thus remain more prone to data manipulation or theft. Centralized servers also introduce a single point of failure and are venerable to Denial-of-Service attacks. If the centralized system is compromised, it may make the network completely useless. Thus, a centralized approach always requires an adequate security system with protective, detective, and corrective measures to protect against different security threats. Therefore, decentralized methods are being proposed in [12–14] to ensure data security and privacy.

For remote eHealth applications, it remains essential to provide a decentralized IdM. What is required is a facility that empowers users to manage their identities independently from their eHealth provider. Blockchain technology allows distributed storage of records with cryptography protection to ensure security [15]. It facilitates decentralization and stores time-stamped data in an immutable, auditable, and secure manner. These features can be used to facilitate the owner-driven identity. In the survey in Reference [16], a blockchain-based IdM is suggested for eHealth consumers to control their identity fully. There are several examples of blockchain-based IdM, including ShoCard [17], uPort [18], Sovrin [19], and Blockstack [20]. However, these solutions are not directly applicable to telehealth as they fail to provide adequate identity proofing for patients and healthcare providers. Identity proofing is the process of verifying that the claimed identity of a person matches their actual identity. For healthcare providers, it is essential to verify their practice licenses before allowing them to authenticate themselves to other entities in the network. The verification can only be done by the regulatory authorities who have issued the practice license. At present, remote healthcare applications rely on a centralized IdM where subscribers are forced to trust their service providers in the authentication of other participants. Researchers who have utilized blockchain to provide a decentralized health record system [21–25] also rely on the centralized IdM of hospitals. Therefore, it remains essential to provide a decentralized IdM that allows patients and healthcare providers to authenticate and validate each other in a trusted and reliable manner.

We propose a blockchain-based decentralized identity management for remote healthcare. Health-ID harnesses the power of blockchain technology to safeguard patient information and help ensure regulatory compliance. For that, we invest the automated nature of smart contracts and transparency of the blockchain to provide an IdM with capabilities such as automated provisioning and de-provisioning, user-centric identity governance across domain boundaries, and robust audit and reporting. In this paper, we have three significant contributions that are as follows:

- The architecture of Health-ID is presented, which consists of four actors, namely user, healthcare regulator, blockchain, and cloud storage. The owner can control their own identity by using web tokens for identity attributes. The healthcare regulators provide their attestation after conducting identity proofing. In order to maintain data integrity and auditability, the hash of the identity attribute is uploaded on the blockchain.
- Two smart contracts Health_SC and Registry_SC are deployed to facilitate the authentication and identification process. The health_SC allows users to manage their identity, whereas the registry_SC allows regulators to store the attestations.
- A consortium blockchain is used to implement healthID. The blockchain's performance effectiveness and computational efficiency are computed using transaction gas cost, transaction per second, number of blocks lost, and block propagation time.

2. Related Work

Identity management is described as a set of policies and technologies to control entities' identities and ensure that the right entities are authorized to utilize relevant resources. The IdM is broadly categorized into centralized, federated, user-centric, and decentralized. In centralized IdM, the identity provider has complete control to manage the identity of users and provide them authentication services. Most of the current services and applications use centralized IdM to create a silo of users where users identified in a specific domain cannot authenticate themselves to other domains [6]. Federated IdM, on the other hand, is an arrangement between two or more organizations to allow users from one domain to authenticate and access services of other domains [26], for instance, single-sign-on systems such as Facebook connect [27]. However, current centralized and federated digital identity models do not allow for complete independence or control by the user. This leads to a privacy issue as users do not know where their data are being utilized. On the other hand, a user-centric identity tries to give control of identity to its owners while reducing identity information disclosure of personal information [27].

The recent emergence of blockchain technology has allowed the development of decentralized IdM. Decentralized IdM will enable consumers to manage and maintain their identity on a blockchain that is not controlled by a single central authority. This allows users to decide what, when, and with whom they want to share their information. Recently, there have been various proposed solutions based on blockchain technology. The decentralized IdM can be broadly categorized into self-sovereign identity and decentralized trusted identity. Self-sovereign identity is a type of user-centric model that requires no central authority, which may lead to the possibility of identity disclosure. In this approach, a unique identifier is used to represent an entity, whereas the attributes of user identity are stored on the blockchain [28]. For instance, uPort is built on Ethereum, which allows its users to manage and keep their identity by using a self-sovereign wallet [18]. In addition, an uPort registry smart contract is used to store the identifiers and their identity attributes. SelfKey [29] is also built on top of the Ethereum blockchain and uses a claim protocol to share identity information with third parties. Sovrin [19] is a decentralized IdM solution that uses a permissioned blockchain network Hyperledger Indy. In Sovrin, only trusted authorities, such as governments, universities, or banks, manage the blockchain by running the consensus protocol [17]. It uses virtual chains to pin the state machine on the network. Evernym [30] uses Sovrin and IOTA blockchain to support a self-sovereign trusted identity for enterprises and organizations. Whereas Blockstack [20] provides a decentralized public-key infrastructure using the Bitcoin blockchain. The major limitation of the self-sovereign approach is that the identities are self-asserted. The user provides identity information with no means to verify its authenticity.

In contrast, the decentralized trusted identity supports identity proofing by allowing trusted third parties to provide identity attestation by verifying public credentials, such as a passport, national identity card, and driving license. ShoCard [17] is the most prominent solution based on a decentralized trusted identity approach. It provides multi-factor authentication without the need to use a password or a username. It uses the bitcoin blockchain and a centralized server to exchange identity information between two parties. However, ShoCard has two major limitations. Firstly, it remains centralized as it relies on a ShoCard server that stores identity certification. Without the centralized server, users are not able to authenticate themselves to third parties. Secondly, based on the bitcoin blockchain, the waiting time for a transaction to be mined is very high, which causes delays to the authentication process. None of these solutions are designed and applied to healthcare scenarios for identity authentication and verification purposes to the best of our knowledge. Furthermore, they do not address the challenges and issues of healthcare applications. Therefore, the eHealth applications that support telehealth still depend upon a centralized IdM [31]. This creates silos of users restricting inter-operable identification between different eHealth applications. Our motivation is to investigate the potential of blockchain technology for the use of IdM in remote healthcare applications.

The most prominent adoption of blockchain technology in healthcare is electronic health records (EHR), aiming to resolve data management, security, and interoperability challenges. For instance, BlocHIE, a blockchain-based medical data exchange platform, is proposed in [32] that uses loosely coupled blockchains to store different types of healthcare data. The system provides on-chain verification to ensure security, privacy, and authentication. An attribute-based signature scheme for multiple users in EHR management is presented in [21], whereas BIoTHR is a novel privacy-preserving IoT-based EHR scheme [33]. In [34], a healthcare management framework is suggested for emergency scenarios that use blockchain technology to ensure access control, authentication, and audibility. Blockchain has enabled an efficient method of data authentication in electronic health records. For instance, a blockchain-based key management scheme is proposed in [22] that provides an efficient mechanism for protecting sensitive medical data in the health blockchain. In [23], a blockchain-based cloud-assisted eHealth system is proposed, which aims to avoid outsourced EHR from malicious modification. A two-way authentication scheme developed in [24] allows data sharing between hospitals. Similarly, Ref. [25] provides cross-platform authentication schemes between hospital networks while ensuring security and privacy. However, these blockchain-based EHR systems are assumed to have a decentralized IdM or rely on a centralized IdM of hospitals. None of these solutions provide an implementation of IdM that allows patients and healthcare providers to authenticate and verify each other irrespective of their healthcare application. Therefore, in this paper, we aim to provide an IdM solution for remote healthcare applications. Patients and healthcare providers will remain in control of their identity by managing and storing their identity attributes. The consortium of healthcare regulators will work the blockchain and provide identity attestation by conducting identity proofing of patients and healthcare providers.

3. Blockchain Overview

A Blockchain is a replicated database, managed by a consensus mechanism, in a peer-to-peer network of non-trusting parties. Blockchain can be simply defined as a time-stamped series of data records that are managed by a cluster of nodes [35]. Nodes are computers that are connected in a peer-to-peer network and have an identical copy of the data. A new data entry is validated and transmitted to the entire network to maintain the identical copy of the database. The blockchain data structure consists of a chain of blocks. Each block records transactions validated in a particular period and has not yet been recorded in any prior blocks. These blocks are linked to one another through a cryptographic hash such that each subsequent block contains the hash of the previous block (also called parent) header and hence constitutes a chain. The first block, known as the genesis block, has no reference to a previous block since it has no parent block. This linkability is a cryptographic mechanism that maintains data integrity and immutability in the network. A transaction goes through multiple steps in a blockchain network before it ends up validated by the network. Firstly, a user digitally signs and submits its information as a transaction. Secondly, the transaction is broadcasted to the entire network, where each neighboring node conducts validation for the transaction before relaying it to the next node. Thirdly, the transaction is collected and validated by a validator who includes it in a new proposed block. Fourthly, the consensus mechanism determines the validator who has the right to propose his block to the network. Fifthly, once other nodes validate the block, the block will be added to the chain, and the block will be propagated to all nodes to allow these nodes to update their database. Sixthly, after being recorded in the blockchain, the transaction is considered complete and henceforth consumed by its new owner.

Blockchains can be classified into public, private, and consortium blockchain based on their settings. A public blockchain is permissionless if the platform is publicly open for users without permission from any authority. Generally, in a public blockchain, all transactions are visible to the public. Bitcoin is a well-known example of a public blockchain. On the other hand, a private blockchain is not entirely open for the public to use—a centralized authority controls and defines who has the right to join the network. Thus, a private blockchain is considered to be centralized due to the fact because a single authority maintains the network. In addition, data in a private blockchain is prone to tampering. Prevalent examples of private blockchain include Corda, Hyperledger Fabric, and Hyperledger Sawtooth. A consortium blockchain has different organizations involved to manage a shared blockchain [36]. The authority is distributed among different organizations, and thus, the consortium blockchain is considered to have semi-decentralized management and governance. In a consortium blockchain, only a preselected set of nodes participate in the consensus process. A consortium blockchain is best suited for organizational collaboration. In a consortium blockchain, a limited number of trusted participants are required to validate the block. This is what makes the consortium blockchain highly scalable and guarantees high throughput.

Ethereum is a stateful blockchain-based computing platform with smart contract functionality that lets users build decentralized applications running on blockchain technology. In addition to the distributed ledger, Ethereum provides a virtual machine, called the Ethereum Virtual Machine (EVM), which can execute scripts written in a high-level programming language (e.g., Solidity). In Ethereum, the blockchain data structure is more complex than in its predecessor, Bitcoin. The block's header comprises metadata, and its body comprises multiple types of data, namely, transactions, receipts, and system states (account states). Each of these data types is organized into a Merkle tree or a Patricia tree (Radix tree) in the state tree. The state tree (or the account storage tree) is an essential component in the Ethereum ledger. It is used to implement the account model, whereby each account is linked to its related states (account balances, smart contract states, etc.). Any node can parse the tree using the account address and get the updated state without any overhead calculation. The state tree grows each time a change occurs in a state. It grows by adding new nodes (stored in the new block)—holding new states—which points to the nodes (stored in the previous block) containing the old value for the same state (Figure 1). To enforce immutability, Ethereum keeps its root hash in the block header. This tree manages two accounts: the externally owned account (EOA) and the smart contract account. The first type is an account controlled by a private key held by a given user, whereas the second is an account controlled by a smart contract Bytecode. Both accounts are represented by a cryptographically generated address of 20 bytes. To prevent Denial-of-Service (DoS) attack, EVM adopts the gas system, whereby every computation of a program must be paid for upfront in a dedicated unit called gas as defined by the protocol. If the provided amount of gas does not cover the cost of execution, the transaction fails.

The block size is controlled by the gas-limit, which the miners define, and a constant rise of the gas-limit happens.

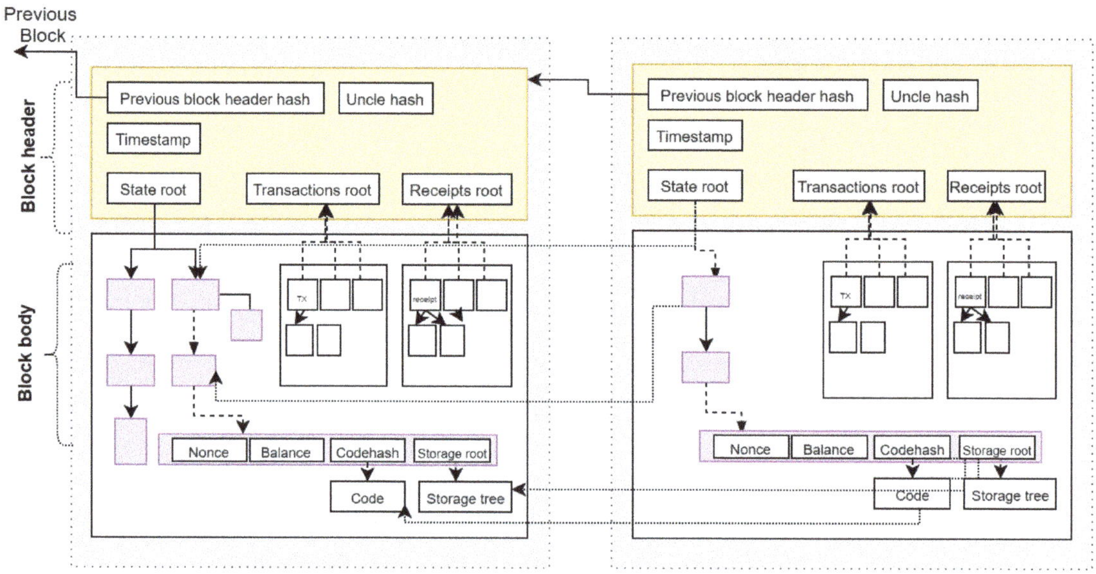

Figure 1. Structure of Ethereum's chain of blocks.

4. Remote Healthcare Identity Management System

In this section, we present an IdM solution for remote healthcare services using a consortium Ethereum blockchain. The consortium is managed by healthcare regulators, whereas patients and healthcare providers are the consumers of the IdM identified by a unique health identifier (healthID). Firstly, we define the actors involved and our proposed architecture. Secondly, we discuss the two smart contracts and their functions required for creating, using, and validating healthID. Lastly, we demonstrate the workflow for the healthID registration and authentication process.

4.1. Actors

The remote healthcare IdM framework involves five entities. Each entity is briefly described as follows:

1. **User:** A user is the owner of the identity. A user in healthID can be a patient or a healthcare provider. The patient is a consumer of healthcare services, such as diagnosis, treatment, and therapy, whereas a healthcare provider is a professional that is licensed by regulatory authorities to provide healthcare services. Healthcare providers include doctors, nurses, pharmacists, dentists, opticians, midwives, psychologists, and psychiatrists, etc.
2. **Healthcare Regulator:** A regulator is responsible for registering and administrating healthcare providers. Examples of healthcare regulators include the department of health and social care professionals, nursing council, and midwife council, pharmaceutical council, optical council. They are responsible for registering, renewing, and revoking the license of healthcare providers of their respective fields. On the other hand, public hospitals can register patients by verifying their public identity.
3. **Blockchain:** A consortium blockchain is utilized to provide a secure and distributed identity management service for healthcare. The blockchain platform should support smart contracts such as Etherum and Hyperledeger. A piece of code known as the smart contract is deployed over Ethereum to ensure identity management. Two types

of smart contracts are deployed, namely Health SC and Registry SC. The healthID of patients and providers is the address of their deployed smart contract over the Ethereum blockchain.

4. **Cloud storage:** The cloud storage system is used to store the identity attributes of patients and healthcare providers. The identity attributes are stored in a JSON object and attested by a regulatory authority to create a JSON Web Token (JWT). The hash of the identity attribute can be used to locate and download a particular identity attribute. The identity owner may select a centralized storage system (such as dropbox) or a distributed cloud storage (such as IPFS) to store their identity attributes.

4.2. Proposed Architecture

The overview of the remote healthcare IdM is illustrated in Figure 2. The patient, regulator, and provider use their applications to register to the blockchain. The application contains a secure inbuilt wallet having public and private key pairs. The application stores the private key in the secure enclave of the user device that can be utilized by biometric or password authentication. The private key is used to sign attestations and transactions sent to the blockchain. The public key is used to generate an account on the blockchain. The account is further used to deploy smart contracts over the blockchain. Each patient and healthcare provider deploys their smart contract. The healthID is the address of the smart contract deployed by each entity. The unique healthID is used for the identification and authentication process. Healthcare regulators register it by performing off-block identity proofing. The identity proofing of healthcare providers is conducted using their practice license, whereas patients can prove their identity using public identification such as passports, national identity cards, and driving licenses. For instance, the pharmaceutical council will be able to register the healthID of a pharmacist by verifying their practice license. In contrast, a public hospital will be able to register the healthID of a patient by verifying their public identity document. A consortium of healthcare regulators will manage the blockchain. Each member of the consortium will manage a node of the blockchain. When the blockchain is initialized, a specific predefined authority node would be used to validate new blocks on the network. New authority nodes can be included at any time based on the majority decision of existing authority nodes.

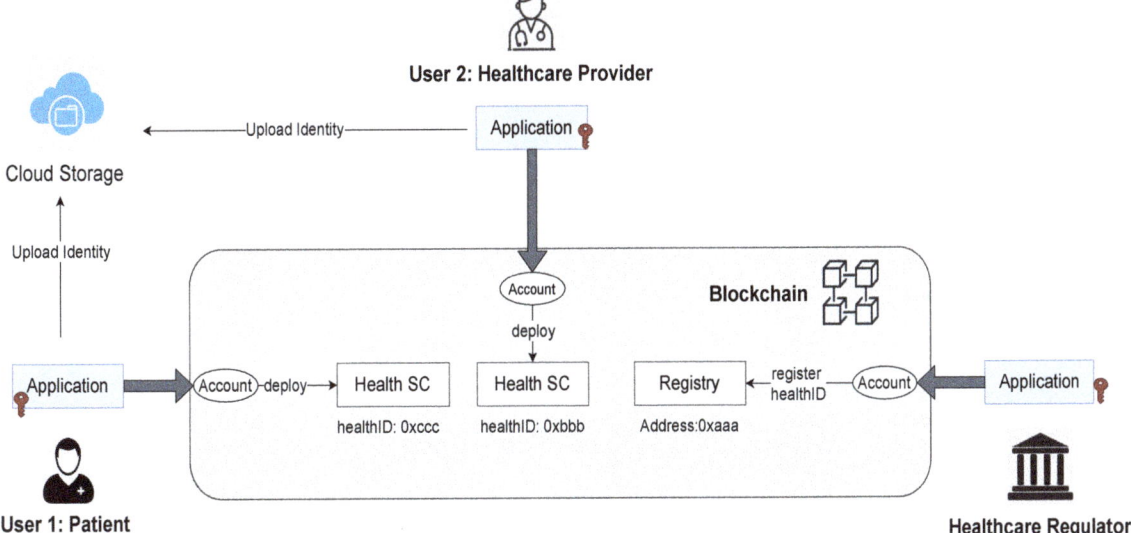

Figure 2. Architecture of the smart healthcare identity management system.

In our proposed architecture, the owner can control their own identity. Figure 3 shows how the owner of healthID creates, stores, and manages the identity. The identity is a set of identity attributes describing the owner. We use a JSON (https://www.json.org/json-en.html (accessed on 1 May 2021)) object to define identity attributes, for instance, name, profile picture, license number, and public citizenship number, etc. The JSON attributes are digitally signed by a regulator to create a JSON Web Token (JWT). A JWT (https://jwt.io/ (accessed on 1 May 2021)), which is an open standard to securely transmitting information as a JSON object. The JWT identity token is an attested identity attribute of the owner. It can be used as proof that a particular regulator attests to the claim about the identity of a specific patient or healthcare provider. Attestation can also be a self-signed JSON token. The owner uploads the encrypted JWT identity attributes over a cloud service (Dropbox, IPFS). The hash of the identity attribute is used to ensure the integrity of the data. Each hash is identified by its hashID, which is a unique random number assigned to a particular hash. The hash and hashID are uploaded over the blockchain using the owner's smart contract.

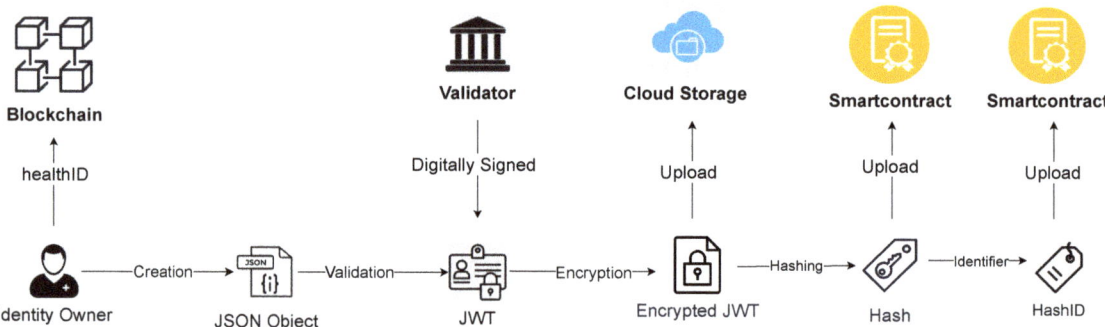

Figure 3. An overview of digital health identity.

An example of the JWT having an identity attribute of a doctor's practice license is provided. The encoded and decoded JWT token is shown below:

```
 1  encoded token:
 2  "eyJ0eXAiOiJKV1QiLCJhbGciOiJFUzI1NksifQ.eyJhdHRyaWJ1dGUiOnsibmFtZSI6IkNocmlzdGl
 3  hbiBMdW5ka3Zpc3QifSwic3ViamVjdCI6IjB4N2RiNTM1ZmFjOGEyNTg2OWE3YWViNWY3ODQyYzcxZD
 4  U5ODI0ODcyMyIsImlzc3VlciI6IjB4Y2I4NTE4ZTFhYjQyMmM4NjQ1ODQ3ZTYzYmQ1N2Q4YTcwYWFhY
 5  jY0YyIsImlzc3VlEF0IjoiMjAxNi0wMS0yN1QyMjo0ODoyOS42MzlaIiwiZXhwaXJlcOF0IjoiMjAx
 6  NyOwMS0yN1QyMjo0ODoyOS42MzlaIn0.L0_rHNSq_Piow3kLTqks86BVsYLIWpUoN7LMBXqD8q3YR2I
 7  v6q9BWjvtPKao34H1ZKqPDZeXtjOVFPXmH5eRMg"
 8
 9  decoded token
10  {
11  header: { typ: 'JWT', alg: 'HS256' },
12  payload:
13  {
14  Identity Attribute:
15  {
16  "Name": "Dr Annmarie",
17  "Speciality": "General practitioner",
18  "Licence": 1516239022,
19  "Picture": "image.jpg",
20  "Date of Issue": 2020-10-01,
21  "Date of Expiry": 2025-10-01
22  },
```

```
23  subject:
24  {"healthID": "0x7db535fac8a25869a7aeb5f7842c71d598248723"},
25  issuer:
26  {"publickey": "0xcb8518e1ab422c8645847e63bd57d8a70aaab64c"},
27  token issued : {'2021-02-01 T22:48:29.639Z'},
28  token expires: {'2025-10-01 T22:48:29.639Z'}
29  signature: "L0_rHNSq_Piow3kLTqks86BVsYLIWpUoN7LMBXqD8q3YR2Iv6q9BWjvtPKao34H1ZKq
30  PDZeXtjOVFPXmH5eRMg",
31  encrypted: True,
32  publicKey:
33  '02e8a9b0aeee81f80ca32eb09d97319d61b5df9485bdf6f726465155ca778f69f1'
34  }
```

The encoded JWT consists of three parts separated by dots (xxx.yyy.zzz): header, payload, and signature. The header consists of the token type and the signing algorithm such as HMAC, SHA256, or RSA. The payload contains the data about the entity. The signature is created by using an encryption algorithm over the encoded header and payload. In the above example, the JWT is created using the HMAC SHA256 algorithm to create the signature. The payload consists of the license attribute, subject healthID, issuer public key, token issue date, and token expiry date.

4.3. Smart Contract

The healthcare IdM consists of two types of smart contracts (Health SC and Registry SC). The Health SC consists of five functions, including set_public_key, retrieve_public_key, set_hash, retrieve_hash and pause_SC, whereas the registry SC consists of functions, register_regulator, verify_regulator, register_attestation, verify_attestation, and revoke_attestation. The algorithm of each function is provided in Algorithms 1–10, respectively. The complete code of the smart contract is available in the github repository (https://github.com/ibrahimtariqjaved/healthid (accessed on 1 May 2021)).

Algorithm 1: set_publickey(*publickey*)

if *sender==owner* then
| Store *publickey*;
else
| return false;
end

Algorithm 2: retrieve_public_key

if *publickey exists* then
| return *publickey*;
else
| return false;
end

Algorithm 3: set_hash(*hash_id, hash, url*)

if *sender==owner* then
| Map *hash* and *url* to *hash_id*;
else
| return false;
end

Algorithm 4: retrieve_hash(*hash_id*)

if *hash_id exists* then
  | return *hash* and *url*;
else
  | return false;
end

Algorithm 5: pause_smartcontract()

if *sender==owner* then
  | Pause owner's smart contract
else
  | return false;
end

Algorithm 6: register_regulator(*public_key*)

if *sender==enodeaddress* then
  | Map *public_key* to *msg.sender*
else
  | return false;
end

Algorithm 7: verify_regulator(*address*)

if *address exist* then
  | return *public_key* mapped to *address*;
else
  | return false;
end

Algorithm 8: register_attestation(*healthid, verify_attestation*)

if *sender==registered regulator* then
  | Map *public_key* to *healthid*;
else
  | return false;

Algorithm 9: verify_attestation(*healthid*)

if *healthid exist* then
  | return *public_key* mapped to *healthid*;
else
  | return false;

Algorithm 10: revoke_attestation(*healthid, public_key*)

if *sender==enode address* then
  | Remove *healthid*'s *public_key*;
else
  | return false;

The description of each function is provided as follows:

1. *set_public_key:* This function allows the owner of the smart contract to upload and store its public key over the Ethereum network. Only the owner of the smart contract will be allowed to upload their public key.
2. *retrieve_public_key:* This function allows anyone to retrieve the public key of the owner by using their healthID. Retrieving the public key from this function ensures that the public key belongs to the entity having the healthID.
3. *set_hash:* This function allows the owner to store the hash and hashID of their identity attribute. The function stores the hash with the corresponding hashID of the identity attribute. Only the owner of the smart contract is allowed to upload the hash.
4. *retrieve_hash:* This function is used to extract the hash by using the hashID of the identity attribute required. The function uses the hashID to locate and return the corresponding hash of the required identity attribute.
5. *pause_SC:* This function allows the owner of the smart contract to pause and unpause the contract. If the smart contract is paused, no one will access the hash of the identity attribute.
6. *register_regulator:* This function allows regulators to register themselves and upload their public key. The public key is stored with their corresponding Ethereum address. This function will only register the regulator who is operating as a node of the blockchain.
7. *verify_regulator:* This function allows anyone to retrieve the public key of regulators using their Ethereum address. In addition, this function ensures that the regulator having a particular Ethereum address is registered on the network.
8. *register_attestation:* This function allows regulators to register the healthID and public key of patients and healthcare providers. The Ethereum address of the regulator is also stored with it. Only the registered regulators will be able to use this function.
9. *verify_attestation:* This function allows anyone to extract the public key of the registered healthID. In addition, the function returns the public key and Ethereum address of the regulator who provided the attestation.
10. *revoke_attestation:* This function allows the regulator to revoke the attestation of a particular patient or healthcare provider using their healthID.

4.4. Identification and Authentication Workflow

Identity management consists of the identification and authentication process. In identification, the patients and providers would register and identify themselves to the system using their applications. In the authentication step, the identity owner would prove their identity to a third party using their validated healthID and identity token. The system supports single-sign-on, in which the individual, once logged into its application, would be able to authenticate itself to different entities. The workflow of each process is described using a sequence diagram. The process of identification is presented in Figure 4. The identification process of patients and healthcare providers is the same. In the Figure, we take the example of a healthcare provider registering to the remote healthcare IdM by following the identification process. The identification process consists of the followings steps:

1. Deployment: In the first step, the healthcare provider will use the EoA account to deploy a smart contract on the Ethereum blockchain using their application. The address of the smart contract would be the digital healthID of the healthcare provider.
2. Registration: In the registration step, a request along with the owner's healthID is sent to the regulator by the provider. The regulator will use the healthID to request the public key from the provider's health SC using *retrieve_publickey* function. Using the public key, the regulator will encrypt a challenge message and send it to the provider. If the provider decrypts using its private key and responds successfully, this ensures that the provider is the real owner of the healthID and public key.
3. Identity proofing: In this step, the provider would be required to prove their identity by presenting their practice license. The provider may be required to physically or remotely present their license based on the policy of the healthcare regulator.

After proofing is conducted successfully, the regulator registers the healthID and public key of the provider in the registry SC using the *register_attestation* function. The regulator further signs the identity attribute and provides an identity token (JWT) to the provider.

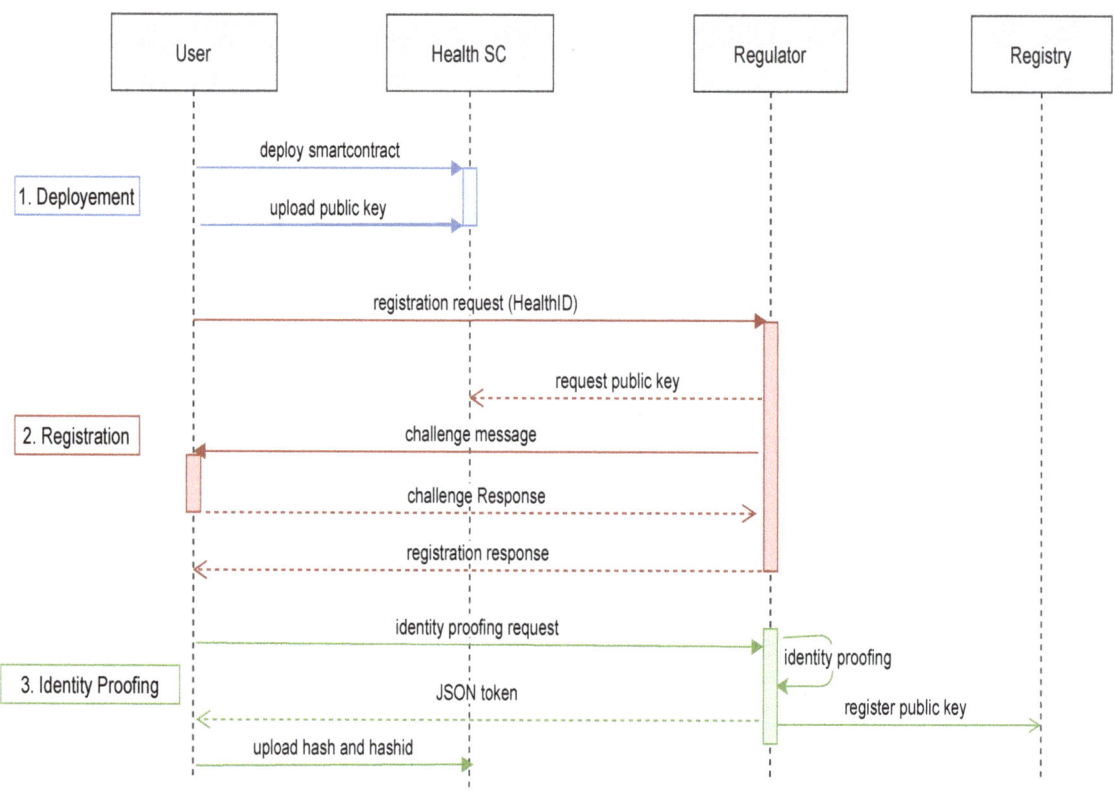

Figure 4. Identification sequence diagram.

After identification, the healthID is registered, and the owner receives a signed identity token. The provider stores the identity token on its device or uploads it to the cloud. The hashID and hash of the identity token are uploaded to the provider's Health SC using *set_hash*. Now the healthcare provider can authenticate themself to anyone before providing their healthcare services. The process of authentication is presented in Figure 5. The authentication process for a provider and a patient is similar. We present how a provider authenticates itself to a patient. The steps for the authentication process are discussed below:

1. HealthID Verification: In the first step, the healthcare provider sends the healthID to the patient. The patient uses the healthID to extract the public key from registry SC using the *verify_attestation* function. This ensures that the attested healthID is verified and registered by a particular regulator. The Ethereum address of the regulator providing the attestation is also provided. Next, the provider's public key is used to send a challenge message to the healthcare provider. If the response is correct, this guarantees that the public key and healthID belong to the healthcare provider.
2. Identity Assertion: In this step, identity assertion is used by the patient to authenticate the provider. The provider sends the hashID of the required identity token. The patient uses the hashID to receive the corresponding hash from the provider's

Health SC using the *retrieve_hash* function. This allows the blockchain to keep a record of each authentication taking place. The patient then uses the hash to retrieve the identity token (JWT) from cloud storage.
3. Attribute Verification: The provider shares the symmetric key securely, which is used to decrypt the identity token received from the cloud. To verify the signature of the regulator, the public key of the regulator is requested using its Ethereum address from the *verify_regulator* function of Registry SC. This allows the patient to verify that the regulator is registered. The public key received is used to verify the identity token. This proves that the identity assertion is validated and attested by the regulator.

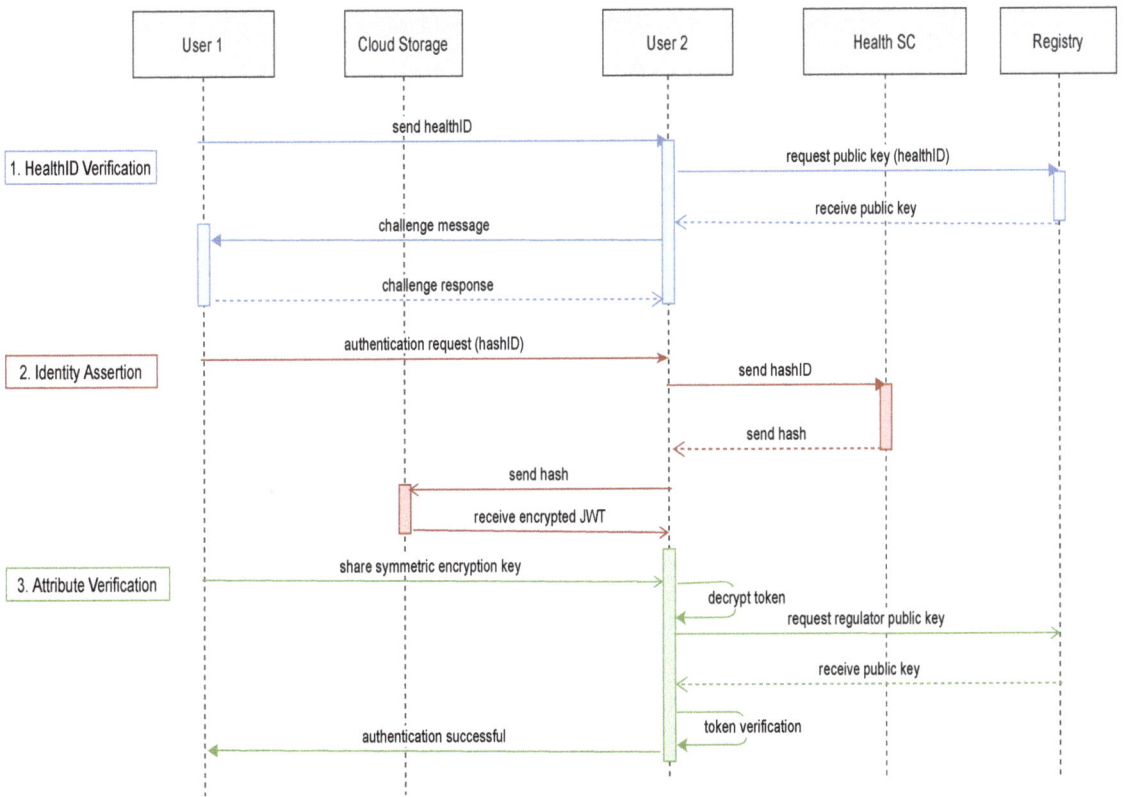

Figure 5. Authentication sequence diagram.

4.5. Discussion

The healthcare solutions presented in [21–25,32–34] only focus on decentralized healthcare record management systems. These solutions either assume to have a decentralized IdM or rely on a centralized IdM of hospitals. None of these solutions provide a detailed implementation of an IdM system where patients and healthcare providers can authenticate and verify each other irrespective of their healthcare application. On the other hand, the existing blockchain-based IdM solutions, such as [17–20,29,30], provide a single sign-on authentication system where users have self-asserted identities by creating their profiles. These systems lack adequate identity proofing to validate the identity information. It is essential to conduct identity proofing in healthcare applications before allowing patients and healthcare providers to authenticate each other. In the healthcare sector, healthcare providers are licensed by regulatory authorities to provide healthcare services. For instance, a doctor would be certified by healthcare professionals, whereas the pharmaceutical council would approve a pharmacist. Therefore, the identity attestation should be conducted by the relevant regulatory authority. Compared to the existing solutions, the healthID facilitates patients and healthcare providers to authenticate each other without depending on their eHealth provider. HealthID harnesses the power of blockchain technology to safeguard patient information and help ensure regulatory compliance by allowing identity proofing. The complete implementation of the solution is presented in the next section.

5. Implementation and Evaluation

In this section, we implement the smart healthcare identity framework on a consortium Ethereum network. We explain the setup that is used to deploy a smart contract over the blockchain. We further present and discuss the performance of deployed consortium blockchain.

5.1. Blockchain Deployment

We choose a consortium blockchain to implement healthID. Consortium removes the centralized control as a group of healthcare regulators manages it in contrast to a single entity in a private blockchain. Furthermore, it is more privacy-ensuring and efficient due to the smaller node count compared to the public blockchain. We deployed the consortium blockchain using the Ethereum network on five nodes. Each node is set up on an EC2 virtual machine using an AWS cloud service. The virtual machine has 1 GB RAM and 20 GB storage with a Linux Ubuntu operating system. Each virtual machine is configured with the Go Ethereum client (Geth (https://github.com/ethereum/go-ethereum/wiki/geth (accessed on 1 May 2021))) that is implemented in Go language. The five nodes running the Geth client are connected using their eNode addresses. After initializing the blockchain, we used Remix IDE (https://remix.ethereum.org/ (accessed on 1 May 2021)) to compile healthID smart contracts implemented in solidity language. We further used the Metamask (https://metamask.io (accessed on 1 May 2021)) wallet to deploy the smart contract onto our consortium blockchain. After deploying our smart contacts, we submit dummy transactions over the blockchain. The commands used to set up and initialize the Ethereum blockchain are provided in the GitHub repository (https://github.com/ibrahimtariqjaved/healthid (accessed on 1 May 2021)).

The PoA consensus agreement is used to deploy the consortium blockchain. The PoA blockchain in Ethereum is named the Clique network. The nodes that validate the block are called sealers. In PoA, the network consensus is achieved by a majority agreement among the sealer nodes. The genesis JSON file configures the network and initializes the first block on the blockchain network. A sample JSON genesis file is presented in Listing 1. The genesis file contains several parameters that are essential to configure the PoA consensus. The *chainID* is used to allocate an identifier to the network. The *parentHash* parameter defines the hash of the previous block, which is set to 0 as the genesis block has no parent block. The *gasLimit* is used to set the limit of gas that can be used per block. Gas refers to the cost required to perform a transaction on the network. The *gasLimit* defines how many transactions can be part of each block. The *Epoch Period* defines the size of each block as it is the time set between two successive blocks. The block-time is used to determine the size of each block. The *extraData* is used to set the addresses of sealers when initializing the blockchain. Sealers are nodes that can validate and include a transaction on a block. In our case, healthcare regulators are set as sealers of the network. A consortium is deployed by initializing a set of sealers in the genesis block. The majority voting of existing sealers can include a new sealer. The genesis file is used to set the initial parameters necessary for the blockchain. We analyze the performance of blockchain by using three parameters (i) Block-Time, (ii) Gas-Limit, and (iii) Sealers Number. The consortium blockchain is tested by varying these three parameters. For each configuration, we run the blockchain for one hour to compute the performance.

Listing 1. JSON genesis.

5.2. Performance Evaluation

We compute the performance of the healthcare identity framework on a consortium blockchain using the Ethereum network. We use four metrics to compute the performance of the Ethereum blockchain:

1. *Transaction gas cost (TGS):* TGS is the amount of gas needed to run a smart contract transaction on the Ethereum blockchain network. It represents the efficiency of the smart contract in terms of its execution. TGS needs to be minimized to achieve higher efficiency and lower delays in the network as each transaction is executed over all nodes of the blockchain.
2. *Transaction Per Second (TPS):* TPS is the total transactions that can be carried out on the blockchain in one second. It is computed using the $gasLimit$ divided by the TGS and $Block-time_{measured}$. Where The $Block-time_{measured}$ is the actual block-time recorded from the geth console. The $Block-time_{measured}$ may differ from the block-time set in genesis due to synchronization and network delays.
3. *Number of Blocks Lost (NBL):* The NBL is the number of blocks lost in the network. The NBL can be measured directly from the geth console. A block is lost when the sealer delays broadcasting the signed block for a specific time. After that, the block is replaced by a new block proposed by a backup sealer. The block that was required to be added to the blockchain is considered lost. Therefore, the number of blocks lost produces lag in the blockchain network. To reduce the delay of block generation, the NBL needs to be minimized.
4. *Block Propagation Time (BPT):* BPT is the time that is needed for a new block to be distributed to the majority set of nodes present in the network. Each block is propagated to all nodes in the network after validation using a defined broadcast protocol. Thus, for a block to reach the entire network, it passes through approximately seven intermediary nodes. The propagation time for each block can be extracted from the geth console.

In order to compute the performance, we ran the blockchain for one hour for each setting. The information regarding each block is extracted from the geth console. The screenshot of the geth console is shown in Figure 6. The $Block-time_{measured}$, NBL and BPT are directly extracted from the geth console.

5.2.1. Transaction Gas Cost of HealthID Smart Contract

In this subsection, we compute the performance of our smart contracts in terms of their complexity. We compute the TGS for deploying smart contracts and their functions, as presented in Table 1. However, PoA does not require any cost to be paid. The TGS is a good metric to check the complexity of the smart contract. The higher the gas cost, the more time it will take to execute the function on the blockchain. The TGS for deploying Health SC requires 485561 gas, as shown in Table 1 (a). The deployment cost of the registry smart contract is almost similar, as seen in Table 1 (b). This cost is required only once upon deployment of the smart contract. Regarding the smart contract functions, we can observe that none of the functions has TGS above 50,000 gas. The TGS of *set_publickey* and *set_hash, register_ regulator* and *register_attestation* functions are above 40,000 gas as they require mapping of 32 bytes addresses. From Section 4.4, we can observe that for the identification process, five smart contract functions are required, namely *Patient_SC deployment, set_publickey, get_publickey, register_attestation* and *set_hash*. Therefore, for the identification process, a total of 485,561 + 44,538 + 22,351 + 66,327 + 46,887 = 623,465 gas is required. The cost of identification is high due to smart contract deployment. However, this cost is required only once for initializing the smart contract on the blockchain. After the smart contract is deployed, the process of identity proofing will only require a *TGS* of 135,565 gas. On the other hand, the authentication process requires only three functions *verify_attestation, get_hash* and *verify_regulator*. For which a *TGS* of 24,911 + 22,351 + 23,920 = 71,182 gas is required. This shows that the authentication process requires very little computational power and can be executed quickly.

Table 1. Gas cost for healthcare identity smart contracts.

(a) Gas Cost for Health Smart Contract		
No	Contract Transaction	TGS
1	Deploy Health_SC	485,561
2	set_publickey	44,538
3	get_publickey	22,351
4	set_hash	46,887
5	get_hash	24,434
6	pause_smartcontract	43,436
(b) Gasgas Cost for Registry Smart Contract		
No	Contract Transaction	TGS
1	Deploy Registry_SC	474,939
2	register_regulator	43,757
3	verify_regulator	23,920
4	register_attestation	66,327
5	verify_attestation	24,911
6	revoke_attestation	14,492

5.2.2. Effect of Block-Time and Gas-Limit on Blockchain Performance

In this subsection, we evaluate the effect of block-time and gas-limit on the performance of the blockchain. To determine the effect of these two parameters on blockchain performance, we compute TPS and NBL. As discussed earlier, *TPS* represents the number of transactions processed by the blockchain in a second, whereas NBL represents the number of blocks lost during block creation. Figure 7a shows *TPS* with respect to block-time. We can observe that *TPS* decreases rapidly when block-time is increased. To achieve a high *TPS*, a small value of block-time is required. However, we further observed that lower values of block-time have a high number of *NBL*, as shown in Figure 7b. The lost blocks introduce delay in the network as new blocks are required to replace them. A large decrease in NBL is observed for block-time between 1 to 5. This is because, at high block-time, sealers have additional time to validate the transactions. Therefore, we suggest a block-time between 5 and 10. For a block-time of 7, *TPS* of around 100 can be achieved with a low number of lost blocks. We further computed the effect of gas-limit on the TPS. From Figure 7c, we can observe the effect of gas-limit on the TPS. For a block-time of 7, we varied the gas-limit from 60,000,000 to 200,000,000. Currently, the public Ethereum blockchain [37] uses a gas-limit of 20,000,000. However, we can use higher gas-limits for a private blockchain as there are a limited number of nodes present in the network. To achieve higher TPS in a private blockchain, we can increase the gas-limit. This will allow a high number of transactions to be accommodated inside the block-time. For a gas-limit of 200,000,000, we observed that TPS reached above 130. We also experimented with the effect of gas-limit on NBL. However, we did not found any effect.

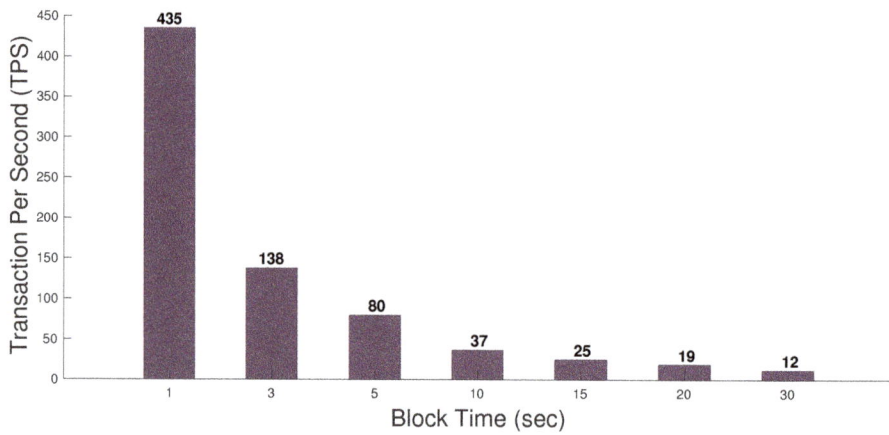

(a) Transaction per Second as a function of block-time

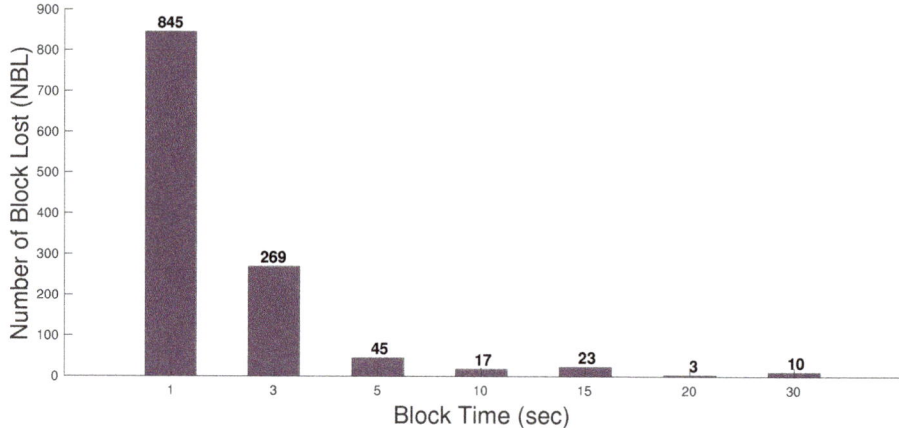

(b) Number of blocks lost as a function of block-time

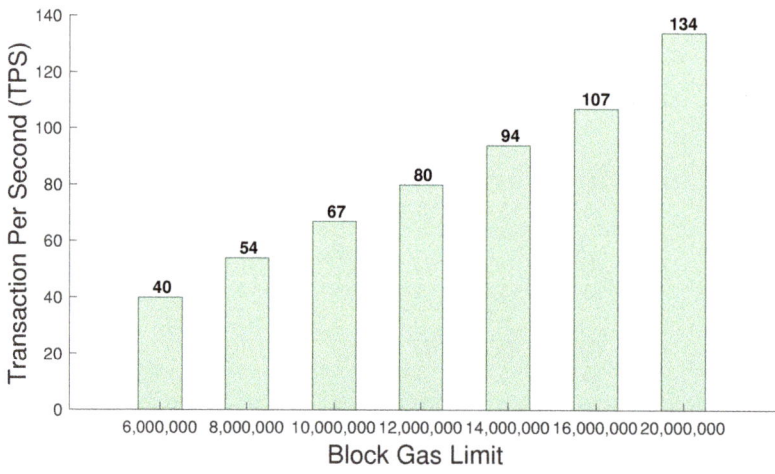

(c) Transaction Per Second as a function of Gas-limit

Figure 7. Effect of block-time and Gas-limit on blockchain performance.

5.2.3. Effect of Sealers on Blockchain Performance

In this subsection, we observe the effect of sealers on blockchain performance. In the five-node network, we set the number of sealers from one to five and observed their effect on NBL and BPT. First, we tried to observe the NBL in one hour for sealers in the network, as shown in Figure 8a. It can be seen that there were no lost blocks until three sealers were selected. However, when more than three sealers were selected from five nodes, a high number of NBL were observed. The high number of NBL is caused due to synchronization between sealers. In order to validate the block as at least 51%, sealers need to verify it. Therefore if more nodes are made sealers, this may cause NBL to increase. Therefore the sealers should not be more than half the number of nodes present in the network. We further observed the BPT in the network concerning the number of sealers, as shown in Figure 8b. As discussed earlier, BPT is the time required for a block to be distributed to most nodes in the network. It can be observed from the Figure that the BPT is strongly dependent on the number of sealers. More synchronization issues were observed when the number of sealers was added to the network, which was the reason behind the higher propagation delay. As seen from the Figure, increasing the number of sealers to five, the BPT is increased by around 381.88. Therefore, to reduce the network minimum possible number, several sealers should be selected to run the network.

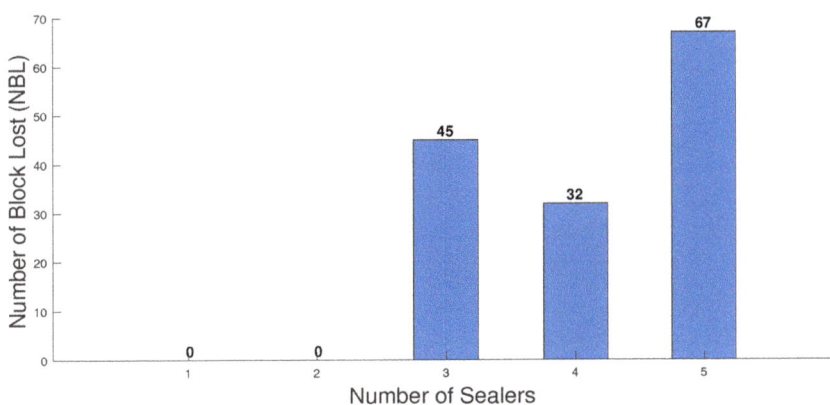

(a) Blocks lost as a function of sealers.

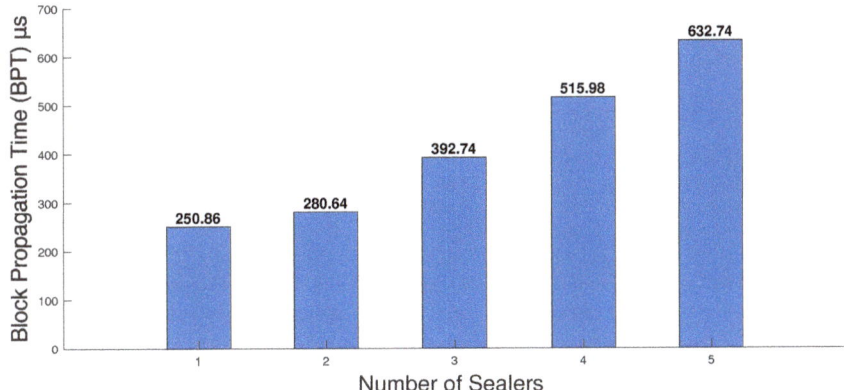

(b) Block propagation time as a function of sealers.

Figure 8. Effect of sealers on blockchain performance.

6. Conclusions and Future Work

Identity management has gained significant attention in recent years. However, the interoperability, regulation compliance, and security of identity management solutions are still complex challenges yet to be solved. The end-user can only trust the eHealth service provider regarding the safety and protection of its data and attributes. This paper presented a portable and privacy-preserving decentralized identity management solution with an application for remote healthcare services that shifts the control over identity information from service provider to end-user. The proposed system allows patients and healthcare providers to authenticate themselves across different eHealth domains without relying on a central service provider. The healthID approach harnesses a set of smart contracts to tokenize the identity of the network's entities and end-users, such that a unique healthID identifies each entity. A healthcare regulator digitally signs the identity attributes to create a JSON Web Token, which the owner stores. The identity attributes are further indexed on the blockchain using the owner's smart contract to ensure immutability and traceability.

To evaluate the performance of the proposed system, we implemented the smart contracts over an Ethereum blockchain managed by a consortium of healthcare regulators and assessed its efficiency in terms of gas cost and speed. We observed that a throughput higher than 100 TPS could be achieved over the consortium blockchain, which is around eight times greater than the throughput of a public blockchain. Moreover, we evaluated the blocks lost in the presence of a different number of sealers. We found out that the number of sealers should be less than half the network number to minimize propagation and synchronization delays for optimized performance. We intend to extend our work to securely manage and store patient's health records by using zero-knowledge proofs for future work. Our proposed IdM solution would be applied to the real health ecosystem using a cancer patient health record database. We also plan to integrate the blockchain with a distributed storage system, such as IPFS, and measure its performance.

Author Contributions: Conceptualization, I.T.J.; methodology, I.T.J. and B.B.; validation, I.T.J.; writing—original draft preparation, F.A. and B.B.; writing—review and editing, T.M., N.C. and K.N.Q.; visualization, I.T.J.; project administration, T.M.; funding acquisition, T.M., F.A. and N.C. All authors have read and agreed to the published version of the manuscript.

Funding: This work is partly supported with the financial support of the Science Foundation Ireland grant 13/RC/2094_P2 and partly funded from the European Union's Horizon 2020 research and innovation programme under the Marie Skłodowska-Curie grant agreement No. 754489.

Conflicts of Interest: The authors declare no conflict of interest.

References

1. Stowe, S.; Harding, S. Telecare, telehealth and telemedicine. *Eur. Geriatr. Med.* **2010**, *1*, 193–197. [CrossRef]
2. Wootton, R.; Craig, J.; Patterson, V. *Introduction to Telemedicine*; CRC Press: Boca Raton, FL, USA, 2017.
3. *Digital Health Global Market Trajectory & Analytics*; Technical Report; Global Industry Analysts Inc.: San Jose, CA, USA, 2020.
4. eHealth Market-2027 | Global Industry Analysis By Development, Size, Share and Demand Forecast. Available online: https://www.marketwatch.com/press-release/ehealth-market--2027-global-industry-analysis-by-development-size-share-and-demand-forecast-2021-04-05?tesla=y (accessed on 1 May 2021).
5. Seh, A.H.; Zarour, M.; Alenezi, M.; Sarkar, A.K.; Agrawal, A.; Kumar, R.; Ahmad Khan, R. Healthcare Data Breaches: Insights and Implications. *Healthcare* **2020**, *8*, 133. [CrossRef]
6. Javed, I.T.; Copeland, R.; Crespi, N.; Emmelmann, M.; Corici, A.; Bouabdallah, A.; Zhang, T.; El Jaouhari, S.; Beierle, F.; Göndör, S.; et al. Cross-domain identity and discovery framework for web calling services. *Ann. Telecommun.* **2017**, *72*, 459–468. [CrossRef]
7. Javed, I.T.; Toumi, K.; Alharbi, F.; Margaria, T.; Crespi, N. Detecting Nuisance Calls over Internet Telephony Using Caller Reputation. *Electronics* **2021**, *10*, 353. [CrossRef]
8. Javed, I.T.; Toumi, K.; Crespi, N. TrustCall: A Trust Computation Model for Web Conversational Services. *IEEE Access* **2017**, *5*, 24376–24388. [CrossRef]
9. Bouras, M.A.; Lu, Q.; Zhang, F.; Wan, Y.; Zhang, T.; Ning, H. Distributed Ledger Technology for eHealth Identity Privacy: State of The Art and Future Perspective. *Sensors* **2020**, *20*, 483. [CrossRef]
10. Truong, N.B.; Sun, K.; Lee, G.M.; Guo, Y. GDPR-Compliant Personal Data Management: A Blockchain-Based Solution. *IEEE Trans. Inf. Forensics Secur.* **2020**, *15*, 1746–1761. [CrossRef]

11. Rathee, T.; Singh, P. A systematic literature mapping on secure identity management using blockchain technology. *J. King Saud Univ. Comput. Inf. Sci.* **2021**. [CrossRef]
12. Javed, I.T.; Alharbi, F.; Margaria, T.; Crespi, N.; Qureshi, K.N. PETchain: A Blockchain-Based Privacy Enhancing Technology. *IEEE Access* **2021**, *9*, 41129–41143. [CrossRef]
13. Alamri, B.; Javed, I.T.; Margaria, T. Preserving Patients' Privacy in Medical IoT Using Blockchain. In Proceedings of the Edge Computing—EDGE 2020, Honolulu, HI, USA, 18–20 September 2020; Katangur, A., Lin, S.C., Wei, J., Yang, S., Zhang, L.J., Eds.; Springer International Publishing: Cham, Switzerland, 2020; pp. 103–110.
14. Alamri, B.; Javed, I.T.; Margaria, T. A GDPR-Compliant Framework for IoT-Based Personal Health Records Using Blockchain. In Proceedings of the 2021 11th IFIP International Conference on New Technologies, Mobility and Security (NTMS), Paris, France, 19–21 April 2021; pp. 1–5. [CrossRef]
15. Belotti, M.; Božić, N.; Pujolle, G.; Secci, S. A Vademecum on Blockchain Technologies: When, Which, and How. *IEEE Commun. Surv. Tutor.* **2019**, *21*, 3796–3838. [CrossRef]
16. Houtan, B.; Hafid, A.S.; Makrakis, D. A Survey on Blockchain-Based Self-Sovereign Patient Identity in Healthcare. *IEEE Access* **2020**, *8*, 90478–90494. [CrossRef]
17. Liu, Y.; He, D.; Obaidat, M.S.; Kumar, N.; Khan, M.K.; Choo, K.K.R. Blockchain-based identity management systems: A review. *J. Netw. Comput. Appl.* **2020**, *166*, 102731. [CrossRef]
18. Lundkvist, C.; Heck, R.; Torstensson, J.; Mitton, Z.; Sena, M. Uport: A Platform for Self-Sovereign Identity. 2017. Available online: https://whitepaper.uport.me/uPort_whitepaper_DRAFT20170221.pdf (accessed on 1 May 2021).
19. Windley, P.; Reed, D. *Sovrin: A Protocol and Token for Self-Sovereign Identity and Decentralized Trust*; The Sovrin Foundation: Provo, UT, USA, 2018.
20. Ali, M.; Nelson, J.; Shea, R.; Freedman, M.J. Blockstack: A global naming and storage system secured by blockchains. In Proceedings of the 2016 USENIX Annual Technical Conference, Denver, CO, USA, 22–24 June 2016; pp. 181–194.
21. Guo, R.; Shi, H.; Zhao, Q.; Zheng, D. Secure Attribute-Based Signature Scheme With Multiple Authorities for Blockchain in Electronic Health Records Systems. *IEEE Access* **2018**, *6*, 11676–11686. [CrossRef]
22. Zhao, H.; Bai, P.; Peng, Y.; Xu, R. Efficient key management scheme for health blockchain. *CAAI Trans. Intell. Technol.* **2018**, *3*. [CrossRef]
23. Wang, H.; Song, Y. Secure Cloud-Based EHR System Using Attribute-Based Cryptosystem and Blockchain. *J. Med. Syst.* **2018**, *42*, 1–9. [CrossRef]
24. Cao, S.; Zhang, G.; Liu, P.; Zhang, X.; Neri, F. Cloud-assisted secure eHealth systems for tamper-proofing EHR via blockchain. *Inf. Sci.* **2019**, *485*, 427–440. [CrossRef]
25. Yazdinejad, A.; Srivastava, G.; Parizi, R.M.; Dehghantanha, A.; Choo, K.K.R.; Aledhari, M. Decentralized Authentication of Distributed Patients in Hospital Networks Using Blockchain. *IEEE J. Biomed. Health Inform.* **2020**, *24*, 2146–2156. [CrossRef]
26. Haddouti, S.E.; Kettani, M.D.E.C.E. Towards an interoperable identity management framework: a comparative study. *arXiv* **2019**, arXiv:1902.11184.
27. Mell, P.; Dray, J.; Shook, J. Smart Contract Federated Identity Management without Third Party Authentication Services. *arXiv* **2019**, arXiv:1906.11057.
28. Dunphy, P.; Petitcolas, F.A. A first look at identity management schemes on the blockchain. *IEEE Secur. Priv.* **2018**, *16*, 20–29. [CrossRef]
29. Self-Sovereign Identity for More Freedom and Privacy. Available online: https://selfkey.org/ (accessed on 7 December 2020).
30. Evernym | The Self-Sovereign Identity Company. Available online: https://www.evernym.com/ (accessed on 7 December 2020).
31. Copyright. *e-Health Systems*; Rodrigues, J.J.P., Sendra Compte, S., de la Torra Diez, I., Eds.; Elsevier: Amsterdam, The Netherlands, 2016; p. iv. [CrossRef]
32. Jiang, S.; Cao, J.; Wu, H.; Yang, Y.; Ma, M.; He, J. BlocHIE: A BLOCkchain-Based Platform for Healthcare Information Exchange. In Proceedings of the 2018 IEEE International Conference on Smart Computing (SMARTCOMP), Taormina, Italy, 18–20 June 2018; pp. 49–56. [CrossRef]
33. Ray, P.P.; Chowhan, B.; Kumar, N.; Almogren, A. BIoTHR: Electronic Health Record Servicing Scheme in IoT-Blockchain Ecosystem. *IEEE Internet Things J.* **2021**. [CrossRef]
34. Rajput, A.R.; Li, Q.; Ahvanooey, M.T. A Blockchain-Based Secret-Data Sharing Framework for Personal Health Records in Emergency Condition. *Healthcare* **2021**, *9*, 206. [CrossRef]
35. Wu, J.; Tran, N. Application of Blockchain Technology in Sustainable Energy Systems: An Overview. *Sustainability* **2018**, *10*, 3067. [CrossRef]
36. Dib, O.; Brousmiche, K.L.; Durand, A.; Thea, E.; Ben Hamida, E. Consortium blockchains: Overview, applications and challenges. *Int. J. Adv. Telecommun.* **2018**, *11*, 51–64.
37. Werner, S.M.; Pritz, P.J.; Perez, D. Step on the Gas? A Better Approach for Recommending the Ethereum Gas Price. *arXiv* **2020**, arXiv:2003.03479.

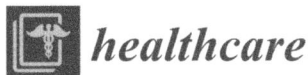 healthcare

Opinion

Medical Apps and the Gray Zone in the COVID-19 Era: Between Evidence and New Needs for Cybersecurity Expansion

Giovanni Maccioni and Daniele Giansanti *

Centre Tisp, Istituto Superiore di Sanità, 00161 Rome, Italy; gvnnmaccioni@gmail.com
* Correspondence: daniele.giansanti@iss.it; Tel.: +39-06-49902701

Abstract: The study focuses on emerging problems caused by the spread of medical apps. Firstly, it reviews the current role of cybersecurity and identifies the potential need to widen the boundaries of cybersecurity in relation to these apps. Secondly, it focuses on the pivotal device behind the development of mHealth: the smartphone, and highlights its role and current potential for hosting wearable medical technology. Thirdly, it addresses emerging issues regarding these apps, which are in a gray zone. This is done through an analysis of the important positions of scholars, and by means of a survey report on the increased use of various categories of apps during the COVID-19 pandemic, highlighting an accentuation of the problem. The study ends by explaining the reflections and proposals that emerged after performing the analysis.

Keywords: eHealth; medical devices; digital health; mHealth; cyber-risk; pacemaker; artificial pancreas; app; regulation; wearable device

1. Purpose of the Prospective Study

The proposed study is based on problems identified some time ago in relation to medical apps with regard to correct use by both the citizen and the medical actor, the clear identification of the intended use, and quality control and certification (when necessary).

As a prospective study, the first objective is to review the current role of cybersecurity and identify new needs to be covered in these medical apps.

The second objective is to highlight the opportunities of the smartphone device in mHealth, which has become a medium for wearable medical technology through dedicated apps and appropriate sensors.

The third objective, without the aim of performing a review, is to highlight the main problems found on these medical apps by the research world, which are considered to be in a gray zone.

The fourth objective is to highlight how the COVID-19 pandemic has exacerbated these problems. This is achieved through the development and submission of a targeted survey to investigate the increase in the use of these apps during the pandemic.

In line with the highlights of the Special Issue "Cybersecurity and the Digital Health: An Investigation on the State of the Art and the Position of the Actors" [1], this study ends with the expression of an opinion on how these issues are to be addressed (in particular with regard to how cybersecurity should act on these issues) and the role and positions that the various actors should have in order to act effectively in relation to the problem. It is in fact basic to understand [1] whether and how it is appropriate to expand and better generalize the role of cybersecurity in new border areas of the health sector, for example, with regard to nonmedical apps that can be confused with medical devices and for which noncompliant use could put patient safety at risk, especially during the COVID-19 pandemic. From a general point of view, this contribution aims to respond to this.

2. The Boundaries of the Cybersecurity Today and the Gray Zone of Medical Apps

2.1. The Boundaries of the Cybersecurity

Cybersecurity has applications in four main areas of the cybersystem, and can be used either in complex medical devices and/or complex interoperable and heterogeneous systems (involving elaboration systems, informatics, biomechatronics, bioengineering, electronics, networks, eHealth, and mHealth [1]). These four areas are data preservation, data access and modification, data exchange, and interoperability and compliance. The following systems have cybersecurity issues in health care:

2.1.1. Wearable Medical Devices

Wearable medical devices [2–6], particularly implantable ones, are part of a heterogeneous system (e.g., pacemakers, artificial pancreases). In these systems, the wireless connection creates an environment that is potentially susceptible to cyberattacks.

2.1.2. Picture Archiving and Communication Systems

Picture Archiving and Communication Systems (PACSs) [7] represent a form of medical device software (defined by the FDA as a Class II medical device) that is dedicated to the management of a diagnosis reached using medical imaging. A PACS embeds several parts such as elaborators, workstations, digital databases, digital data-stores, and digital applications that are subject to potential cyberattacks.

2.1.3. Health Networks

As is well known, hospital companies today are strongly reliant on digital technologies. The cyber-risk is rapidly increasing with [1,7]:
1. The so-called dematerialization of administrative processes; and
2. The increased dependence on computerized biomedical and nonbiomedical technologies.

Hospital Information Systems (HIS) have been attacked and breached in some cases in terms of both privacy and activities [7].

2.2. The App in Health Care: The Gray Zone

Today, we are witnessing a diffusion in the market of apps that in some way have a correlation with aspects relating to health, in particular:
- *Apps certified as medical devices;*
- *Apps not certified as medical devices, whose manufacturers have decided by choice not to follow articulated certification processes, but which in any case have the potential to provide consistent physiological parameters;*
- *Apps that do not require certification based on intended use;*
- *Noncertified apps that have an intended use that would require a certification process and that do not have the potential to provide consistent physiological parameters.*

There is no doubt that in medical use, strict regulations and protocols that have broad implications ranging from diagnostics to therapy to legal aspects must be respected.

The way these apps are used (for example in telemonitoring or telemedicine) therefore has important implications that must be seriously considered.

At the moment, these implications do not seem to fall completely within the boundaries of cybersecurity, and include aspects of cybersecurity that are oriented towards the *cybersafety* of the patient and citizen, with strong correlations with market surveillance. A Google search with the words "Best Apps Health" returns millions of sites that support certain apps. However, this can disorient the patient and/or ordinary citizen when they face with this. It is therefore evident how a strong response is needed.

3. The Smartphone: New Opportunities as a Wearable Device Today in mHealth

Before the development of the smartphone, the monitoring and sending of physiological parameters took place through specially developed wearable devices, and the worlds of cell phones and telemonitoring remained separate [8].

As we know it today, the smartphone, with its development since 2008, has established itself first as a mediator between these two worlds and then consequently as a pivotal tool in mHealth for monitoring parameters, i.e., wearable with both sensor and processing potential. In general, the smartphone as [9] we know it today differs from the mobile phone due to the simultaneous presence of the following features:

1. The increased memory, a higher computing capacity, and a much more advanced data connection capacity due to the presence of dedicated operating systems;
2. A great potential for the production and management of multimedia content, such as taking high-resolution photos and producing video clips;
3. The ability to easily install free and/or paid features and/or applications (apps);
4. The provision of a high-resolution touch screen;
5. The possibility of using/maneuvering a virtual keyboard to interact with the various functions of the device (from the address book to the notepad), with the web, with the various applications installed, and with the so-called social networks;
6. Integration with sensors such as accelerometers, gyroscopes, magnetometers, thermometers, and even, in the most advanced models, photoelectric sensors, depth laser sensors, hall effect sensors, proximity sensors, and barometers;
7. The possibility of tethering (i.e., providing internet access to other devices such as access points) over the wireless network, e.g., Wi-Fi or Bluetooth, to devices such as other smartphones or mobile phones, laptops, or fixed computers;
8. The availability of GPS sensors.

In parallel to the development of the smartphone, dedicated operating systems have been spreading, some have consolidated (Android and IOS), while others have gone into obsolescence (Windows for example). Other new operating systems are emerging that also offer compatibility with consolidated operating systems; an example of this is the Harmony operating system from Huawei (Shenzhen, China), which seems to offer compatibility with Android.

Since the development of these devices and related devices, so-called virtual stores have proliferated, from which one can extract dedicated free and/or paid apps. Today, the most famous of these are connected to the two dominant OSs: Google Play (for Android) and App store (for IOS).

Initially, smartphones were not equipped with apps for health purposes.

Today, some smartphones already come with preinstalled apps for this purpose, which generally allow:

(1) Monitoring of some physiological parameters and activities related to wellness and fitness;
(2) Compatibility with other third-party apps and/or other sensors (piloted through the app) and/or smartwatches.

The examination of these case studies goes beyond the scope of this work, which is certainly not aimed at finding the best solutions in this regard.

Two well-known examples are the Samsung smartphone health app [10] on the Android operating system and the iPhone health app on the IOS operating system [11].

Harmony for Huawei, the new operating system that was previously mentioned, is also moving in this direction [12].

Recently, as a result of COVID-19, we have also seen a further push to search for new solutions and to verify the reliability of the physiological parameters provided by smartphones.

An noteworthy example is one of the most important physiological parameters considered in the pandemic: pulse oximetry [13]. Pulse oximetry is used to assess the severity of

COVID-19 infection and to categorize the risk. Browne et al. [14]: (a) highlighted that over 100 million Samsung smartphones that contain dedicated biosensors (Maxim Integrated Inc, San Jose, CA) and preloaded apps to perform pulse oximetry are in use globally; and (b) successfully tested the Samsung S9 smartphone to determine if this integrated hardware meets the full FDA/ISO requirements for clinical pulse oximetry [14].

4. The Gray Zone of Apps That Provide Physiological Parameters and/or Suggest Therapies and/or Medical Support

In addition to any basic equipment that may concern health aspects, smartphones can be populated with apps for monitoring physiological parameters, medical support, and medical therapy.

It is now possible to find all kinds of apps in virtual stores. There are so many that regulation has become particularly complex, especially in the medical field. As far as we are concerned and in line with the objectives of the Special Issue "Cybersecurity and the Digital Health: An Investigation on the State of the Art and the Position of the Actors" in the journal *Healthcare* [1], this is the area that is most worrying. For this reason, we must pay attention to apps confounding the citizen and/or physician with respect to the related use [15].

App stores are now full of apps that can confuse the citizen.

The world of research has mobilized and has begun to address the problem of the quality and reliability of these apps with reference to all the players. It is in fact possible, for practically every medical sector, to find a great many reviews of such apps.

In the following, in line with the objectives of the study, we report some converging outcomes, regardless of the topic under consideration. Jones et al. focused on plastic surgery apps [16] and their review found that most applications with a medical purpose were not certified as a medical device, had not been validated in any peer-reviewed research, and did not have any documented involvement of medical professionals. They concluded that the potential consequences of such applications operating incorrectly are stark and represent a risk to patient safety. Trecca et al. [17] focused on otolaryngology apps and found that the apps that are currently available need further development and further dialogue between physicians and patients, and that formal support from professional and scientific associations should be encouraged. Knitza et al. analyzed German rheumatology apps [18] for patients and physicians available in German app stores and found a lack of supporting clinical studies, use of validated questionnaires, and involvement of academic developers. They concluded that to create high-quality apps, closer cooperation led by patients and physicians is vital. Tabi et al. [19] reviewed apps for medication management and identified detailed characteristics of the existing apps with the aim of informing future app development. They highlighted the need for improved standards for reporting on app stores and underlined the need for a platform to offer health app users an ongoing evaluation of apps by health professionals and other users and to provide them with tools to easily select an appropriate and trustworthy app. Haskins et al. published a systematic review of smartphone applications for smoking cessation [20]. Adhering to the Preferred Reporting Items for Systematic Reviews and Meta-Analyses (PRISMA) guidelines, apps were reviewed in four phases, in which they: (1) identified apps from the scientific literature; (2) searched app stores for apps identified in the literature; (3) identified top apps available in leading app stores; and (4) determined which top apps available in stores had scientific support. They highlighted that among the top 50 apps suggested by each of the leading app stores, only two (4%) had any scientific support.

Mandracchia et al. published a review [21] regarding mobile phone apps for food allergies or intolerances in app stores. They used the mobile app rating scale. They found that the included apps should be tested in trials and identified some critical points that can help improve the innovativeness and applicability of future food allergy and intolerance apps. Xie et al. reviewed cardiovascular disease mobile apps [22] and found that they are insufficient in providing comprehensive health information, high-quality information, and interactive functions to facilitate self-management. They concluded that: (a) end users should exercise caution when using existing apps; (b) health care professionals and app developers should collaborate to better understand end users' preferences and follow evidence-based guidelines to develop mHealth apps. Nicholas et al. focused on psychiatry apps and, in particular, mobile apps for Bipolar Disorder (BD) [23]. In their systematic review they found that, in general, the content of the currently available apps for BD is not in line with practice guidelines or established self-management principles. Apps also fail to provide important information to help users assess their quality, with most lacking source citation and a privacy policy. Therefore, they conclude that: (a) both consumers and clinicians should exercise caution with app selection; (b) while mHealth offers great opportunities for the development of quality evidence-based mobile interventions, new frameworks for mobile mental health research are needed to ensure the timely availability of evidence-based apps to the public.

Huckvale et al. reviewed apps for asthma self-viewed management [24] and found that: (a) no apps for people with asthma combined reliable comprehensive information about the condition with supportive tools for self-management; (b) health care professionals considering recommending apps to patients as part of asthma self-management should exercise caution, recognizing that some apps may be unsafe. The COVID-19 pandemic itself has led to the development of a great many apps in the medical field. This development only further highlights the need for greater attention to the phenomenon. Ming et al. reviewed COVID-19 mobile health apps launched in the early days of the pandemic [25]. They highlighted that: (a) it can be difficult for health care professionals to recommend a suitable app for COVID-19 education and self-monitoring purposes; (b) it is important to evaluate the contents and features of COVID-19 mobile apps to guide users in choosing a suitable mobile app based on their requirements.

In light of the above, it is clear to see that we are witnessing the phenomenon of a gray zone in relation to these apps.

On the one hand, there are the needs of the actors in health processes, from doctors to citizens and, on the other hand, we have the rightly strict and rigorous rules of certification bodies such as the FDA.

Looking online, we are witnessing a proliferation of offers of incredible solutions. The scholars that analyze these offers with scientific rigor conclude that these solutions often represent a wild west [16]. Furthermore, these offers often do not adhere to the reality and what is published online is practically never supported by adequate scientific documentation and/or proof of what is being declared [16–25].

5. Highlighting the Problem during the COVID-19 Pandemic through an Electronic Survey

Examples that both intrigue and worry, when looking at the laypeople, especially those left alone in the COVID-19 era, are those represented by apps published online that promise solutions at your fingertips.

There are a multitude of apps that presumably saw an increase in popularity due to isolation, for example those that:

(a) Promise weight loss through dietetic programs;
(b) Promise to help you quit smoking;
(c) Promise to aid in the gym and/or with pseudo-rehabilitation motion programs;
(d) Support a fitness regime;
(e) Promise certain types of therapy (for example, psychological).

It is clear that the citizen when confronted with such an offer can become confused, relying on the app, and not seeking the advice of experienced professionals.

The COVID-19 pandemic has left many citizens isolated and lonely at home, so the problem has been further accentuated. On the one hand, there was a great opportunity for eHealth and mHealth to support the citizen; on the other, the offers available were very broad and often unclear. Many individuals have started to exercise, follow diets, quit smoking, etc. by relying on these apps in a self-taught way.

Herein, we have reported a few examples; however, by browsing the virtual stores, it is clearly evident that the problem is considerable and certainly worthy of attention. We developed a survey using established methods of electronic survey development, offering the opportunity to provide a useful measure of the acceptance and/or opinion of the citizen actor. Moreover, this modality, in the middle of the COVID-19 pandemic, allows for the maintenance of social distancing.

Recently, using social networks, we submitted an anonymous survey to a sample of 1150 young subjects; among them 1122 agreed to participate. The sample is represented by:
- Men: 580; with an average age of 25.7 years; a maximum age of 30 years; a minimum age of 19 years; a minimum of secondary school level education;
- Women: 542; with an average age 25.4 years; a maximum age of 30 years; a minimum age of 18 years; a minimum of secondary school level education.

The submission is still active and datamining will be further expanded. Here, with the aim of the study, we present the outcome on the first sample.

Figure 1 shows the answers to the Likert A question: "Please indicate the intensity of use of the following apps during the COVID-19 pandemic."

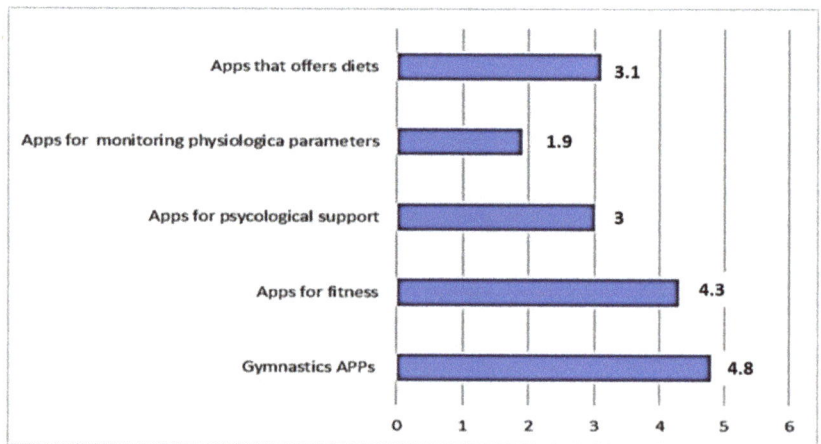

Figure 1. The answers to the Likert A question.

For each subquestion of the Likert question, it was possible to assign a score from 1 (for nothing or never used) to 6 (very large use). Therefore, the threshold of average use (TA) was set at 3.5.

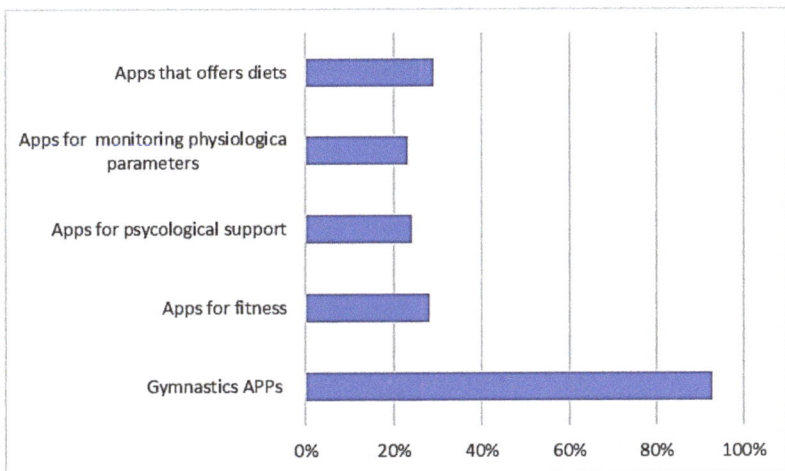

Figure 2. The answers to the Likert B question.

For each subquestion of the Likert question, it was possible to assign a percentage according to these indications (0%, 5%, 10%, ... 100%, more than 100%).

The Likert A question results highlight that:

- All the apps proposed have on average recorded use with an average score greater than 1;
- The apps for gymnastics and fitness had an average use greater than 3.5 = TA;
- Psychological and dietary therapeutic apps were also used, even if the score was not higher than TA.

The Likert B question results highlight that, in general, the average increase in use was always higher than 23%. Gym apps saw an increase in usage of over 90%. It is clear that before the pandemic, these apps had very little use when gyms were open and exploded during the pandemic.

A basic question was "In general, do you think that you have such knowledge of these Apps that allows you to distinguish the difference between medical apps and non-medical Apps?" This question could be answered with an evaluation ranging from one star (no knowledge) to six stars (a lot of knowledge). Therefore, the threshold of average use (TA) was set at 3.5. The average value obtained was 1.4, indicating a very low perception of knowledge << TA.

6. Conclusions

6.1. Highlights of the Study

Thanks to the astonishing development of mobile technologies, we are witnessing an enormous boom in mHealth technology.

This development is today conveyed by the smartphone device, which has gradually allowed the integration of wearable technology that once needed separate solutions [8].

Today, smartphones arrive configured with apps dedicated to health and with sensors that have the potential to provide measurements of important physiological parameters, such as oxygen saturation [14,15]. This applies to both of the dominant operating systems (Android and IOS) [10,11], and to new operating systems under development such as Harmony OS [12]. At the same time, apps dedicated to medical use are developed with the possibility of connecting to sensor devices and/or device kits.

This development has been so disruptive that it makes accurate regulation difficult if not impossible: some have defined it as regulating infinity [26]. The offer of these apps is impressive. For example, type "best App cardiology en" and you are diverted to a huge number of blog sites that promise you a list of the best cardiology apps. This is why the problem is relevant.

Currently, cybersecurity has well-defined and identified boundaries; these are more identified by concepts that revolve around the security of IT systems and data through solutions that prevent malicious attacks or the clumsy actions of operators [1].

Here, as regards apps that somehow fall into the sphere of medical applications, the concept of safe use must be understood with a different and broader meaning.

First of all, it must be said that an app with a medical destination, as dictated by the intended use, must be certified according to strict experimental protocols, strict documentation management [15], and by resorting to certification bodies. In some cases, the developers choose for their own reasons not to certify their apps; however, they must be aware that a doctor and/or medical specialist using mHealth/eHealth solutions, for example in telemedicine, is strongly bound by regulations and obligations in the use of certified devices and must defer to certification bodies.

The study proposed herein was developed according to various lines of thought.

A first step was to reassess the current boundaries of cybersecurity [1] to take into account the new needs concerning medical apps that fall in the gray zone.

In a second step, the evolution of the pivotal device of the great development of mHealth was analyzed: the smartphone, which today: (a) in the factory configuration, includes applications for health and openings to third-party apps in this area; (b) includes important sensorial integrations that allow, at least potentially, for the reliable measurement of physiological parameters important in the COVID-19 era [13,14].

The third step focused on the gray zone of these apps and explored the positions of various scholars who have published reviews of important categories of these apps, highlighting relevant problems.

In summary, the following criticalities emerge from these studies [16–24]:

- Most applications with a medical purpose were not certified as a medical device, had not been validated in any peer-reviewed research, and did not have any documented involvement of medical professionals; therefore, the potential consequences of such applications operating incorrectly are stark and represent a risk to patient safety;
- Most apps that are currently available need further development and dialogue between physicians and patients, and formal support from professional and scientific associations should be encouraged;
- There is a lack of supporting clinical studies, the use of validated questionnaires, and involvement of academic developers;
- To create high-quality apps, closer cooperation led by patients and physicians is vital;
- There is a low general level of scientific support;
- Apps are insufficient in providing comprehensive health information, high-quality information, and interactive functions to facilitate self-management;
- In general, the content of currently available apps is not in line with practice guidelines or established self-management principles.

Concerning the merits of the fabulous development of apps during the COVID-19 pandemic, the overall opinion is similar. It is clear [25] that it can be difficult for health care professionals to recommend a suitable app for coronavirus disease (COVID-19) education and self-monitoring purposes and that it is important to evaluate the contents and features of COVID-19 mobile apps to guide users in choosing a suitable mobile app based on their requirements.

After identifying various categories of apps of evident potential use during these great periods of isolation, the fourth step involved presenting a survey, the results of which generally highlighted both an increase in the use of these apps compared to the prepandemic period and a general lack of knowledge of the medical aspects in relation to their use. It is clear that an increase in the use of these apps combined with a lack of knowledge of the information aspects only reaffirms a potential increase in the problems highlighted above.

6.2. Final Reflections

It is evident that the problems that have emerged require wide-ranging and articulated solutions. Surely, the role of cybersecurity could be expanded and rethought to support solutions to the problems that have emerged. Many tools are available.

Tools to highlight the validity of an app exist, such as the mobile app rating scale [21].

Tools and methodologies that allow a community engaged approach to develop robust apps with close collaboration between potential users and developers also already exist [15].

Acceptance techniques through dedicated surveys such as the Technology assessment model (TAM) have already shown robustness [27]. Accessible databases through which to check the presence of certified apps exist and there is the possibility of creating online registers for apps that have followed qualification and validation paths, as was suggested by various authors [19]. However, it is extremely necessary to understand both: (a) why today some developers of these applications are not interested in having them validated by specialized entities in the medical, fitness, or nutrition fields; and (b) why there is an apparent poor lack or no interest from some of these entities in analyzing and validating that the applications meet the necessary requirements, e.g., that they do not harm the physical or mental health of users. All this is important and serves to explain why we are witnessing a wild west in the field of App production, and why we are seeing a proliferation of blog sites, that in some cases seem to support this or that App as if they were a cooking product.

In all probability, the answer must be sought in the pressures of the market: the same pressures that should guarantee better control, from clearer and more understandable indications in app stores, to surveillance policies and blanket monitoring of these apps in order to stimulate entities and developers to better collaborate, to the intensification of the supply and demand of support and services from development to training. It is evident that cybersecurity can help us, but it must be reassessed to include a concept of security that is not merely IT, and is more an expansion of citizen safety. Cybersecurity can certainly intervene in various ways, for example:

1. Through monitoring policies and regulation initiatives;
2. Through citizen training and information policies, perhaps offered in an e-learning format.

The first initiative should start from the supranational surveillance and regulation of virtual stores for all operating systems. It should also include the monitoring of public sites and supporting the advertising of platforms with certified apps and/or those that have followed a qualification path. It should ensure that the developers are motivated to follow these paths as well as the entities that offer the services.

The second initiative should also begin in virtual stores with the inclusion of clear and understandable information, not only to health care professionals but to laypeople. It should then continue with initiatives that involve school-aged citizens that help them understand and explore the situation [28].

Author Contributions: Conceptualization, D.G.; methodology, D.G.; software, G.M and D.G; validation All.; formal analysis, D.G and G.M.; investigation, All.; resources, D.G.; data curation, D.G.; writing—original draft preparation, D.G.; writing—review and editing, All.; supervision, D.G.; project administration, D.G. All authors have read and agreed to the published version of the manuscript.

Funding: This research received no external funding.

Institutional Review Board Statement: Not applicable.

Informed Consent Statement: Not applicable.

Data Availability Statement: Data sharing not applicable.

Conflicts of Interest: The authors declare no conflict of interest.

References

1. Giansanti, D. Cybersecurity and the *Digital-Health*: The Challenge of This Millennium. *Health* **2021**, *9*, 62. [CrossRef]
2. O'Keeffe, D.T.; Maraka, S.; Basu, A.; Keith-Hynes, P.; Kudva, Y.C. Cybersecurity in Artificial Pancreas Experiments. *Diabetes Technol. Ther.* **2015**, *17*, 664–666. [CrossRef] [PubMed]
3. Baranchuk, A.; Alexander, B.; Campbell, D.; Haseeb, S.; Redfearn, D.; Simpson, C.; Glover, B. Pacemaker Cybersecurity. *Circulation* **2018**, *138*, 1272–1273. [CrossRef] [PubMed]
4. Baranchuk, A.; Refaat, M.M.; Patton, K.K.; Chung, M.K.; Krishnan, K.; Kutyifa, V.; Upadhyay, G.; Fisher, J.D.; Lakkireddy, D.R.; American College of Cardiology's Electrophysiology Section Leadership. Cybersecurity for cardiac implantable electronic devices: What should you know? *J. Am. Coll. Cardiol.* **2018**, *71*, 1284–1288.
5. Kramer, D.B.; Fu, K. Cybersecurity concerns and medical devices: Lessons from a pacemaker advisory. *JAMA* **2017**, *318*, 2077–2078. [CrossRef] [PubMed]
6. Ransford, B.; Kramer, D.B.; Foo Kune, D.; Kune, D.M.; de Medeiros, J.A.; Yan, C.; Xu, W.; Crawford, T.; Fu, K. Cybersecurity and medical devices: A practical guide for cardiac electrophysiol-ogists. *Pacing Clin. Electrophysiol.* **2017**, *40*, 913–917. [CrossRef] [PubMed]
7. Giansanti, D.; Grigioni, M.; Monoscalco, L.; Gulino, R.A. Chapter: A Smartphone Based Survey to Investigate the Cyber-Risk Perception on the Health-Care Professionals. In *Mediterranean Conference on Medical and Biological Engineering and Computing, Proceedings of the XV Mediterranean Conference on Medical and Biological Engineering and Computing—MEDICON 2019, Coimbra, Portugal, 26–28 September 2019*; Henriques, J., Neves, N., de Carvalho, P., Eds.; Springer: Berlin, Germany, 2019; Volume 76, pp. 914–923.
8. Bonato, P. Wearable sensors/systems and their impact on biomedical engineering. *IEEE Eng. Med. Boil. Mag.* **2003**, *22*, 18–20. [CrossRef]
9. Giansanti, D. *Health in the Palm of Your Hand: Between Opportunities and Problems, Rapporti ISTISAN 19/15*; Istituto Su-Periore di Sanità: Roma, Italy, 2019; pp. 1–60.
10. Available online: https://www.samsung.com/it/apps/samsung-health/ (accessed on 7 April 2021).
11. Available online: https://www.apple.com/ca/ios/health/ (accessed on 7 April 2021).
12. Available online: https://www.huaweicentral.com/huawei-harmonyos-2-2/ (accessed on 7 April 2021).
13. Neto, A.S.; Checkley, W.; Sivakorn, C.; Hashmi, M.; Papali, A.; Schultz, M.J. COVID–LMIC Task Force and the Mahidol–Oxford Research Unit (MORU), Bangkok, Thailand. Pragmatic Recommendations for the Management of Acute Respiratory Failure and Mechanical Ventilation in Patients with COVID-19 in Low- and Middle- Income Countries. *Am. J. Trop. Med. Hyg.* **2021**, *104*, 60–71. [CrossRef]
14. Browne, S.H.; Bernstein, M.; Bickler, P.E. Accuracy of Smartphone Integrated Pulse Oximetry Meets Full FDA Clearance Standards for Clinical Use. *medRxiv*. in press. [CrossRef]
15. Giansanti, D. Introduction of Medical Apps in Telemedicine and e-Health: Problems and Opportunities. *Telemed. J. E Health* **2017**, *23*, 773–776. [CrossRef]
16. Jones, O.; Murphy, S.H.; Durrani, A.J. Regulation and validation of smartphone applications in plastic surgery: It's the Wild West out there. *Surgeon* **2021**. (ahead of print). [CrossRef]
17. Trecca, E.M.C.; Lonigro, A.; Gelardi, M.; Kim, B.; Cassano, M. Mobile Applications in Otolaryngology: A Systematic Review of the Literature, Apple App Store and the Google Play Store. *Ann. Otol. Rhinol. Laryngol.* **2021**, *130*, 78–91. [CrossRef]
18. Knitza, J.; Tascilar, K.; Messner, E.-M.; Meyer, M.; Vossen, D.; Pulla, A.; Bosch, P.; Kittler, J.; Kleyer, A.; Sewerin, P.; et al. German Mobile Apps in Rheumatology: Review and Analysis Using the Mobile Application Rating Scale (MARS). *JMIR mHealth uHealth* **2019**, *7*, e14991. [CrossRef]
19. Tabi, K.; Randhawa, A.S.; Choi, F.; Mithani, Z.; Albers, F.; Schnieder, M.; Nikoo, M.; Vigo, D.; Jang, K.; Demlova, R.; et al. Mobile Apps for Medication Management: Review and Analysis. *JMIR mHealth uHealth* **2019**, *7*, e13608. [CrossRef]
20. Haskins, B.L.; Lesperance, D.; Gibbons, P.; Boudreaux, E.D. A systematic review of smartphone applications for smoking cessation. *Transl. Behav. Med.* **2017**, *7*, 292–299. [CrossRef]
21. Mandracchia, F.; Llauradó, E.; Tarro, L.; Valls, R.M.; Solà, R. Mobile Phone Apps for Food Allergies or Intolerances in App Stores: Systematic Search and Quality Assessment Using the Mobile App Rating Scale (MARS). *JMIR mHealth uHealth* **2020**, *8*, e18339. [CrossRef]
22. Xie, B.; Su, Z.; Zhang, W.; Cai, R. Chinese Cardiovascular Disease Mobile Apps' Information Types, Information Quality, and Interactive Functions for Self-Management: Systematic Review. *JMIR mHealth uHealth* **2017**, *5*, e195. [CrossRef] [PubMed]
23. Nicholas, J.; Larsen, M.E.; Proudfoot, J.; Christensen, H. Mobile Apps for Bipolar Disorder: A Systematic Review of Features and Content Quality. *J. Med Internet Res.* **2015**, *17*, e198. [CrossRef] [PubMed]
24. Huckvale, K.; Car, M.; Morrison, C.; Car, J. Apps for asthma self-management: A systematic assessment of content and tools. *BMC Med.* **2012**, *10*, 144. [CrossRef]
25. Ming, L.C.; Untong, N.; Aliudin, N.A.; Osili, N.; Kifli, N.; Tan, C.S.; Goh, K.W.; Ng, P.W.; Al-Worafi, Y.M.; Lee, K.S.; et al. Mobile Health Apps on COVID-19 Launched in the Early Days of the Pandemic: Content Analysis and Review. *JMIR mHealth uHealth* **2020**, *8*, e19796. [CrossRef]
26. Baldani, G. Regolamentare l'infinito: La sfida della Food and Drug Administration. *Salute E Soc.* **2014**, 171–175. [CrossRef]

27. Knox, L.; Gemine, R.; Rees, S.; Bowen, S.; Groom, P.; Taylor, D.; Bond, I.; Rosser, W.; Lewis, K. Using the Technology Acceptance Model to conceptualise experiences of the usability and acceptability of a self-management app (COPD.Pal®) for Chronic Obstructive Pulmonary Disease. *Health Technol.* **2021**, *11*, 111–117. [CrossRef]
28. Giansanti, D.; Maccioni, G. Health in the palm of your hand—part 2: Design and application of an educational module for young people on the risks from smartphone abuse and the opportunities of telemedicine and e-Health. *mHealth* **2021**. ahead of print. Available online: https://mhealth.amegroups.com/article/view/61063/44616 (accessed on 7 April 2021).

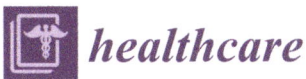

Review

A Quantitative and Qualitative Review on the Main Research Streams Regarding Blockchain Technology in Healthcare

Yong Sauk Hau [1,2] and Min Cheol Chang [2,3,*]

1. Department of Business Administration, School of Business, Yeungnam University, Gyeongsan 38541, Korea; augustine@yu.ac.kr
2. Medical Management Research Center, School of Business, Yeungnam University, Gyeongsan 38541, Korea
3. Department of Physical Medicine and Rehabilitation, College of Medicine, Yeungnam University, Taegu 38541, Korea
* Correspondence: wheel633@ynu.ac.kr; Tel.: +82-53-620-4682

Abstract: (1) Background: Blockchain technology has been gaining high popularity in the healthcare domain. This has brought about a spate of recent studies regarding blockchain technology in healthcare, creating high demand for quantitative or qualitative reviews on the main research streams thereof. In order to contribute to satisfying the high demand, this research presents a quantitative and qualitative review on studies regarding blockchain technology in healthcare. (2) Methods: A quantitative review was performed by searching the Web of Science database for articles published until 10 March in 2020, and a qualitative review was conducted by using the content analysis based on the integrative view of Leavitt's diamond model. (3) Results: The quantitative review identified five research streams. The number of articles about blockchain technology in healthcare has dramatically increased since 2016, with a compound annual growth rate of 254.4%. English is the most dominant language used in the articles, and the USA and China are the top two countries of origin of the articles, representing overwhelming portions. The IEEE Access, Journal of Medical Systems, Journal of Medical Internet Research, Applied Sciences Basel, and Sensors are the top five journals in terms of publication. The articles showed an L-shaped distribution in terms of their annual average numbers of citations. The qualitative review revealed two research streams. Most of the top 10 articles ranked by their annual average numbers of citations concentrated on developing or proposing new technological solutions using blockchain technology to effectively revolutionize the current methods of managing data in the healthcare domain. The majority of the top 10 articles pursued the convergence of blockchain technology with cloud technology or IoT. (4) Conclusions: This article illuminates the main research streams about blockchain technology in healthcare through a quantitative and qualitative review, providing implications for future research on blockchain technology.

Keywords: blockchain; healthcare; review; electronic medical record; cloud; internet of things; technology convergence

Citation: Hau, Y.S.; Chang, M.C. A Quantitative and Qualitative Review on the Main Research Streams Regarding Blockchain Technology in Healthcare. *Healthcare* **2021**, *9*, 247. https://doi.org/10.3390/healthcare9030247

Academic Editors: Daniele Giansanti and Pedram Sendi

Received: 8 January 2021
Accepted: 19 February 2021
Published: 1 March 2021

Publisher's Note: MDPI stays neutral with regard to jurisdictional claims in published maps and institutional affiliations.

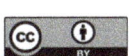

Copyright: © 2021 by the authors. Licensee MDPI, Basel, Switzerland. This article is an open access article distributed under the terms and conditions of the Creative Commons Attribution (CC BY) license (https://creativecommons.org/licenses/by/4.0/).

1. Introduction

Blockchain technology, a distributed ledger based on peer to peer networks [1], has been gaining high popularity in healthcare [2,3]. This high popularity has resulted from the innovative advantages of blockchain technology in managing medical data when compared to conventional methods. For example, blockchain technology can enhance not only the security of patients' medical data in hospitals [4,5], but also the safety of their medical data transfer between hospitals [6,7]. It can ensure that patients have unrestricted access to their own medical data whenever and wherever they require [6].

Furthermore, blockchain technology can provide innovative medical services for both patients and healthcare organizations through technological convergence with cutting edge information technology (IT) such as cloud technology [7,8], internet of things (IoT) [9,10], big data [11], and smart devices [10]. Therefore, more and more researchers and practitioners in healthcare are paying special attention to blockchain technology. This interest has recently brought about many studies on blockchain technology in healthcare, creating high demand for quantitative or qualitative reviews on the main research streams thereof. In order to contribute to satisfying this high demand for the reviews, this research conducts not only a quantitative review but also a qualitative review on studies about blockchain technology in healthcare. For the quantitative review, this research analyzes the main research streams in terms of their distribution by publication year, language, country of origin, journal, and the annual average numbers of citations. For the qualitative review, this research examines the contents of the top ten studies ranked by their annual average numbers of citations through the lens of Leavitt's diamond model [12]. Leavitt's diamond model [12] is a widely used theoretical framework for analyzing the impact of new technology on an organization by considering its impact on the inter-relationships between the four major factors of the organization—technology, people, structure, and task—in an integrative view.

In this article, we present a quantitative and qualitative review on prior studies about blockchain technology in healthcare and illuminate the main research streams thereof with a view to providing useful implications for future research.

2. Methods

This study conducts a quantitative and qualitative review to effectively illuminate the main research streams regarding blockchain technology in healthcare. Our quantitative review aims at not only revealing the main research streams in terms of the distribution of relevant studies by their publication year, language, country of origin, journal, and the annual average numbers of citations, but also identifying the top ten articles ranked by their annual average numbers of citations. Our qualitative review focuses on analyzing the main content trends in the top ten articles using the solid theoretical basis of Leavitt's diamond model [12]. The following two subsections describe the quantitative and qualitative methods used for this review, and Figure 1 summarizes our review flow.

2.1. Quantitative Method

We searched the Web of Science database for studies published until 10 March in 2020. Studies on blockchain technology in healthcare were observed to be published not only in medical journals but also in other journals from various domains, including IT, law, engineering, economics, and business administration. Therefore, we adopted the Web of Science database as the source of articles for this review, considering its extensive coverage of a variety of journals in both the natural and social sciences.

In order to perform a rigorous quantitative review, we used four steps, including identifying potential studies, filtering out irrelevant studies, confirming relevant studies, and analyzing selected articles.

In the first step of identifying potential studies, we performed an initial search for studies containing a keyword such as "blockchain" in their titles, abstracts, or keywords. This step identified a total number of 2472 potential studies. In another search, we narrowed down these studies to those containing key phrases, such as "blockchain" combined with "medic~", "health~", "biomedi~", "clinic~", or "hospital~" in their titles, abstracts, or keywords. This yielded a total number of 287 potential studies.

In the second step of filtering out irrelevant studies in terms of the document types, the 287 potential studies were filtered into a total number of 200 articles which belonged to the article or early access in the document types classified by the Web of Science database. According to this database, the early access indicated articles published online ahead of official publication.

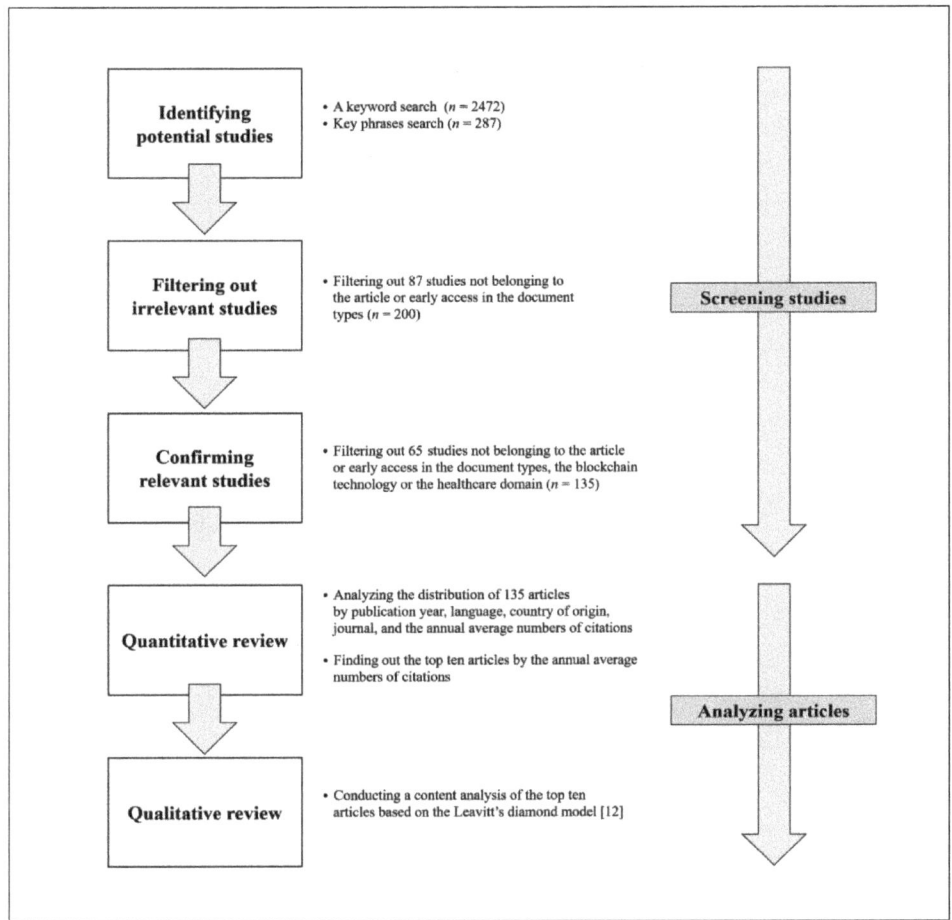

Figure 1. Review flow chart.

In the third step of confirming the relevancy of the 200 remaining studies by their document types and contents, we examined their document types, titles, abstracts, and keywords and filtered out 65 studies that satisfied the criterion of our search with the key phrases but did not belong to the article or early access in the document types, the blockchain technology or the healthcare domain. This step confirmed a total number of 135 articles, including the early access, which were used for our review.

In the fourth step of analyzing the 135 articles, we investigated their distribution by publication year, language, country of origin, journal, and the annual average numbers of citations. The countries of origin of the articles were examined by identifying the nationalities of the organizations to which the authors belonged. The country of origin of an article was evaluated to be two countries if the article had two authors working for organizations in two different countries. The annual average numbers of citations of the 135 articles were used to identify the top ten articles. The annual average numbers of citations can more effectively show the degree of influence of each article on other research than the total number of citations, by controlling the impact of time after publication. For example, an article published in 2016 is likely to have been cited more frequently than articles published in 2019. Therefore, we used the annual average numbers of citations to determine the ranks of the 135 articles.

2.2. Qualitative Method

We conducted a content analysis of the top ten articles under the integrative view of Leavitt's diamond model [12]. Leavitt's diamond model [12] is well-known for its integrative perspective of the influence of new technology on an organization, based on the inter-relationships between the four factors of an organization such as structure, task, technology, and people, as illustrated in Figure 2. The diamond model [12] has been widely used to analyze the impact of new technology on organizations since it was introduced by Harold J. Leavitt, a psychologist in organizational behavior in the field of management.

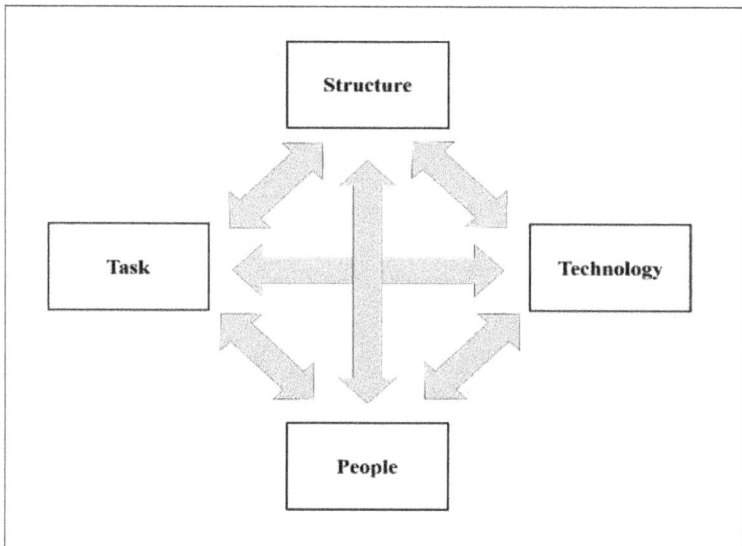

Figure 2. Leavitt's diamond model [12] (note: the source of this figure is page 1145 of [12]).

According to Leavitt's diamond model [12] in Figure 2, in the healthcare domain, the structure is the organizational hierarchy or the subsystem of work process and communication in healthcare organizations. The task refers to the work necessary to produce healthcare services or goods [12]. The technology indicates the IT programs or resources to support the processes of healthcare [12]. Finally, the people include the medical or administrative staff in healthcare organizations [12]. Leavitt's diamond model [12] considers healthcare organizations as complex systems wherein their structure, task, technology, and people have significant interactions with one another. This interaction can mean that the application of blockchain technology to healthcare organizations influences not only their technology but also other factors such as structure, task, and people in these organizations [12]. According to Leavitt [12], major approaches applied to the change in healthcare organizations on the adoption of blockchain technology can be classified into three approaches by using three of the four factors in the diamond model: the people approach, the structural approach, or the technological approach. Therefore, this study performs a content analysis of the top ten articles under the integrative perspective of Leavitt's diamond model [12] by examining which approach, among the people, structural, and technological approaches, has been adopted in the articles to reveal the main research streams therein.

The content analysis was performed by the two authors of this article, who are experts in IT and medicine, respectively. One author has a Ph.D. in IT management, and the other is a professor in the School of Medicine. We examined which approach, among the people, structural, and technological approaches according to Leavitt [12], was adopted in the contents of the top ten articles to analyze the main streams therein.

3. Results

The following two subsections report our review results according to the two review methods used in this study. The first subsection presents the results using the quantitative method, and the second subsection provides the results using the qualitative method.

3.1. Quantitative Review Results

Our quantitative review revealed five major research streams in the 135 articles about blockchain technology in healthcare in terms of their distribution by publication year, language, country of origin, journal, and the annual average numbers of citations as follows.

First, the number of articles has dramatically increased since 2016. These articles began being published in 2016. In 2016, only two articles were published. Since then, however, the number of published articles has grown rapidly, with a high compound annual growth rate of 254.4%, as shown in Figure 3. In greater detail, 6 and 30 articles were published in 2017 and 2018, respectively. In 2019, 89 articles were published, further showing the rapid growth in publication volume.

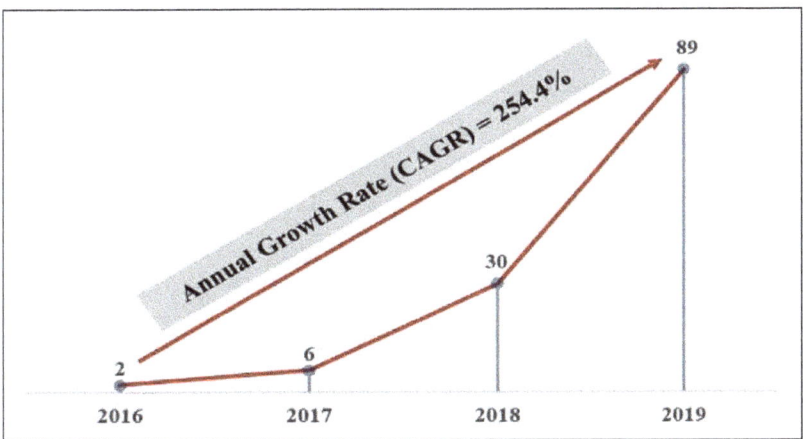

Figure 3. Distribution of the articles by publication year (2016~2019) (note: CAGR: Compound Annual Growth Rate; As of 10 March in 2020, 8 articles were published in 2020 but they were not included in this figure).

Second, English is the most dominant language used across the 135 articles. A total of 131 articles were written in English (97%). The other four articles included three in German (2.2%) and one (0.8%) in Spanish, as summarized in Figure 4.

Third, the USA, China, England, South Korea, and India are the top five countries of origin. A total of 41 articles could be traced to researchers in the USA (30.4%), 40 from China (29.6%), 11 from England (8.1%), 11 from South Korea (8.1%), and 10 from India (7.4%), as shown in Figure 5. Appendix A reports the distribution by country of origin for all 135 articles.

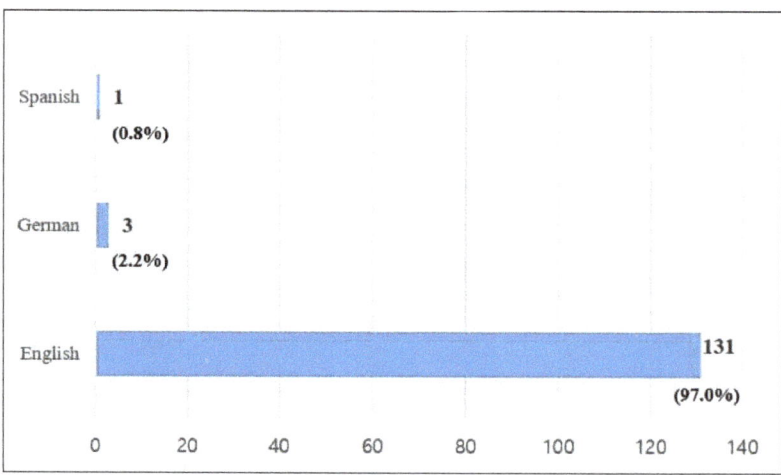

Figure 4. Distribution of the articles by language.

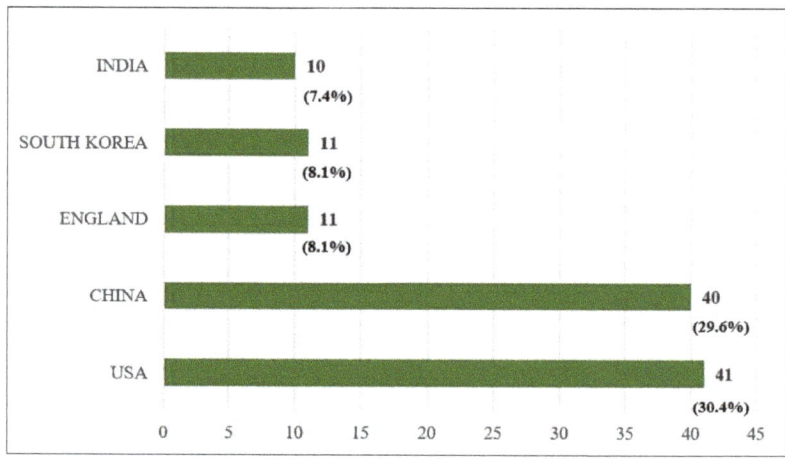

Figure 5. Top five countries of origin.

Fourth, the IEEE Access, Journal of Medical Systems, Journal of Medical Internet Research, Applied Sciences Basel, and Sensors are the top five journals in terms of their share among 61 journals in which the 135 articles were published. A total of 23 articles were published in the IEEE Access (17.0%), 16 articles in the Journal of Medical Systems (11.9%), 14 articles in the Journal of Medical Internet Research (10.4%), 5 articles in the Applied Sciences Basel (3.7%), and 5 articles in the Sensors (3.7%), as summarized in Figure 6. Appendix B reports the specific distribution of all journals.

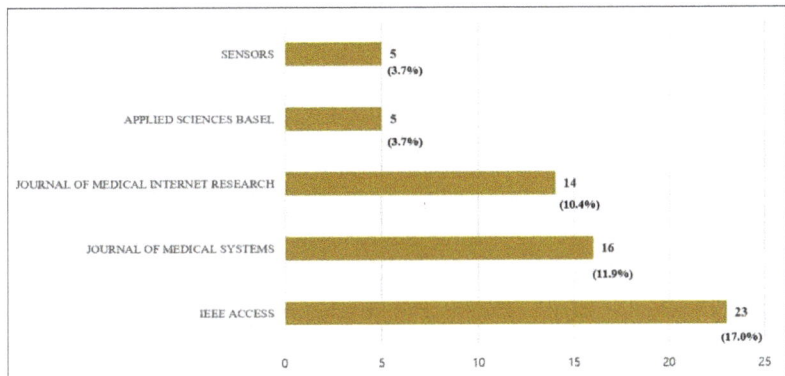

Figure 6. Top five journals in the 135 articles in terms of publication.

Fifth, the 135 articles show an L-shaped distribution as illustrated in Figure 7, arranged by their ranks in terms of the annual average number of citations. The minimum, median, and maximum values of the L-shaped distribution were 0, 0.67, and 34.6, respectively. Table 1 reports the top ten articles regarding the annual average number of citations. Their values all exceeded 12.

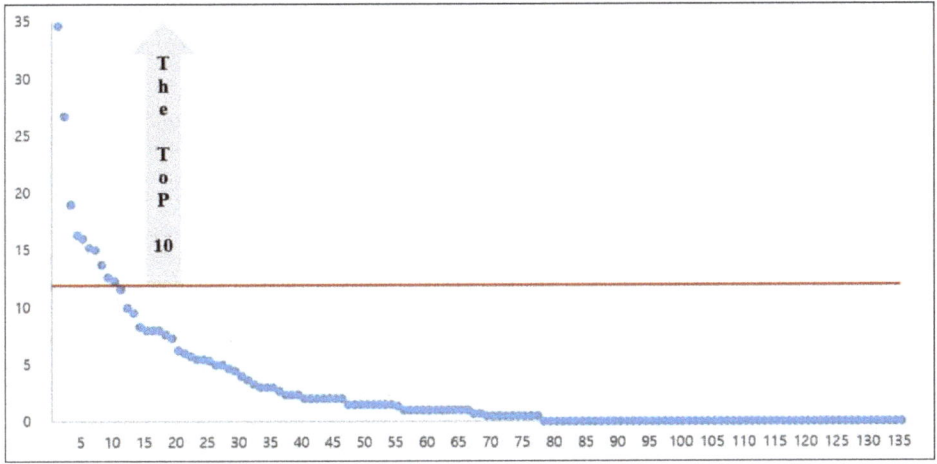

Figure 7. Distribution of the articles by the annual average numbers of citations (note: The blue dots indicate each of the 135 articles; X-axis shows the rank of the 135 articles by the annual average numbers of citations; Y-axis indicates their annual average numbers of citations; The blue dots above the red line are the top ten articles ranked by their annual average numbers of citations).

Table 1. Top ten articles in terms of the annual average numbers of citations.

Rank	Article	Annual Average Numbers of Citations
1	Yue, Wang, Jin, Li, and Jiang [13]	34.6
2	Xia et al. [7]	26.8
3	Esposito, De Santis, Tortora, Chang, and Choo [8]	19.0
4	Guo, Shi, Zhao, & Zheng [5]	16.3
5	Dagher, Mohler, Milojkovic, and Marella [4]	16.0
6	Xia, Sifah, Smahi, Amofa, and Zhang [14]	15.3
7	Dwivedi, Srivastava, Dhar, and Singh [9]	15.0
8	Hussein et al. [15]	13.7
9	Zhang, White, Schmidt, Lenz, and Rosenbloom [16]	12.7
10	Griggs et al. [10]	12.3

3.2. Qualitative Review Results

Our qualitative review identified two major research streams in the contents of the top ten articles as follows. First, the top ten articles overwhelmingly utilized the technological approach among the three approaches according to Leavitt [12], but they paid little attention to the influence of blockchain technology on the people, structure, and task of healthcare organizations in the integrative perspective of Leavitt's diamond model [12]. More specifically, most of the top ten articles focused on developing or suggesting technological solutions with blockchain technology to effectively innovate ways of managing medical data in the healthcare domain. For example, Yue, Wang, Jin, Li, and Jiang [13] developed and suggested a blockchain technology-based app named Healthcare Data Gateway to enable patients to effectively manage their medical data through the use of their smartphones. Xia et al. [7] designed and suggested a medical data sharing system using the blockchain called MedShare to effectively manage shared medical data. Guo, Shi, Zhao, and Zheng [5] proposed a safe attribute-based signature (ABS) scheme to securely protect the privacy of patients' electronic health records with blockchain technology. In line with these studies, the majority of the other studies in Table 1 also adopted the technological approach. However, in the top ten articles, there are few studies that have analyzed the impacts of applying blockchain technology on the people, structure, and task of healthcare organizations under the integrative perspective of Leavitt's diamond model [12].

Second, the convergence of blockchain technology with cloud technology or IoT is revealed to be salient in the contents of the top ten articles. The majority of the top ten articles concerned new ways of managing medical data by integrating blockchain technology with cloud technology or IoT. With regard to the convergence of blockchain technology with cloud technology, Esposito, De Santis, Tortora, Chang, and Choo [8] analyzed the potential pros and cons of using blockchain technology for healthcare data protection in the environment based on cloud technology. Xia, Sifah, Smahi, Amofa, and Zhang [14] suggested a blockchain-based data sharing (BBDS) system for effectively managing electronic medical data in the context of cloud technology. The blockchain cloud composes one of the three layers essential for the Healthcare Data Gateway suggested by Yue, Wang, Jin, Li, and Jiang [13]. The MeDShare suggested by Xia et al. [7] is a system for medical data sharing to control shared data in the medical data repositories with cloud technology. With regard to the convergence of blockchain technology with IoT, Dwivedi, Srivastava, Dhar, and Singh [9] suggested a new blockchain-based system architecture to solve issues of safety and privacy in medical data transfer through IoT healthcare devices for remote patient monitoring. Griggs et al. [10] developed and proposed a healthcare blockchain system for automated real-time patient monitoring through IoT healthcare devices. The contents of more than five of the top ten articles are based on the technology convergence of blockchain technology with cloud technology or IoT.

4. Discussion

Our review results can provide useful implications for future research regarding blockchain technology in the healthcare domain as follows.

First, it is desirable for future studies to pay more attention to the use of the people approach or the structural approach. Our qualitative review results point out that most of the top ten articles adopted the technological approach by concentrating on blockchain-based solutions to current issues in managing medical data without analyzing the impacts of blockchain technology on the people, structure, and task of healthcare organizations in the integrative perspective of Leavitt's diamond model [12]. As emphasized by Leavitt [12], the technology is a major factor that can transform healthcare organizations, but the interrelationships between people, technology, structure, and task can ultimately determine the success of blockchain-based solutions in managing medical data in healthcare organizations. No matter how effective the solutions that blockchain technology may provide to healthcare organizations are, the solutions can hardly succeed without considering the harmony of the blockchain-based solutions with the people, structure, and task of healthcare organizations [12]. Therefore, the scope of the major research streams—which mainly focus on the technological approach—can be widened by illuminating a way to ensure harmony by adopting the people approach or the structural approach in future studies.

Second, it is worthwhile to pay special attention to the technology convergence of blockchain technology with cloud technology or IoT in the contents of the top ten articles, as revealed by this review. The majority of the top ten articles suggested blockchain-based solutions with the convergence of blockchain technology with cloud technology or IoT. Blockchain technology has both strengths and limitations [1], facing potential challenges which must be overcome for successfully managing medical data in the healthcare domain [8]. Therefore, the major research streams in blockchain technology in healthcare can be deepened by illuminating new ways of complementing its limitations with the strengths of other technologies through technology convergence.

Third, there is a high demand for an interdisciplinary approach of future studies on blockchain technology in healthcare. It would be effective for future studies to adopt an interdisciplinary approach, rather than a monodisciplinary approach, to provide innovative ways of managing medical data for healthcare organizations. Various views from multiple experts of not only healthcare but also of IT, human psychology, organizational structure, and task are necessary to more accurately analyze the influences of blockchain technology on the people, structure, and task of healthcare organizations and more effectively create blockchain-based solutions for issues of managing medical data.

5. Conclusions

In the current study, we illuminated the main research streams through a quantitative and qualitative review, providing implications for future research on blockchain technology.

The quantitative review identified five research streams. First, the number of articles about blockchain technology in healthcare has dramatically increased since 2016, with a compound annual growth rate of 254.4%. Second, English is the most dominant language used in the articles. Third, the USA and China are the top two countries of origin of the articles, representing the overwhelming portions. Fourth, the IEEE Access, Journal of Medical Systems, Journal of Medical Internet Research, Applied Sciences Basel, and Sensors are the top five journals in terms of publication. Fifth, the articles showed an L-shaped distribution in terms of their annual average numbers of citations.

The qualitative review revealed two research streams. First, most of the top 10 articles ranked by their annual average numbers of citations concentrated on developing or proposing new technological solutions using blockchain technology to effectively revolutionize the current ways of managing data in the healthcare domain. Second, the majority of the top 10 studies pursued the convergence of blockchain technology with cloud technology or IoT.

This study provides three implications for future research on blockchain technology in healthcare based on the quantitative and qualitative review. First, it is desirable for future studies to pay more attention to the use of the people approach or the structural approach. The scope of the major research streams mainly focusing on the technological approach can be widened by illuminating a way to ensure harmony by adopting the people approach or the structural approach in future studies. Second, it is worthwhile for future studies to pay special attention to the technology convergence of blockchain technology with cloud technology or IoT. The major research streams in blockchain technology in healthcare can be deepened by illuminating new ways of complementing its limitations with the strengths of other technologies through technology convergence. Third, there is a high demand for future studies to adopt an interdisciplinary approach for blockchain technology in healthcare. It would be effective for future studies to adopt an interdisciplinary approach, rather than a monodisciplinary approach, to provide innovative ways of managing medical data for healthcare organizations.

Our review has limitations that must be overcome in future review papers on blockchain technology in healthcare. It would be desirable to review studies on applying blockchain technology to more specific domains of healthcare. It would be valuable to analyze the contents of more than the top ten articles ranked by the annual average numbers of citations.

Author Contributions: Conceptualization, Y.S.H. and M.C.C.; formal analysis, Y.S.H. and M.C.C.; investigation, Y.S.H. and M.C.C.; writing—original draft preparation, Y.S.H. and M.C.C.; writing—review and editing, Y.S.H. and M.C.C. All authors have read and agreed to the published version of the manuscript.

Funding: This work was supported by the 2019 Yeungnam University Research Grant. The present study was supported by a National Research Foundation of Korea grant that was funded by the Korean Government (grant no. NRF-2019M3E5D1A02069399).

Institutional Review Board Statement: Not applicable.

Informed Consent Statement: Not applicable.

Data Availability Statement: The data presented in this study are available on request from the corresponding author.

Conflicts of Interest: The authors declare no conflict of interest.

Appendix A

Table A1. Distribution of articles by country of origin.

Rank	Country	Frequency	Portion (%)
1	USA	41	30.4
2	China	40	29.6
3	England	11	8.1
3	South Korea	11	8.1
5	India	10	7.4
6	Saudi Arabia	8	5.9
7	Australia	6	4.4
7	Canada	6	4.4
7	Spain	6	4.4
10	Japan	5	3.7
10	Malaysia	5	3.7
10	Taiwan	5	3.7
13	Pakistan	4	3.0
14	Brazil	3	2.2
14	Germany	3	2.2
14	Iraq	3	2.2

Table A1. Cont.

Rank	Country	Frequency	Portion (%)
14	Italy	3	2.2
14	Norway	3	2.2
19	France	2	1.5
19	Greece	2	1.5
19	Netherlands	2	1.5
19	New Zealand	2	1.5
19	Poland	2	1.5
19	Portugal	2	1.5
19	United Arab Emirates	2	1.5
26	Austria	1	0.7
26	Bangladesh	1	0.7
26	Belgium	1	0.7
26	Bulgaria	1	0.7
26	Colombia	1	0.7
26	Croatia	1	0.7
26	Denmark	1	0.7
26	Ecuador	1	0.7
26	Jordan	1	0.7
26	Libya	1	0.7
26	North Ireland	1	0.7
26	Palestine	1	0.7
26	Philippines	1	0.7
26	Qatar	1	0.7
26	Scotland	1	0.7
26	Thailand	1	0.7
26	Wales	1	0.7

Appendix B

Table 2. Distribution of articles in journal.

Rank	Journal	Frequency	Portion (%)
1	IEEE Access	23	17.0
2	Journal of Medical Systems	16	11.9
3	Journal of Medical Internet Research	14	10.4
4	Applied Sciences Basel	5	3.7
4	Sensors	5	3.7
6	Computational and Structural Biotechnology Journal	3	2.2
6	Electronics	3	2.2
6	Future Generation Computer Systems The International Journal of Escience	3	2.2
6	Wireless Communications Mobile Computing	3	2.2
10	Healthcare Informatics Research	2	1.5
10	Information	2	1.5
10	International Journal of Advanced Computer Science and Applications	2	1.5
10	International Journal of Distributed Sensor Networks	2	1.5
10	Internet Technology Letters	2	1.5
10	Journal of Digital Imaging	2	1.5
10	Journal of The American Medical Informatics Association	2	1.5
10	Pneumologe	2	1.5

Table 2. *Cont.*

Rank	Journal	Frequency	Portion (%)
18	3c Tecnologia	1	0.7
18	Academic Medicine	1	0.7
18	Applied Health Economics and Health Policy	1	0.7
18	Australasian Journal of Information Systems	1	0.7
18	Big Data Society	1	0.7
18	Bmc Medicine	1	0.7
18	Bmj Global Health	1	0.7
18	Business Process Management Journal	1	0.7
18	Clinics in Dermatology	1	0.7
18	Cognitive Systems Research	1	0.7
18	Computers	1	0.7
18	Concurrency and Computation Practice Experience	1	0.7
18	Cryptologia	1	0.7
18	Future Internet	1	0.7
18	Health Informatics Journal	1	0.7
18	IBM Journal of Research and Development	1	0.7
18	IEEE Cloud Computing	1	0.7
18	IEEE Consumer Electronics Magazine	1	0.7
18	IEEE Internet of Things Journal	1	0.7
18	IEEE Network	1	0.7
18	IEEE Transactions on Computational Social Systems	1	0.7
18	Industrial Management Data Systems	1	0.7
18	Information Sciences	1	0.7
18	International Journal of Cardiology	1	0.7
18	International Journal of Engineering Business Management	1	0.7
18	International Journal of Environmental Research and Public Health	1	0.7
18	International Journal of Healthcare Information Systems and Informatics	1	0.7
18	International Journal of Healthcare Management	1	0.7
18	International journal of Networked and Distributed Computing	1	0.7
18	JMIR Mhealth and Uhealth	1	0.7
18	JMIR Research Protocols	1	0.7
18	Journal of Biomedical Informatics	1	0.7
18	Journal of Information Assurance and Security	1	0.7
18	Journal of Information Processing Systems	1	0.7
18	Journal of Information Security and Applications	1	0.7
18	Journal of the American College of Radiology	1	0.7
18	Nature Communications	1	0.7
18	Neural Computing Applications	1	0.7
18	Parkinsonism Related Disorders	1	0.7
18	Procesamiento Del Lenguaje Natural	1	0.7
18	Security and Communication Networks	1	0.7
18	Sustainable Cities and Society	1	0.7
18	Technology Innovation Management Review	1	0.7
18	Unfallchirurg	1	0.7

References

1. Bashir, I. *Mastering Blockchain*; Packt: Birmingham, UK, 2017.
2. Agbo, C.C.; Mahmoud, Q.H.; Eklund, J.M. Blockchain technology in healthcare: A systematic review. *Healthcare* **2019**, *7*, 56. [CrossRef] [PubMed]
3. Khezr, S.; Moniruzzaman, M.; Yassine, A.; Benlamri, R. Blockchain technology in healthcare: A comprehensive review and directions for future research. *Appl. Sci.* **2019**, *9*, 1736. [CrossRef]
4. Dagher, G.G.; Mohler, J.; Milojkovic, M.; Marella, P.B. Ancile: Privacy-Preserving framework for access control and interoperability of electronic health records using blockchain technology. *Sustain. Cities Soc.* **2018**, *39*, 283–297. [CrossRef]
5. Guo, R.; Shi, H.; Zhao, Q.; Zheng, D. Secure attribute-based signature scheme with multiple authorities for blockchain in electronic health records systems. *IEEE Access* **2018**, *6*, 11676–11686. [CrossRef]
6. Hau, Y.S.; Lee, J.M.; Park, J.; Chang, M.C. Attitudes toward blockchain technology in managing medical information: Survey study. *J. Med. Internet Res.* **2019**, *21*, e15870. [CrossRef]
7. Xia, Q.; Sifah, E.B.; Asamoah, K.O.; Gao, J.; Du, X.; Guizani, M. MeDShare: Trust-Less medical data sharing among cloud service providers via blockchain. *IEEE Access* **2017**, *5*, 14757–14767. [CrossRef]
8. Esposito, C.; De Santis, A.; Tortora, G.; Chang, H.; Choo, K.R. Blockchain: A panacea for healthcare cloud-based data security and privacy? *IEEE Cloud Comput.* **2018**, *5*, 31–37. [CrossRef]
9. Dwivedi, A.D.; Srivastava, G.; Dhar, S.; Singh, R. A decentralized privacy-preserving healthcare blockchain for IoT. *Sensors* **2019**, *19*, 326. [CrossRef] [PubMed]
10. Griggs, K.N.; Ossipova, O.; Kohlios, C.P.; Baccarini, A.N.; Howson, E.A.; Hayajneh, T. Healthcare blockchain system using smart contracts for secure automated remote patient monitoring. *J. Med. Syst.* **2018**, *42*, 130. [CrossRef] [PubMed]
11. Dhagarra, D.; Goswami, M.; Sarma, P.R.S.; Choudhury, A. Big Data and blockchain supported conceptual model for enhanced healthcare coverage The Indian context. *Bus. Process Manag. J.* **2019**, *25*, 1612–1632.
12. Leavitt, H.J. Applied organizational change in industry: Structural, technological and humanistic approaches. In *Handbook of Organizations*, 1st ed.; (Reprinted from the first version published in 1965 by Rand McNally & Company); March, J.G., Ed.; Routledge: London, UK; New York, NY, USA, 2013; pp. 1144–1170.
13. Yue, X.; Wang, H.; Jin, D.; Li, M.; Jiang, W. Healthcare data gateways: Found healthcare intelligence on blockchain with novel privacy risk control. *J. Med. Syst.* **2016**, *40*, 218. [CrossRef] [PubMed]
14. Xia, Q.; Sifah, E.B.; Smahi, A.; Amofa, S.; Zhang, X. BBDS: Blockchain-Based data sharing for electronic medical records in cloud environments. *Information* **2017**, *8*, 44. [CrossRef]
15. Hussein, A.F.; ArunKumar, N.; Ramirez-Gonzalez, G.; Abdulhay, E.; Tavares, J.M.R.S.; de Albuquerque, V.H.C. A medical records managing and securing blockchain based system supported by a Genetic Algorithm and Discrete Wavelet Transform. *Cogn. Syst. Res.* **2018**, *52*, 1–11. [CrossRef]
16. Zhang, P.; White, J.; Schmidt, D.C.; Lenz, G.; Rosenbloom, S.T. FHIRChain: Applying blockchain to securely and scalably share clinical data. *Comp. Struct. Biotechnol. J.* **2018**, *16*, 267–278. [CrossRef] [PubMed]

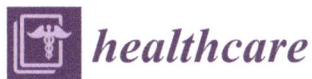

Article

A Blockchain-Based Secret-Data Sharing Framework for Personal Health Records in Emergency Condition

Ahmed Raza Rajput [1,*], Qianmu Li [1,2,*] and Milad Taleby Ahvanooey [3]

1. School of Computer Science and Engineering, Nanjing University of Science and Technology, Nanjing 210094, China
2. School of Cyber Science and Engineering, Nanjing University of Science and Technology, Nanjing 210094, China
3. School of Information Management, Nanjing University, Nanjing 210023, China; M.Taleby@nju.edu.cn
* Correspondence: Ahmedrajput@njust.edu.cn (A.R.R.); Qianmu@njust.edu.cn (Q.L.); Tel.: +86-139-5164-0290 (A.R.R.); +86-025-8431-5732 (Q.L.)

Citation: Rajput, A.R.; Li, Q.; Ahvanooey, M.T. A Blockchain-Based Secret-Data Sharing Framework for Personal Health Records in Emergency Condition. *Healthcare* **2021**, *9*, 206. https://doi.org/10.3390/healthcare9020206

Academic Editors: Tin-Chih Chen and Daniele Giansanti

Received: 31 December 2020
Accepted: 10 February 2021
Published: 14 February 2021

Publisher's Note: MDPI stays neutral with regard to jurisdictional claims in published maps and institutional affiliations.

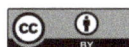

Copyright: © 2021 by the authors. Licensee MDPI, Basel, Switzerland. This article is an open access article distributed under the terms and conditions of the Creative Commons Attribution (CC BY) license (https://creativecommons.org/licenses/by/4.0/).

Abstract: Blockchain technology is the most trusted all-in-one cryptosystem that provides a framework for securing transactions over networks due to its irreversibility and immutability characteristics. Blockchain network, as a decentralized infrastructure, has drawn the attention of various startups, administrators, and developers. This system preserves transactions from tampering and provides a tracking tool for tracing past network operations. A personal health record (PHR) system permits patients to control and share data concerning their health conditions by particular peoples. In the case of an emergency, the patient is unable to approve the emergency staff access to the PHR. Furthermore, a history record management system of the patient's PHR is required, which exhibits hugely private personal data (e.g., modification date, name of user, last health condition, etc.). In this paper, we suggest a healthcare management framework that employs blockchain technology to provide a tamper protection application by considering safe policies. These policies involve identifying extensible access control, auditing, and tamper resistance in an emergency scenario. Our experiments demonstrated that the proposed framework affords superior performance compared to the state-of-the-art healthcare systems concerning accessibility, privacy, emergency access control, and data auditing.

Keywords: personal health record; emergency access; access control; blockchain; hyperledger fabric; hyperledger composer; auditability; privacy & security

1. Introduction

The Healthcare management system has traditionally been involved with information exchange between patients, business entities such as different hospital systems, pharmaceutical companies, etc. Nevertheless, there has been recent attention towards patient-driven personal health record (PHR), in which health information exchange is patient-mediated. In general, the PHR interoperability involves new requirements and challenges concerning technology, incentives, security and privacy, and governance which should be solved for data sharing issues. Technically, the use of blockchain technology in healthcare management system can provide five mechanisms including: (i) patient identity, (ii) data aggregation, (iii) data liquidity, (iv) digital access rules, and (v) data immutability, which might address such challenges [1–3]. However, several management systems exist for healthcare, which controls PHR, incredibly delicate data such as PHR entities [1–3]. An ever-increasing selection of medical data estimates actions such as creation, creating, exchanging, and modifying information objects, creating difficulties in tracing malicious activities and security breaches. A PHR is a mechanism for digitally storing a patient's health data. It needs to allow appropriate access control for manage, track, and restrict their health data [4]. The PHR contains comprehensive health information related to a particular patient like visit dates, prescription drug plans, allergy reports, immunization records, lab results, and so on [5]. Healthcare data sharing is crucial to perform an adequate cooperative manner and care options for patients. In an emergency, the staff requires some essential elementary and relevant health data concerning the patient to enhance the possibility of saving his/her life in sympathetic situations [6]. Some distinct access control policies become limited because no specific policy would admit an emergency staff to obtain the patients' records. Misuse of the PHR accessing in the emergency is one of the remaining issues in security and privacy [7,8]. In the traditional PHR emergency circumstances, the state-of-the-art frameworks did not confirm the entity's credentials, unless a single person or group posted a request for the PHR. During the conventional emergency access of the PHR practice, while the Emergency Team (EMT) do actions on the medical records, the malicious users can capture the patient's health information [9,10]. Most importantly, in the traditional system, it is needed an auditing trail or activity tracking system where the patient can assign some permissions for accessing the PHR. Because when the patient is in an emergency, he/she cannot engage in the access permission approval [11,12]. In the following, we briefly summarized the research objectives of our study.

I. Where a traditional emergency system is used to manage the PHRs, it lacks a sufficient control policy tool to limit the access permissions of any third-party person (e.g., doctor/intruder). Therefore, we address this problem by considering security policies using smart contracts which can limit the access permissions to PHRs in an emergency condition.

II. Since there is a lack of tracking PHRs in traditional emergency systems, we utilized the audit trails in blockchain technology to provide a tracking option that patients can monitor the history of activities to their records.

III. In the traditional emergency system, the PHR access permission should be inquired from one or a number of trustworthy individuals (e.g., family members/friends), where an emergency condition occurs, i.e., it takes much time for contacting such persons. Hence, we solve this issue by defining security policies that a patient can assign which type of users (e.g., family doctor) can access the PHR without requiring any inquiry from other persons.

To address such obstacles and ensure the reliability of PHR, we propose a novel management system based on a blockchain network [13,14] that leverages the shared and changeless distributed ledger. Blockchain is a technology to achieve a valid, challenging to tamper ledger over shared servers. Because of the blockchain network-based system's capability, when the transaction is endorsed, then the transaction is arduous to alter validly. It utilizes several consensus algorithms to reach approval on the new event for the blockchain. In general, blockchain considers the security as mentioned earlier policies to ensure the reliability of generated records, containing events, termed as blocks. Besides, it empowers authoritative participant's entry and access control and needs to support accountability. Auditing is the significant property of the blockchain. When the transaction is performed, the current block records the transaction with a timestamp, and the participant of the system trails the previous event actions. It records a history of all transactions. This strategy is beneficial for individual persons or medical organizations that require to obtain tamper-proof account records.

Our system uses the Hyperledger composer [15] based blockchain, which could provide an efficient tool for solving malicious access to the PHR, i.e., This is an extensible and scalable data storage in the off-chain and a person-centered mobile and web edge. In this framework, the blockchain is employed to maintain non-repudiation, accountability, and tamper-proof attributes [16]. The delegate re-encryption method is applied to recommend an access control tool that can help granular access authority. The proposed system utilizes the smart contracts [17,18], which allows the owner of the PHR to assign the rules for an EMT or staff member (certified physician) who can obtain permission to access the current information from the PHR by considering the time restriction. In the normal condition, the patient and their family physician can undoubtedly enter the system through a web browser and mobile interface in an application-based hyperledger composer.

The rest of the article is arranged as follows. Section 2 briefly describes the blockchain Network, Hyperledger Fabric, and Composer. Section 3 explains related works. Section 4 introduces the architecture of our proposed framework. In Section 5, we experiment with the proposed framework by implementing it using the JavaScript Object Notation (JSON) in the Eclipse platform. In Section 6, we discuss our experiments by considering various types of attacks and exhibiting the performance analysis. Finally, Section 7 concludes the remarks of our contributions.

2. Blockchain Network

Blockchain is a decentralized distributed technology (DDT) [16]. In blockchain, a collection of records that close share or transfer of value and digital assets such as transactions, goods, and services, is designed and managed by a distributed system of computing nodes in the peer-to-peer network. Blockchain is originated from the bitcoin, a technology that is a distributed database and with the continuously growing records regarded as a block, and these records cannot be changed or altered [19]. The main idea of blockchain is to stabilize the integrity, traceability, and accountability of shared data. Distributed Ledger constrains methods including preservation and authentication, which are executed in a network of interacting nodes. These nodes implement and audit software that harmonizes the shared Ledger images between a peer-to-peer network of shareholders, presenting all accountable activities via digital fingerprints or hash codes. Ledger is classified as pervasive and determined in data recording. In the blockchain, each node member has its shared ledger. It generates a transparent, immutable record [20]. A blockchain logs present accuracy for communication acceptance over the health IT environment and audit logs for following inquiries into such permissions and access models' performance. Based on this functionality, the framework works as a consistent description of authorization to access the electronic health information (EHI). Over the last decade, the researchers have introduced several healthcare management systems based on blockchain for assuring various security purposes [21,22]. Blockchain guarantees that data was not tampered with by malicious attacks and verified multiple data provenance aspects [23]. This technology involves cryptographic techniques, and the blockchain network's distributed environment ensures all information distribution, which affords the visible, trustworthy digital fingerprint and auditable paths [24].

There are two primary kinds of blockchain, Permissionless and Permissioned Blockchain. A public blockchain is also called Permissionless Blockchain. The first invention of the permissionless blockchain is Bitcoin. A permissionless blockchain is easily accessible and open for reading and writing actions by all participants on the system [25]. It implies that everybody can participate in the system with pseudonymous identification. The user could also read the information or broadcast them and is identified as a part of the consensus mechanism [26,27]. Ethereum also applies a permissionless Blockchain, and anyone can evolve and combine smart contracts over the network, with no limitation forced by the developers. A permissioned blockchain is also called private blockchain. An individual organization performs a permissioned blockchain [28]. Unlike permissionless blockchain, the permissioned blockchain is designed where participants in the network are predefined for read/write actions and forever identify within the system. So, the main difference between permissionless and permissioned blockchain is how a user can have access to the network. In the permissioned blockchain network, implement Byzantine Fault Tolerance (BFT) [29]. The Hyperledger Fabric is sketched for providing the safety of shared ledger technology and empower permissioned.

2.1. Hyperledger Fabric

The Hyperledger Fabric is a type of permissioned blockchain technology that works based on an open-source blockchain enterprise entertained by the Linux Foundation [30]. Hyperledger is a constantly prevalent, collective permissioned or private blockchain that attempts at improving blockchain technology through industry applications. Generally,

Hyperledger Fabric is a distributed network formulating a peer-to-peer system where every peer has a replicated, consistent copy of the blockchain data structure, particularly a chained index of transaction describing invocation and executions of chain codes. Hyperledger Fabric gives the chance to increase the application range of blockchain technology beyond cryptocurrency trades which distinct various relational database application domains, comprising the management of healthcare information [31].

2.2. Hyperledger Composer

The Linux Foundation entertained Hyperledger Fabric projects which the Hyperledger Composer is one of such examples. The business network archive (BNA) is the functional production of Hyperledger Composer, which is inherited from the blockchain Hyperledger Fabric [15].

The business network comprises participants, and they are combined through their identifications, as well as, assets that generate on the system; transactions define the exchange of assets. These rules involve executing the transactions called smart contracts, and eventually, all the transactions are saved in the ledger. Figure 1 illustrates the general architecture of Hyperledger Composer. The model file contains three main components: participants, assets, and transactions. The participants are the end-users of the system and can deal with the assets and communicate with other ones by transactions. Assets are usually the variables saved in the network. Transactions are the purposes of the system and are invoked to bring up-to-date the setup. The Script file in the business network determines multiple transaction functions in the system. It is composed of the Java Script (JS) and deals with the business logic, containing which standards of users act and which types of assets are shared. The access control list (ACL) outlines the distinct ranges of participants' access own in the network. In the ACL file, the participants' goal is fixed, determining their performance in creating, reading, updating, or deleting the assets. The Query file explains the composition and employment of queries from the system. These remain fixed to extrapolate transactions of the historian, which all of the previous transactions' records in the network. The Historian record is a registry list fed by the historian record that includes the history of transactions and events performed on the system. While the transaction is processed, the historian record is updated, saving a history of all transactions within a business network. The participants with their identities are involved in submitting the transactions, and historian record assets can be retrieved utilizing composer queries to require particular records.

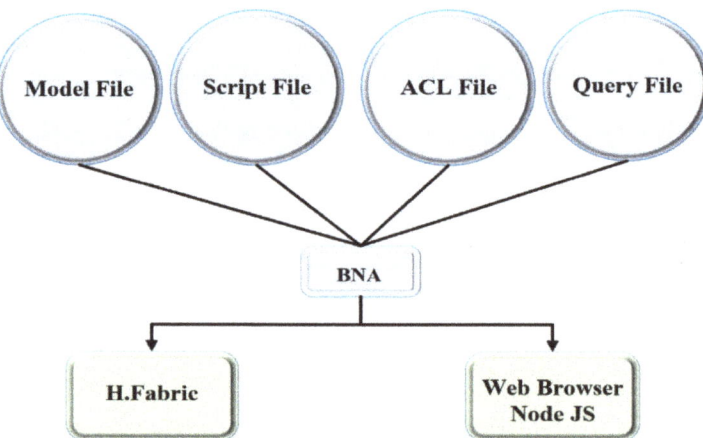

Figure 1. A global architecture for hyperledger composer.

3. Related Works

In this section, we summarize the state-of-the-art healthcare management systems by considering their merits and limitations. Table 1 also shows the merits and limitations of the existing methods.

Guy Zyskind et al. [32] presented the Enigma privacy platform based on blockchain to manage access control and auditing log, privacy, and security objectives, such as a tampered proof record of transactions. Enigma utilizes a multi-party computational model and guarantees data privacy by employing a verifiable secret sharing mechanism. In this platform, researchers claimed that Enigma eliminates the necessity to provide a trusted third-party platform, enabling personal data control anonymously.

Table 1. Existing blockchain healthcare systems.

Blockchain Systems	Health Data	Merits	Limitations
Xia et al. [33]	Electronic Medical Record	To adequately pursue the execution of the information and revoke access to offending nodes on the exposure of breach of permissions on information.	Participants' transactions are intended to support various, but limited events for user transaction instances not considered for.
Xiao et al. [34]	Healthcare data	Affords anonymization, productive interaction among HDGs, and data reinforcement and improvement utilizing cloud.	It is inadequate to process information and executes computations without exposing information.
Azaria et al. [35]	Electronic Medical Record	Provides reliable access, perpetual log, and complete services. It also eludes a single point of failure	Does not recognize contract encryption, obfuscation, scalability, and auditability. The scheme demands to be extended for complicated situations concerning healthcare data.
Ichikawa et al. [36]	Electronic Medical Record	Hardy against network faults such as assigned node down.	Vulnerable to attack.
Xia et al. et al. [37]	Medical data	Ensures data provenance, security, and user verification. It provides remote access and data access revocation.	Omitted data revealing concerns.
Hussein et al. [38]	Electronic Medical Record	Enhances overall security and access control, allows fast verification process, and further accountability.	This would support expand system devices and enhance security.
Dagher et al. [39]	Electronic Health Record	Concentrates on protecting patient's security and privacy utilizing cryptographic techniques and allows access control.	Absorbs computational energy due to a large number of applied smart contracts.
Chen et al. [40]	Personal Medical Data	Patients control their personal medical data.	Interoperability is not examined across various healthcare companies.
Zhang et al. [41]	Personal Health Information	Protected records of PHI are traced employing the consortium blockchain, while the private blockchain reserves the PHI.	The data location might be modified so the old URL cannot be altered, and a novel URL needs to be created.

Xia et al. [33] presented a framework using the blockchain for protecting data privacy. In this work, the authors suggested a permissioned blockchain system that permits access to data requests by affording knowledge to the information stored in the cloud repository. They employed the data grantors, which authorize the aggregation and review of information, leading to value derivation. Their experimental analysis demonstrated that the system is lightweight, dynamic, and scalable.

A decentralized risk-control system based on blockchain called healthcare data gateways (HDG) system, presented by Xiao Yue et al. [34]. In this system, the patient can own, manage, and distribute his data securely without involving complicated actions, which presents a different latent approach to develop healthcare systems' ability while preserving patient data confidentiality. From HDG results, it can be concluded that this system is trustable and auditable due to utilizing a decentralized network of peers accomplished by a public ledger.

Azaria et al. [35] developed a medical record sharing prototype called MedRec, the first and only model proposed utilizing some smart contracts to assign appropriate permissions for confidential data sharing. They considered various metadata domains in a single record that distributes individually and may comprise additional limitations such as termination time for data viewership. MedRec provides record versatility and fine-grained, which facilitates patient data sharing and motivations for health data reviewers to maintain the network. In this work, the researchers employed the ledger to maintain an auditable record of medical interactions for patients, healthcare providers, and researchers.

Ichikawa et al. [36] proposed a tamper-resistant mHealth system based on blockchain technology, which provides auditable computing and trustable policies. In this system, they suggested a mHealth network system for cognitive-behavioral medicine in the somnolence ("sleepiness") disease by developing a smartphone app. Furthermore, they collected the Electronic Medical Records (EMR) from the patients voluntarily via the app saved in JSON format, which was successfully transferred to a permissioned blockchain network called Hyperledger Fabric. Next, the authors analyzed the tamper resistance of the EMRs generated by artificial flaws. Merging blockchain Hyperledger Fabric with mHealth may present an innovative clarification that empowers approachability and data clarity without engaging a third-party.

Xia et al. [37] proposed a new blockchain-based scheme for the trust-less medical data sharing called MeDShare, which protects data records between big-data servers in a trust-less location. In the MeDShare, they utilize a strategy to perform all the events and transmit them into a permanent system, ensuring trust-less and regular auditing policies. Moreover, the authors employed smart contracts and access control policies to efficiently trace the data sharing behavior and prevent access to violated permissions and rules on data.

A data-sharing scheme based on blockchain has been introduced by Hussein [38] for addressing the problems of access control with the blockchain, such as autonomy properties and immutability. In this study, the authors utilized a Discrete Wavelet Transform (DWT) and a genetic algorithm for optimizing the queuing optimization technique. Therefore, it generates a cryptography key for affording access control and immunity, allowing authenticating users in the speedy action.

Dagher et al. [39] introduced a blockchain-based model for providing dynamic, interoperable, and secure access to medical records while protecting patients' sensitive information. In this system, researchers employed the Ethereum blockchain by defining smart contracts for affording access control and obfuscation of data and applied the cryptographic methods for extra security.

Chen et al. [40] designed a storage system to maintain blockchain-based personal medical data and cloud storage. They employ blockchain as a storage supply chain in which all operations are verified, immutable, and accountable. This system defined the permissions of three types of transactions and composed the block formation and the medical blockchain's primary function. Furthermore, they introduced a service framework for sharing medical records, which protects medical data management applications without violating privacy policies.

Zhang et al. [41] proposed a secure and privacy-preserving personal health information sharing protocol for diagnosis improvements in the e-Health system based on Blockchain. Moreover, they described the blockchain consensus mechanism, which is the proof of conformance and devised to build validated blocks. Moreover, researchers employed public-key encryption using the keyword search based on the blockchain. A doctor allows to search and access the expected history of health records to enhance the diagnosis after receiving trapdoors from the patient. Besides, they claimed that this eHealth system achieves security, privacy preservation, and a secure search of medical data.

The above state-of-the-art studies are based on blockchain sharing the health record and access control policies. Still, they do not access PHR in an emergency condition. We used a Hyperledger Composer and Fabric for securing the data privacy and auditing trial in emergency access for PHR.

4. System Architecture

In this section, we present the proposed emergency access control management system, which utilizes blockchain technology for preserving PHR data privacy. All the data on the blockchain network are shared between the nodes. We develop a system that generates a time-stamped log for all the transactions on the network without engaging a PHR owner or any third party utilizing the Hyperledger Composer-SDK and NodeJS. Moreover, we demonstrate the proposed architecture in Figure 2, which facilitates access control scenario of PHR data by using Hyperledger composer blockchain in an emergency. We first specify the following entities, which involve the process of construction. All the activities are controlled with permissions and the smart contracts that affect data retrieval from the Ledger. In this situation, the patient's permissions can allow the EMT access to the PHR data. The assumed entities are as follows.

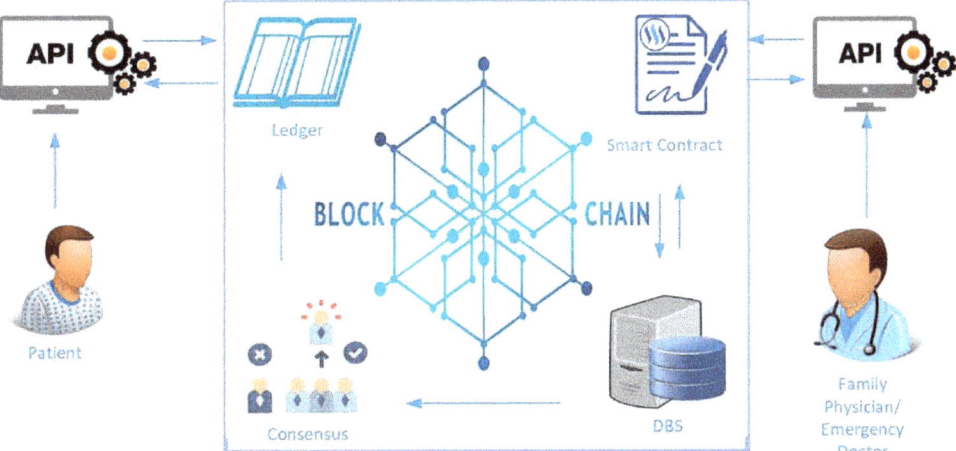

Figure 2. Proposed framework for personal health record (PHR) access control in Emergency.

- Patient is a participant who is the owner of the PHR data. A patient defines the access control policies for the PHR data.
- Doctor is a participant, who can log into the system if the patient has granted the permission to him. The PHR owner has to define the policy of access control permission in a smart contract as a family doctor or primary physician.
- Emergency Doctor is a participant who requests emergency access permission while the patient is in an emergency. The proposed framework utilizes an API for granting access according to patients' rules to the emergency doctor whether he is allowed to access the PHR data or not.
- Rest API, Composer Rest Server creates an Application Programming Interface (API) from the blockchain network that can be efficiently employed by Hypertext Transfer Protocol (HTTP) client for evaluating the permissions.
- Smart Contracts are some transaction protocols that automatically perform, control, and register relevant actions and events according to an agreement's rules [42]. These are executed on blockchain and administered by a system of peers. They also spontaneously run when specific predefined policies are met. In such a case, the data owner (patient) specifies the access permission in smart contracts.

- Consensus is a mechanism that provides the following core functions in our framework for approving the transaction verifying the patient's policies. When the transaction is completed, the Consensus accepts the performance and upgrades the main shared ledger to achieve consistent outcomes.
- Ledger is an outcome, tamper confidential records for all the transactions. Transactions are consequences of the smart contracts or requests transmitted from users. Each transaction's completion is a k-v pair bounded to the state as creates, updates, or delete.

5. System Implementation

In this section, we implement the proposed model using Hyperledger Fabric and Hyperledger Composer. During our experiments, we suppose that the user (client) information is retrieved from the JSON, and requested information by utilizing the Rest Client, i.e., Postman server. Every server was formed in the virtual environment Elastic Compute Cloud (EC2) instance on Amazon Web Server (AWS), which operates in the same local personal computer with Ubuntu Linux 18.04.1, single vCPU @ 2.00 GHz, and 32 GB RAM as the details of configuration summarized in Table 2. We employed the Hyperledger composer playground to develop the Business Network Definition. We used Hyperledger Fabric (version 1.2) an open-source project hosted by the Linux foundation. Moreover, we utilized Docker (version 1.12.1), Oracle Virtual Box (version 5.1.22), and Docker compose (version 1.5.2) to set up Docker execution environment. In our framework, ledger's state is the key-value store database that stores the transaction logs.

Table 2. Implementation Development Environment.

Component	Description
CPU	Single vCPU @ 2.00 GHz
Operating System	Ubuntu Linux 18.04.1 LTS
Memory	32 GB
Hyperledger Fabric	Version 1.2
Docker	Version 1.12.1
Oracle Virtual Box	Version 5.1.22
Docker-Compose	Version 1.5.2

Our proposed architecture involves three elements: a patient-centric user interface, a permissioned blockchain, and off-chain storage. Furthermore, we utilized the Hyperledger Composer to build the Business Network Archive (BNA), which defines the network's properties and abilities. Hyperledger Composer is further used to archive the business network upon the Hyperledger Fabric instance.

This structure includes three main files: Model, Script, and permission (see Figure 1). The model contains three main elements; (i) participants are the actors that can participate in the network (patient, family physician, and emergency doctor), (ii) assets are the data items of the patient's PHR and some necessary personal information, i.e., they are stored in the variables as regular variables, and (iii) the transactions of participants on the assets through the network. The Script is called "logic.js" which describes several transactions that happened on the system. It maintains the confirmation and validation of the participants, assets, and transactions by considering various system access levels. Moreover, the "permission.acl" contains access control policies in which participants' rules are defined, i.e., the participant can use the patient's data in a particular situation (see Table 3). The patient explains the rules for accessing the family physician to PHR information while the patient is in a normal condition. For the emergency condition, the patient also describes the procedure of how an emergency doctor can access using the certified license number. Emergency doctor triggers the smart contracts and receives PHR items with the "emergency access time constraints" function. When the time limit is completed for allowing which emergency doctor could not have access to the system, another essential aspect of Hyperledger Composer is a query file that expresses the formations and policies. Queries are established to generalize activities or actions from the historian, where all the previous records are available through the PHR in the Ledger.

Table 3. The defined access control policies in the "permission.acl" file.

Permission Rules for Limiting Access to the PHRs
1. rule OwnerHasFullAccessToTheirTreatmentDrugAssets
2. {
3. description: "Allow all participants full access to their assets"
4. participant(p): "org.example.basic.Patient"
5. operation: ALL
6. resource(r): "org.example.basic.TreatmentDrugs"
7. condition: (r.owner.getIdentifier() === p.getIdentifier())
8. action: ALLOW
9. }
10. rule emergencydoctorHassAccessToPatientLabTest {
11. description: "Allow all participants full access to their assets"
12. participant(g): "org.example.basic.EmergencyDoctor"
13. operation: READ
14. resource(r): "org.example.basic.LabTest"
15. condition: (r.emergencyAcces===true)
16. action: ALLOW
17. }
18. rule emergencydoctorHassAccessToPatientTreatmentDrugs {
19. description: "Allow all participants full access to their assets"
20. participant(g): "org.example.basic.EmergencyDoctor"
21. operation: READ
22. resource(r): "org.example.basic.TreatmentDrugs"
23. condition: (r.emergencyAcces===true)
24. action: ALLOW
25. }

As depicted in Figure 3, after defining the participant cards in the "My Business Networks" section, we executed the BNA on the Hyperledger Composer. In this case, each network card is utilized to join the system, and identify the kind of participant. These cards regularly have a further organized range of permissions in the network. However, the patient could also complete high-clearance functions (adding or deleting) for participants such as family physician and emergency doctor. This kind of cards determines the node that correlates the identifications to the network and permits to authorize participants.

In our system, new users (family physician and Emergency doctor) with proper identification information can join as a participant at different times. To accomplish an appropriate position, admin manages the participants' permissions using an alignment of Hyperledger Composer consortium. During the access control management, the characteristics or duties are performed, which kind of transactions specified in "permissions.acl" file. In our proposed framework, the assets are the PHR items such as personal data, test results, and prescribed medicine, etc., which already are stored in the assets registry. In our policies, it is assumed that the transactions are the enrollment processes for the participants and procedures for PHR data item like, "getpatientlabtest" and "getpatienttreatmentdrugs". Besides, each particular record and its details of the PHR data will be shown on the network. There are four services in this network, including three registration procedures (for the patient, family physician, and emergency doctor), and one function for getting patient's data from the system. Participants can utilize these functions as a transaction trigger to access relevant data. Each participant's role depends on the conditions that are predefined by the data owner in the "permission.acl" file.

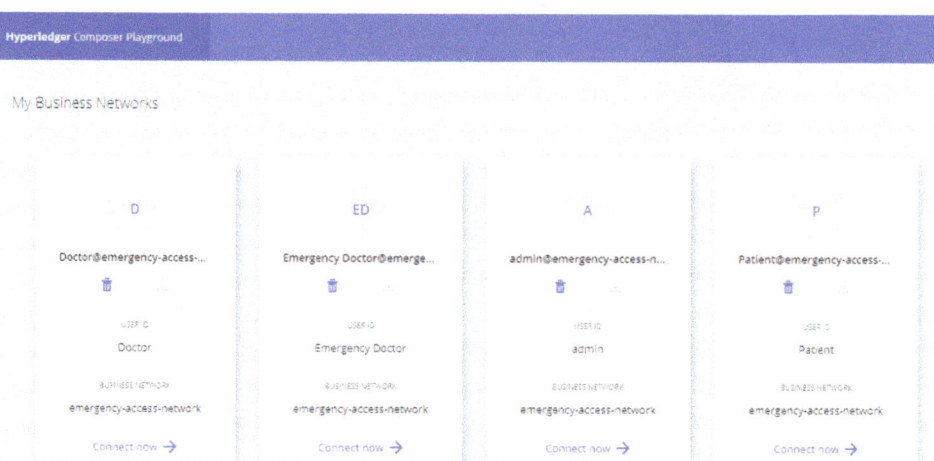

Figure 3. Defined network cards for participants in the hyperledger composer playground.

- Participants Registration: Script file comprises the blockchain transaction processing function (TPF) which is triggered and participant (patient) input parameters consist of the *Card_Id, First_name, Last_name, Address, Patient_Id, Emergency_Access_Time_Costraints*. In the case that the participant is a family doctor, the input parameters include: *Doctor_Id, First_name, Last_name,* and for the emergency doctor input parameters consist of the *Emerency_doctor_id*, and *License_number* only in an emergency situation and requests access permission by using API to the network. When the participant triggers the function from API, then the node server will explore its endpoint matching scheme in the file "app.js". After considering all the parameters of the Transaction Processing Function (TPF) which are already saved in the file "network.js". All TPFs can employ the Hyperledger Composer NodeSDK functions for the registration of patient in the network as a participant. Later, it generates an ID card for the participant and saves it in the ID registry. Query 2 expresses the process of retrieving the PHR records from our system in detail.

- Get Patient Data: This file includes the TPF, which is triggered and obtained from the patient's PHR data, and the emergency doctor input parameters consisting of *Patient_Id* (e.g., current *emergency_doctor_Id* for an emergency condition). When the participant hits the trigger from the *client_side* function named "network.getpatientdata", which is described in the file "app.js.", later, our proposed system considers the mandatory fields of the process body for requesting access permission. Then, it will send certain documents to TPFs "networkgetpatientdata," which is explained in the "network.js" file and is exchanged the data according to prescribed rules. The TPF is again utilized the Hyperledger Composer NodeSDK; first, this verifies whether the participant has permission to access the patient's information and thus delivers PHR data. The smart contracts restrict the access period according to the patient's time limitation considered for a particular participant. Additionally, this function generates an occurrence of "EmergencyTimeConstratints" which participant could observe through the playground utilizing the admin ID card. From the well-defined time limitation, the current emergency doctor can view PHR items. Emergecy_Access_End_Time is only two hours more than Emergency_Access_Start_Time. This function also gets the level and rechecks by triggering the get_patient_data, and the emergency doctor will catch the message "Access Denied." Algorithm 1 shows registering a participant (user) in our system, and Algorithm 2 describes how to get PHR from the system.

Algorithm 1. Participant Registration

1: **Input**: Emergency Doctor ID, License Number
2: **Output**: Emergency Doctor
3:     Emergency doctor ID ← Emergency doctor
4:     License ← Authorized Doctor License Number
5:     Emergency Doctor ID ← Request for the registration to the system
7: **if** (Authorized Doctor License Number match) **then**
8:     Return Success (Register Emergency Doctor)
9: **else**
10:    Return "Unauthorized Person"
11: **end if**

- Get Patient Data: This file includes the TPF, which is triggered and obtained from the patient's PHR data, and the emergency doctor input parameters consisting of *Patient_Id* (e.g., current *emergency_doctor_Id* for an emergency condition) when the participant hits the trigger from the *client_side* function named "network.getpatientdata", which is described in the file "app.js." Later, our proposed system considers the mandatory fields of the process body for requesting access permission. Then, it will send certain documents to TPFs "networkgetpatientdata," which is explained in the "network.js" file, and data is exchanged according to the prescribed rules. The TPF is again utilized the Hyperledger Composer NodeSDK; first, this verifies whether the participant has permission to access the patient's information and thus delivers PHR data. The smart contracts restrict the access period according to the patient's time limitation considered for a particular participant. Additionally, this function generates an occurrence of "EmergencyTimeConstratints," which participants could observe through the playground utilizing the admin ID card. From the well-defined time limitation, the current emergency doctor can view PHR items. Emergecy_Access_End_Time is only two hours more than Emergency_Access_Start_Time. This function also gets the level and rechecks by triggering the get_patient_data, and the emergency doctor will catch the message "Access Denied." Algorithm 1 shows registering a participant (user) in our system, and Algorithm 2 describes how to get PHR from the system.

Algorithm 2. Get PHR

1: **Input**: Emergency Doctor ID, Patient ID
2: **Output**: Display the Patient PHR data items
3: Emergency Doctor ID ← Authorized Emergency Doctor
4: Patient ID ← Discover Registered Patient
5:     Get Patient Data ← Authorized Emergency Doctor request to get patient data
6:     Start time ← get the correct time date
7: **if** (Authorized Emergency Doctor request = true) **then**
8:     Result ← check the Emergency Access Time constraint condition according to the start time
9: **else**
10:    Return "Access Denied"
11: **end if**

Query 1 Patient Data Retrieval

1: { "$class": "org.hyperledger.composer.system.Add Participant",
2: "resources": [{
3: "$class": "org.example.basic.EmergencyDoctor",
4: "emergencyDoctorid": "ED1",
5: "licenceNumber": "A1B2aa444" }],
6: "targetRegistry": "resource:org.hyperledger.composer.system.ParticipantRegistry#org.example.basic.EmergencyDoctor",
7: "transactionId": "f96ff792-b85f-4c9b-b10d-0d02e0b66e91",
8: "timestamp": "2019-10-13T21:53:17.399Z" }

The Historian is a database containing the records that include information about the transactions which occurred on the system. When a transaction is performed, the historian record is updated and timestamp, i.e., a history of transactions in a business network. A Historian record is an asset defined in the Hyperledger Composer network namespace. The Historian registry is updated for all approved transactions. Besides, various operations that the Hyperledger Composer runtime can be classified as transactions.

Query 2 Adding Asset into the System
1: {"$class": "org.hyperledger.composer.system. AddAsset",   2: "resources": [{   3: "$class": "org.example.basic.TreatmentDrugs",   4: "treatmentDrugs": "Special Treatment",   5: "drugName": "Disprine",   6: "formulae": "Asprine",   7: "describption": "High Headache",   8: "result": "Effective",   9: "emergencyAcces": true,   10: "owner": "resource:org.example.basic.Patient#P1",   11: "doctor": "resource:org.example.basic.Doctor#D1"}],   12: "targetRegistry": "resource:org.hyperledger.composer. system.AssetRegistry#org.example.basic.TreatmentDrugs",   "transactionId": "491c6aa6-8d9c-473f-8cdc-bd2fb2fbda68",   13: "timestamp": "2019-10-13T22:09:26.488Z"}

As mentioned earlier, our proposed system utilizes the APIs for querying resources and relationships for registering the historian records. When we call a 'getAll' function, it will likely return a massive amount of data from the historian records. Thus, query capacity is essential for obtaining a subset of records based on time limitations. It utilizes the query capacity to select records where the transaction timestamps a particular position. We have conducted our proposed framework by generating some queries as depicted in Query 1 and Query 2. After recovering from the emergency, the patient can check the system's profile and track all the history records updated on the profile.

6. Discussion

In this section, we discuss the proposed framework's performance concerning auditing, security and privacy, response time, and accessibility.

Does the proposed model provide a secure access control system for PHR data in emergency condition? To answer this question, we applied the Hyperledger Composer based on Hyperledger Fabric, which affords some permissions for participants that allow limited access during an emergency condition. The use of blockchain technology can enhance the security and accessibility of the PHR by different participants in our proposed model while patients are in the emergency concerning confidentiality, non-repudiation, authenticity, and accountability.

Are there any alternatives for malicious attackers to access a patient's PHR? The answer to this question is, our framework guarantees the patient's privacy by presenting expediency for designating well-arranged access control to the PHR. Furthermore, it limits the user's access to the PHR by employing smart contracts. Our mechanism's access rules essentially concentrate on the purpose, what data object, and which activities they have to perform. In our framework, patient predefined access permissions rules such as read, write, update, delete, and period to share their PHR by smart contracts on the blockchain without the lack of control. Smart contracts can be executed on the blockchain network once all the conditions are met. We proposed that patient can empower access to his/her PHR only under predefined conditions of an appropriate type and for a provided time limit. The smart contract stored directly on the blockchain confirms whether data requestors match these circumstances to access the particularized data. If the requestor does not have access permission, the framework will respond with a message unauthorized user. In the proposed framework, we perform security policies according to the specified participant's IDs. Hence, it prevents the PHR data from being accessed by malicious users.

Does the proposed system provide auditing during the PHR access in the emergency department? To answer this question, we utilize the historian record, which provides the auditing facility to trace the registered records and history of the PHR data. The Historian record is used only via the patient after his cure from the hospital. It can track and trace all the activities done with his/her PHR in an emergency condition. In other words, various types of actions through the proposed system can be outlined using the historian records.

Our framework ensures the patient's privacy by affording feasibility for defining granular access control across his/her PHR data. Moreover, it considers access control management by combining smart contracts. In the Hyperledger composer network, the proposed model performs based on the specified participant's identities. Therefore, there are no ways to access the PHR data for malicious users. Channels in the HF are constructed according to access policies that dictate access to the channel's stores, such as smart contracts, transactions, and ledger states. Thus, these channels consist of nodes in which the privacy protection and confidentiality of PHR are defined. Our proposed framework protects the PHR data against ransomware and similar security breaches such as unauthorized access. Because it is the decentralized network topology and does not have a single point of failure or central repository for intruders to infiltrate, the emergency doctor has just short, timely access to the system. After the time limit of his/her access data, the emergency doctor could not access the PHR data. Blockchain technology makes the process of adopting the system much simpler and less costly. The implementation facilitates improved security, privacy availability, and auditing by storing access control lists and logs directly on the blockchain. Each attempt to access a record is verified in the access control list and subsequently logged before access is granted to the user. The system introduces a new standard way of managing access control in the emergency condition and auditing across several participants. The experiments confirm that our framework provides better efficiency compared with the traditional emergency access system. Besides, the patients get the historian records for the audit trail and check the access control policies whether their PHR data have not to breach after recovering from the emergency condition. This work presents an implementation of a blockchain framework for improving auditing and privacy measures of PHR systems.

What is the difference in the response time efficiency between the proposed framework and the traditional emergency system? The answer to this question is, our proposed system preserves the PHR against data violations while being manipulated by malicious users. Figure 4 depicts the evaluation and performance of our system based on time efficiency and memory. Since we used the smart contracts in our proposed framework, it affords various properties such as time control, verification, and classification that reduce the response time during the processing of queries. In References [11,12], researchers introduced a framework based on trusted members in emergency contact for accessing patient's information. However, there is no third party or trusted member in the contact list for an emergency condition in our system because we employed the Hyperledger composer while the patients define the access rules/policies in smart contracts for the emergency doctor. Therefore, the emergency doctor can receive requested information in less than a few seconds from our system. In the traditional system [11,12], the average response time for processing text messages and calls to the trusted members is "7188" minutes. Moreover, trusted member affords the reply to the emergency team for allowing the PHR item access, which is (8 min) for receiving calls and messages response-time. Moreover, average registration time of our system is "6900 ms" and getpatientdata average time is "6000 ms". For responding to the emergency doctor, the average time is "15,000 ms" to "18,000 ms". These results demonstrate that our proposed framework provides accessibility to the PHR data items without approval by trusted members in the contact list for an emergency. In our experiments, the average response time has been decreased in an emergency condition as compared to the aforementioned traditional system for approving the information of PHR. To provide a comparative analysis, we have evaluated the existing blockchain-based health systems [34,39–42] considering their strategies for designing security policies. In other words, we conducted a benchmark study to investigate the capabilities of our framework and other systems regarding immutability, identity management, smart contracts, and data auditing. Table 4 depicts the outcome of the benchmark study. We have chosen the parameters that impact the system performance during our analysis. Since we have developed our framework using the Hyperledger composer using the aforementioned policies, it reduces the system's overall overhead. Note that most of the existing systems work based on EMR functionality (except References [40,41]). Therefore, our framework provides the security policies for PHRs that can improve healthcare system usability in emergency cases.

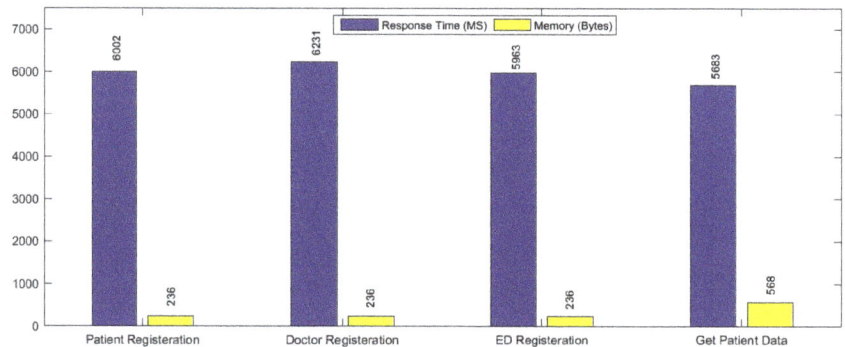

Figure 4. Performance Evaluation of the proposed framework.

Table 4. A comparative analysis of the proposed framework vs the state-of-the-art systems.

Healthcare System Name	Patient Identity	Immutability	Data Auditing	Smart Contracts	Access Control
Our framework	✓	✓	✓	✓	✓
Xiao et al., 2016 [34]	✓	✓	✗	✗	✗
Hussein et al., 2018 [38]	✓	✓	✗	✗	✗
Dagher et al., 2018 [39]	✓	✓	✗	✓	✗
Chen et al., 2019 [40]	✓	✓	✗	✗	✗
Zhang et al., 2018 [41]	✓	✓	✓	✓	✗

7. Conclusions

In this study, we proposed a new access control framework, which preserves PHR data privacy where a patient is in an emergency condition. Systematically, it works based on the permissioned blockchain Hyperledger Fabric and Hyperledger Composer. In this framework, we utilized the smart contracts in blockchain technology to provide security policies that patients can manage the access rules of other participants in the healthcare system using the consortium strategy. Besides, our system affords the historian records for auditing that stores the history of transactions while patients are in an emergency. Moreover, they can trace the history of the records held by other participants (doctors) after recovery. We experienced our framework using the Hyperledger Composer playground to evaluate its performance of our framework. Our experimental results demonstrated that this framework assures the secret data sharing of the PHR by considering the immutability, auditing, and emergency access control policies.

Our proposed framework not only provides security policies for controlling the access permissions to the PHRs during the emergency condition but also enables the health management system to eliminate the time of emergency contact. However, there exist some limitations which should be addressed in future works. Since our framework is at the prototype stage, we should test it by engaging different groups of participants and take their feedback into account during the maintenance stage. Moreover, because the PHRs are exchanged/shared among different participants (or agencies), a standard like HL7 FHIR is needed to guarantee the security of data sharing implementation.

Author Contributions: Conceptualization, A.R.R.; methodology, A.R.R.; software, A.R.R.; formal analysis, M.T.A.; investigation, A.R.R.; data curation, A.R.R.; writing—original draft preparation, A.R.R.; visualization, A.R.R.; review and editing, M.T.A.; supervision, Q.L.; project administration, Q.L.; funding acquisition, Q.L. All authors have read and agreed to the published version of the manuscript.

Funding: This research was funded in part by the Chinese Government Scholarship (CSC), [grant number 2015GXZW13], in part by The 4th project "Research on the Key Technology of Endogenous Security Switches" (2020YFB1804604) of the National Key R&D Program "New Network Equipment Based on Independent Programmable Chips" (2020YFB1804600), the 2020 Industrial Internet Innovation and Development Project from Ministry of Industry and Information Technology of China, 2018 Jiangsu Province Major Technical Research Project "Information Security Simulation System", the Fundamental Research Fund for the Central Universities (30918012204, 30920041112), the 2019 Industrial Internet Innovation and Development Project from Ministry of Industry and Information Technology of China. This work is supported by the National Key R&D Program of China (Funding No. 2020YFB1805503).

Institutional Review Board Statement: Not applicable.

Informed Consent Statement: Not applicable.

Data Availability Statement: Not applicable.

Conflicts of Interest: The other authors have disclosed no conflict of interest.

References

1. Roehrs, A.; Da Costa, C.A.; Da Rosa Righi, R.; De Oliveira, K.S.F. Personal health records: A systematic literature review. *J. Med. Internet Res.* **2017**, *19*, e13. [CrossRef] [PubMed]
2. Ahvanooey, M.T.; Li, Q.; Hou, J.; Rajput, A.R.; Yini, C. Modern text hiding, text steganalysis, and applications: A comparative analysis. *Entropy* **2019**, *21*, 355. [CrossRef] [PubMed]
3. Señor, I.C.; Fernández-Alemán, J.L.; Toval, A. Are personal health records safe? A review of free web-accessible personal health record privacy policies. *J. Med. Internet Res.* **2012**, *14*, e114. [CrossRef] [PubMed]
4. Tang, P.C.; Ash, J.S.; Bates, D.W.; Overhage, J.M.; Sands, D.Z. Personal health records: Definitions, benefits, and strategies for overcoming barriers to adoption. *J. Am. Med. Inform. Assoc.* **2006**, *13*, 121–126. [CrossRef]
5. Krukowski, A.; Barca, C.C.; Rodríguez, J.M.; Vogiatzaki, E. Personal Health Record. *Cyberphys. Syst. Epilepsy Brain Disord.* **2015**. [CrossRef]
6. US Department of Health and Human Services, Office for Civil Rights. Personal Health Records and the HIPAA Privacy Rule. Available online: https://www.hhs.gov/sites/default/files/ocr/privacy/hipaa/understanding/special/healthit/phrs.pdf (accessed on 5 August 2011).
7. Jones, D.A.; Shipman, J.P.; Plaut, D.A.; Selden, C.R. Characteristics of personal health records: Findings of the Medical Library Association/National Library of Medicine Joint Electronic Personal Health Record Task Force. *J. Med. Libr. Assoc.* **2010**, *98*, 243–249. [CrossRef] [PubMed]
8. Fernandez-Luque, L.; Karlsen, R.; Bonander, J.; Mandl, K.; Halkes, R. Review of extracting information from the social web for health personalization. *J. Med. Internet Res.* **2011**, *13*, e15. [CrossRef]
9. Adida, B.; Kohane, I.S. GenePING: Secure, scalable management of personal genomic data. *BMC Genom.* **2006**, *7*, 93. [CrossRef] [PubMed]
10. Zhang, P.; White, J.; Schmidt, D.C.; Lenz, G.; Rosenbloom, S.T. FHIRChain: Applying blockchain to securely and scalably share clinical data. *Comput. Struct. Biotechnol. J.* **2018**, *16*, 267–278. [CrossRef]
11. Thummavet, P.; Vasupongayya, S. A novel personal health record system for handling emergency situations. In Proceedings of the International Computer Science and Engineering Conference, Bangkok, Thailand, 4–6 September 2013; pp. 266–271.
12. Thummavet, P.; Vasupongayya, S. Privacy-preserving emergency access control for personal health records. *Maejo Int. J. Sci. Technol.* **2015**, *9*, 108–120.
13. Benchoufi, M.; Ravaud, P. Blockchain technology for improving clinical research quality. *Trials* **2017**, *18*, 335. [CrossRef] [PubMed]
14. Wang, S.; Zhang, Y.; Zhang, Y. A blockchain-based framework for data sharing with fine-grained access control in decentralized storage systems. *IEEE Access* **2018**, *6*, 38437–38450. [CrossRef]

15. Hyperledger Composer. Available online: https://hyperledger.github.io/composer/latest/introduction/introduction.html (accessed on 6 July 2018).
16. Puthal, D.; Malik, N.; Mohanty, S.P.; Kougianos, E.; Yang, C. The blockchain as a decentralized security framework [future di-rections]. *IEEE Consum. Electron. Mag.* **2018**, *7*, 18–21. [CrossRef]
17. Delmolino, K.; Arnett, M.; Kosba, A.; Miller, A.; Shi, E. Step by Step Towards Creating a Safe Smart Contract: Lessons and Insights from a Cryptocurrency Lab. In Proceedings of the International Conference on Financial Cryptography and Data Security, Christ Church, Barbados, 26 February 2016.
18. Christidis, K.; Devetsikiotis, M. Blockchains and smart contracts for the internet of things. *IEEE Access* **2016**, *4*, 2292–2303. [CrossRef]
19. Nakamoto, S. Bitcoin: A Peer-to-Peer Electronic Cash System. Available online: https://bitcoin.org/bitcoin.pdf (accessed on 1 June 2018).
20. Mettler, M. Blockchain technology in healthcare: The revolution starts here. In Proceedings of the 2016 IEEE 18th International Conference on e-Health Networking, Applications and Services (Healthcom), Munich, Germany, 14–16 September 2016.
21. Gordon, W.J.; Catalini, C. Blockchain technology for healthcare: Facilitating the transition to patient-driven interoperability. *Comput. Struct. Biotechnol. J.* **2018**, *16*, 224–230. [CrossRef]
22. Ouaddah, A.; Elkalam, A.A.; Ouahman, A.A. FairAccess: A new Blockchain-based access control framework for the Internet of Things. *Secur. Commun. Netw.* **2016**, *9*, 5943–5964. [CrossRef]
23. Ouaddah, A.; Elkalam, A.A.; Ouahman, A.A.I.T. Towards a novel privacy-preserving access control model based on blockchain technology in IoT. In Proceedings of the Europe and MENA Cooperation Advances in Information and Communication Technologies, Saidia, Marocco, 3–5 October 2016.
24. Hölbl, M.; Kompara, M.; Kamišalić, A.; Zlatolas, L.N. A systematic review of the use of Blockchain in healthcare. *Symmetry* **2018**, *10*, 470. [CrossRef]
25. Kshetri, N. Blockchain's roles in strengthening cybersecurity and protecting privacy. *Telecommun. Policy* **2017**, *41*, 1027–1038. [CrossRef]
26. Buterin, V.A. Next-generation Smart Contract and Decentralized Application Platform. Available online: https://github.com/ethereum/wiki/wiki/White-Paper (accessed on 31 July 2016).
27. Liang, X.; Shetty, S.; Zhao, J.; Bowden, D.; Li, D.; Liu, J. Towards decentralized accountability and self-sovereignty in healthcare systems. In Proceedings of the 19th International Conference on Information and Communications Security, Beijing, China, 6–8 December 2017; pp. 387–398.
28. Kakavand, H.; Kost De Sevres, N.; Chilton, B. The blockchain revolution: An analysis of regulation and technology related to distributed ledger technologies. *SSRN* **2017**. [CrossRef]
29. Castro, M.; Liskov, B. Practical Byzantine fault tolerance and proactive recovery. *ACM Trans. Comput. Syst.* **2002**, *20*, 398–461. [CrossRef]
30. Thakkar, P.; Nathan, S.; Viswanathan, B. Performance benchmarking and optimizing hyperledger fabric block-chain platform. In Proceedings of the 2018 IEEE 26th International Symposium on Modeling, Analysis, and Simulation of Computer and Telecommunication Systems (MASCOTS), Milwaukee, WI, USA, 25–28 September 2018.
31. Hyperledger. Architecture Explained Read the Docs. 2017. Available online: https://hyperledger-fabric.readthedocs.io/en/release-1.2/archdeep-dive.html (accessed on 3 May 2020).
32. Zyskind, G.; Nathan, O.; Pentland, A. Enigma: Decentralized computation platform with guaranteed privacy. *arXiv* **2015**, arXiv:150603471.
33. Xia, Q.; Sifah, E.B.; Smahi, A.; Amofa, S.; Zhang, X. BBDS: Blockchain-based data sharing for electronic medical records in cloud environments. *Information* **2017**, *8*, 44. [CrossRef]
34. Yue, X.; Wang, H.; Jin, D.; Li, M.; Jiang, W. Healthcare data gateways: Found healthcare intelligence on Blockchain with novel privacy risk control. *J. Med. Syst.* **2016**, *40*, 218–218:8. [CrossRef] [PubMed]
35. Azaria, A.; Ekblaw, A.; Vieira, T.; Lippman, A. MedRec: Using Blockchain for medical data access and permission management. In Proceedings of the 2016 2nd International Conference on Open and Big Data (OBD), Vienna, Austria, 22–24 August 2016; pp. 25–30.
36. Ichikawa, D.; Kashiyama, M.; Ueno, T. Tamper-resistant mobile health using Blockchain technology. *JMIR mHealth uHealth* **2017**, *5*, e111. [CrossRef] [PubMed]
37. Xia, Q.; Sifah, E.B.; Asamoah, K.O.; Gao, J.; Du, X.; Guizani, M. MeDShare: Trust-less medical data sharing among cloud service providers via Blockchain. *IEEE Access* **2017**, *5*, 14757–14767. [CrossRef]
38. Hussein, A.F.; Arunkumar, N.; Ramirez-Gonzalez, G.; Abdulhay, E.; Tavares, J.M.R.; De Albuquerque, V.H.C. A medical records managing and securing blockchain based system supported by a Genetic Algorithm and Discrete Wavelet Transform. *Cogn. Syst. Res.* **2018**, *52*, 1–11. [CrossRef]
39. Dagher, G.G.; Mohler, J.; Milojkovic, M.; Marella, P.B. Ancile: Privacy-preserving framework for access control and interoperability of electronic health records using blockchain technology. *Sustain. Cities Soc.* **2018**, *39*, 283–297. [CrossRef]
40. Chen, Y.; Ding, S.; Xu, Z.; Zheng, H.; Yang, S. Blockchain-based medical records secure storage and medical service framework. *J. Med. Syst.* **2019**, *43*, 5. [CrossRef] [PubMed]

41. Zhang, A.; Lin, X. Towards secure and privacy-preserving data sharing in e-health systems via consortium block-chain. *J. Med Syst.* **2018**, *42*, 140. [CrossRef]
42. Szabo, N. Smart Contracts: Building Blocks for Digital Markets. *EXTROPY J. Transhumanist Thought.* **1996**. Available online: http://www.truevaluemetrics.org/DBpdfs/BlockChain/Nick-Szabo-Smart-Contracts-Building-Blocks-for-Digital-Markets-1996-14591.pdf (accessed on 14 February 2021).

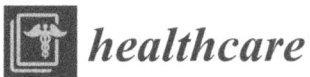

Comment

The Newfound Opportunities of Wearable Systems Based on Biofeedback in the Prevention of Falls. Comment on Tanwar et al. Pathway of Trends and Technologies in Fall Detection: A Systematic Review. *Healthcare* 2022, *10*, 172

Giovanni Morone [1], Giovanni Maccioni [2] and Daniele Giansanti [2,*]

[1] Department of Life, Health and Environmental Sciences, University of L'Aquila, 67100 L'Aquila, Italy; giovanni.morone@univaq.it
[2] Centre Tisp, The Italian National Institute of Health, 00161 Rome, Italy; gvnnmaccioni@gmail.com
* Correspondence: daniele.giansanti@iss.it; Tel.: +39-06-49902701

Citation: Morone, G.; Maccioni, G.; Giansanti, D. The Newfound Opportunities of Wearable Systems Based on Biofeedback in the Prevention of Falls. Comment on Tanwar et al. Pathway of Trends and Technologies in Fall Detection: A Systematic Review. *Healthcare* 2022, *10*, 172. *Healthcare* **2022**, *10*, 940. https://doi.org/10.3390/healthcare 10050940

Academic Editor: Yogesan Kanagasingam

Received: 15 April 2022
Accepted: 12 May 2022
Published: 19 May 2022

Publisher's Note: MDPI stays neutral with regard to jurisdictional claims in published maps and institutional affiliations.

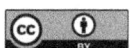

Copyright: © 2022 by the authors. Licensee MDPI, Basel, Switzerland. This article is an open access article distributed under the terms and conditions of the Creative Commons Attribution (CC BY) license (https:// creativecommons.org/licenses/by/ 4.0/).

We are writing to you as the corresponding authors of the interesting *systematic review* study "Pathway of Trends and Technologies in Fall Detection: A Systematic Review" [1].

We found this work to be particularly stimulating, and feel it provides great added value in the field.

Specifically, we believe, first of all, that this review has the great merit of simultaneously focusing both on important key aspects of the integration of systems for fall detection/prediction and prevention in the *health domain*, and on aspects relating to technological innovation and deployment in the three most important fields, where neuromotor problems due to pathologies or aging have a strong impact: falls from bed, falls from sitting, and falls from walking and standing. When the Special Issue "Cybersecurity and the Digital Health: An Investigation on the State of the Art and the Position of the Actors" (https://www.mdpi.com/journal/healthcare/special_issues/cybersecurity_digital_ health (accessed on 1 May 2022)) [2] was launched, one of the objectives [3] was to give scholars the opportunity to broaden the boundaries of studies in this area.

Mainly, studies on cybersecurity turn more toward IT aspects, which is defined as the activity carried out in defending computers, servers, mobile devices, electronic systems, networks, and data from malicious attacks or software defaults. Therefore, what is often addressed is so-called information security and data security.

We very much appreciated your contribution because it has precisely achieved the goal of expanding and exploring new areas in this sector, *enlarging the concept of cyber-systems as tools for the development of physical security approaches for people.*

We found your work particularly interesting, wide-ranging, attractive and full of stimuli for future research. We agree with the findings of the study, that falling is one of the most serious health risks throughout the world for elderly people and for people affected by particular diseases or after recovery from accidents. In the event of a fall, as you have highlighted, considerable expenses are unfortunately necessary for patient management in the health domain. The cyber-systems developed in the field of fall risk, detection/prediction and prevention have the potential to minimize these problems. This is why we believe that your work, that has reviewed papers systematically (publications, projects, and patents), is strategic in this perspective.

As we wrote above, your study, being a review, is also very stimulating toward research initiatives to be undertaken in the future.

We would therefore like to share a reflection on this with you and with the other scholars involved in this field of research.

In the past, there has been much discussion about biofeedback systems for the prevention of falls through training and/or the use of wearable systems. Several studies have been developed based on audio, video, and vibrotactile biofeedback systems [4–19], some involving some of us as authors [8,13]. Many of these wearable systems were considered even before the smartphone boom as we know it today [9–19]. Some recent studies are continuing in this direction [20–23]. The use of inertial sensors, such as accelerometers, for stability control [24–26] integrated in wearable systems equipped with biofeedback [4–23] will certainly provide an increasingly important response in the prevention of falls.

In conclusion, we believe that your review has been a great stimulus for the Special Issue and for the scholars in general regarding future developments. Among these future developments, we also consider important those connected to wearable systems equipped with biofeedback for the prevention of falls.

Funding: This research received no external funding.

Conflicts of Interest: The authors declare no conflict of interest.

References

1. Tanwar, R.; Nandal, N.; Zamani, M.; Manaf, A.A. Pathway of Trends and Technologies in Fall Detection: A Systematic Review. *Healthcare* **2022**, *10*, 172. [CrossRef] [PubMed]
2. Available online: https://www.mdpi.com/journal/healthcare/special_issues/cybersecurity_digital_health (accessed on 1 May 2022).
3. Giansanti, D. Cybersecurity and the Digital-Health: The Challenge of This Millennium. *Healthcare* **2021**, *9*, 62. [CrossRef] [PubMed]
4. Mirelman, A.; Herman, T.; Nicolai, S.; Zijlstra, A.; Zijlstra, W.; Becker, C.; Chiari, L.; Hausdorff, J.M. Audio-biofeedback training for posture and balance in patients with Parkinson's disease. *J. Neuroeng. Rehabil.* **2011**, *8*, 35. [CrossRef] [PubMed]
5. Zijlstra, A.; Mancini, M.; Chiari, L.; Zijlstra, W. Biofeedback for training balance and mobility tasks in older populations: A systematic review. *J. Neuroeng. Rehabil.* **2010**, *7*, 58. [CrossRef]
6. Pirini, M.; Mancini, M.; Farella, E.; Chiari, L. EEG correlates of postural audio- biofeedback. *Hum. Mov. Sci.* **2011**, *30*, 249–261. [CrossRef]
7. Horak, F.B.; Dozza, M.; Peterka, R.; Chiari, L.; Wall, C., 3rd. Vibrotactile biofeedback improves tandem gait in patients with unilateral vestibular loss. *Ann. N. Y. Acad. Sci.* **2009**, *1164*, 279–281. [CrossRef]
8. Giansanti, D.; Dozza, M.; Chiari, L.; Maccioni, G.; Cappello, A. Energetic assessment of trunk postural modifications induced by a wearable audio-biofeedback system. *Med. Eng. Phys.* **2009**, *31*, 48–54. [CrossRef]
9. Dozza, M.; Wall, C., 3rd; Peterka, R.J.; Chiari, L.; Horak, F.B. Effects of practicing tandem gait with and without vibrotactile biofeedback in subjects with unilateral vestibular loss. *J. Vestib. Res.* **2007**, *17*, 195–204. [CrossRef]
10. Dozza, M.; Chiari, L.; Horak, F.B. A portable audio-biofeedback system to improve postural control. *Conf. Proc. IEEE Eng. Med. Biol. Soc.* **2004**, *2004*, 4799–4802. [CrossRef]
11. Dozza, M.; Chiari, L.; Hlavacka, F.; Cappello, A.; Horak, F.B. Effects of linear versus sigmoid coding of visual or audio biofeedback for the control of upright stance. *IEEE Trans. Neural. Syst. Rehabil. Eng.* **2006**, *14*, 505–512. [CrossRef]
12. Dozza, M.; Horak, F.B.; Chiari, L. Auditory biofeedback substitutes for loss of sensory information in maintaining stance. *Exp. Brain Res.* **2007**, *178*, 37–48. [CrossRef]
13. Chiari, L.; Dozza, M.; Cappello, A.; Horak, F.B.; Macellari, V.; Giansanti, D. Audio-biofeedback for balance improvement: An accelerometry-based system. *IEEE Trans. Biomed. Eng.* **2005**, *52*, 2108–2111. [CrossRef]
14. Dozza, M.; Chiari, L.; Horak, F.B. Audio-biofeedback improves balance in patients with bilateral vestibular loss. *Arch. Phys. Med. Rehabil.* **2005**, *86*, 1401–1403. [CrossRef]
15. Dozza, M.; Chiari, L.; Chan, B.; Rocchi, L.; Horak, F.B.; Cappello, A. Influence of a portable audio-biofeedback device on structural properties of postural sway. *J. Neuroeng. Rehabil.* **2005**, *2*, 13. [CrossRef]
16. Wall, C., 3rd; Kentala, E. Control of sway using vibrotactile feedback of body tilt in patients with moderate and severe postural control deficits. *J. Vestib. Res.* **2005**, *15*, 313–325. [CrossRef]
17. Kadkade, P.P.; Benda, B.J.; Schmidt, P.B.; Wall, C., 3rd. Vibrotactile display coding for a balance prosthesis. *IEEE Trans. Neural. Syst. Rehabil. Eng.* **2003**, *11*, 392–399. [CrossRef]
18. Kentala, E.; Vivas, J.; Wall, C., 3rd. Reduction of postural sway by use of a vibrotactile balance prosthesis prototype in subjects with vestibular deficits. *Ann. Otol. Rhinol. Laryngol.* **2003**, *112*, 404–409. [CrossRef]
19. Wall, C., 3rd; Weinberg, M.S.; Schmidt, P.B.; Krebs, D.E. Balance prosthesis based on micromechanical sensors using vibrotactile feedback of tilt. *IEEE Trans. Biomed. Eng.* **2001**, *48*, 1153–1161. [CrossRef]
20. Islam, M.S.; Lim, S. Vibrotactile feedback in virtual motor learning: A systematic review. *Appl. Ergon.* **2022**, *101*, 103694. [CrossRef]
21. Tannert, I.; Schulleri, K.H.; Michel, Y.; Villa, S.; Johannsen, L.; Hermsdorfer, J.; Lee, D. Immediate Effects of Vibrotactile Biofeedback Instructions on Human Postural Control. *Annu. Int. Conf. IEEE Eng. Med. Biol. Soc.* **2021**, *2021*, 7426–7432. [CrossRef]
22. Gao, J.H.; Ling, J.Y.; Hong, J.C.; Yasuda, K.; Muroi, D.; Iwata, H. Investigation of optimal gait speed for motor learning of walking using the vibro-tactile biofeedback system. *Annu. Int. Conf. IEEE Eng. Med. Biol. Soc.* **2021**, *2021*, 4662–4665. [CrossRef]

23. Chen, L.; Feng, Y.; Chen, B.; Wang, Q.; Wei, K. Improving postural stability among people with lower-limb amputations by tactile sensory substitution. *J. Neuroeng. Rehabil.* **2021**, *18*, 159. [CrossRef]
24. Iosa, M.; Bini, F.; Marinozzi, F.; Fusco, A.; Morone, G.; Koch, G.; Martino Cinnera, A.; Bonnì, S.; Paolucci, S. Stability and Harmony of Gait in Patients with Subacute Stroke. *J. Med. Biol. Eng.* **2016**, *36*, 635–643. [CrossRef]
25. Tramontano, M.; Morone, G.; Curcio, A.; Temperoni, G.; Medici, A.; Morelli, D.; Caltagirone, C.; Paolucci, S.; Iosa, M. Maintaining gait stability during dual walking task: Effects of age and neurological disorders. *Eur. J. Phys. Rehabil. Med.* **2017**, *53*, 7–13. [CrossRef]
26. Iosa, M.; Fusco, A.; Morone, G.; Paolucci, S. Development and decline of upright gait stability. *Front Aging Neurosci.* **2014**, *6*, 14. [CrossRef]

MDPI
St. Alban-Anlage 66
4052 Basel
Switzerland
Tel. +41 61 683 77 34
Fax +41 61 302 89 18
www.mdpi.com

Healthcare Editorial Office
E-mail: healthcare@mdpi.com
www.mdpi.com/journal/healthcare

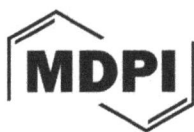

www.ingramcontent.com/pod-product-compliance
Lightning Source LLC
LaVergne TN
LVHW070445100526
838202LV00014B/1672